# THE COMPLETE BOOK OF CORE TRAINING

# THE COMPLETE BOOK OF CORE TRAINING

THE DEFINITIVE RESOURCE FOR SHAPING AND STRENGTHENING THE "CORE"—THE MUSCLES OF THE ABDOMEN, BUTT, HIPS, AND LOWER BACK

KURT, BRETT, & MIKE BRUNGARDT

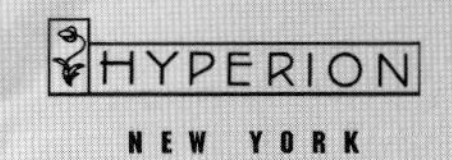


NEW YORK

The recommendations in this book are not intended to replace or conflict with the advice given to you by your physician or other health professionals. All matters regarding your health require medical supervision. Consult your physician before adopting the suggestions in this book. Following these dietary suggestions may impact the effect of certain types of medication. Any changes in your dosage should be made only in cooperation with your prescribing physician. Before using any herbal remedies or vitamins mentioned in this book be sure to consult with the appropriate medical authorities and check the product's label for any warnings or caution. Keep in mind that herbal remedies are not as strictly regulated as drugs.

Pregnant women are advised that special precautions may pertain to any exercise program they undertake. If you are pregnant, talk to your doctor before undertaking any exercises suggested in this book. If you are pregnant, talk to your doctor before taking any herbal remedy or nutritional supplement.

The author and publisher disclaim any liability directly or indirectly from the use of the material in this book by any person.



ISBN 1-4013-0788-4

Hyperion books are available for special promotions and premiums. For details contact Michael Rentas, Assistant Director, Inventory Operations, Hyperion, 77 West 66th Street, 11th floor, New York, New York 10023, or call 212-456-0133.

*Book design by Richard Oriolo*

FIRST EDITION

10 9 8 7 6 5 4 3 2

FOR ZOE

# CONTENTS

## PART FOUR: THE CORE BODY



## PART FIVE: THE COMPLETE CORE PROGRAM



## PART SIX: THE ROUTINES



## PART SEVEN: THE EXERCISES

# ACKNOWLEDGMENTS

We would like to thank everybody who made this book possible. Of course, that's impossible. First of all, Mark Chait, who believed in the book and bought it. Next, Gretchen Young, who took the book when Mark accepted another job offer. It happens in publishing. The new crew never made us feel like orphans. Gretchen Young gave helpful feedback on the manuscript and Ruth Curry worked tirelessly on organization for production. A book of this size with all the different elements and photos can be a production nightmare. The amount of work and effort that goes into production to make the authors look good is mind-boggling. Thanks to the rest of the team, the nameless and faceless production magicians who did the copyediting and design work. I would also like to thank Hyperion for their patience and support when Zoe got cancer.

Thanks to all the trainers who contributed their expertise to the book and the models who held their poses. A special thanks to Steve and Lisa of Birkram Yoga in San Antonio, who let us use their beautiful studio. You are both also great instructors. In Phoenix, special thanks to Scott, who organized the photo shoots and also modeled. Thanks to Dan Hitt, who helped proof the text and assisted in the photos. Thanks to Tracy Rhodes, who also helped in manuscript organization. And to Abigail for proofreading, dog watching, and wine drinking—all at the same time. Thanks to our mother, who came out for a month to help when the dog was sick.

Again, thanks to Laura Katers for her anatomy illustrations. Thank you, Tracy Marx, for the nutrition chapter. And thanks to Karl Osterbuhr for his cover photos and inside pictures. Thanks to Doug Stumpf, who has his hand in many things.

Finally, thanks again to Dan Strone, our agent, for all his work. And Lily, too, for her help.

# FOREWORD
## BY TIM DUNCAN

"Core training" is the big new fitness concept. But it's not new to the Brungardts. Mike has been my strength and conditioning coach for the last eight years. One of the prime objectives in our training, as with all the San Antonio Spurs, is to strengthen the core. The core is the power center of the body. Almost every movement initiates or is transferred through the center of the body. As an athlete, using and strengthening the entire core is key. I need to be strong 360 degrees around my body, not just in my abs. I also need to move with speed and power in all directions. I need to be able to fight and hold my position against a 300-pound center and also be able to explode to the basket at just the right moment. Core training helps my body to work efficiently and with precision. It emphasizes training my muscles to work together in movement sequences, just like they do in a game and in everyday life.

But truly mastering a core routine is hard work. To get even with Mike for taking me through these paces, I started making him tell me a joke before every game. It puts the pressure on him and helps me relax before games. I see him on the plane giggling to himself. He's reading another joke book and he's got his yellow highlighter out.

Soon Mike and I will be approaching the 1,000 joke club. The more championships the Spurs win, the more games we play each season. This means more jokes and the sooner we'll be members of the club. You're probably wondering what types of jokes I've been subjected to. Well, they've crossed all the spectrums you can imagine—some funny, some not funny at all, some clean . . . and a lot of dirty ones. But my favorite is simply a quote of Mike's. It goes, "I've spent all my money on women and beer and the rest of it I've wasted."

But be assured this book is no joke. It will get your entire core in great shape. It will also train these muscles to work efficiently in muscular sequences, and prepare you to use them better in everyday life and in sports. This book will take you to the next level, helping you to achieve your health, fitness, and sports goals.

PART ONE

# INTRODUCING THE CORE

# 1

# CORE CONSULTATION

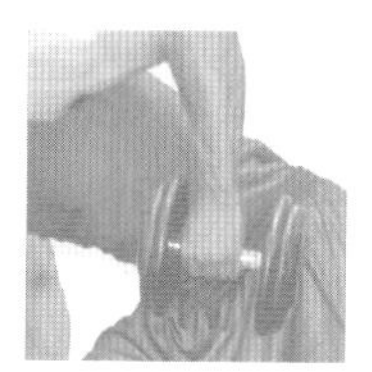

## INTRODUCTION

The goal of this chapter is to get you started on the right track. You've probably heard the quote "A journey of a thousand miles starts with a single step." This is true, but it's important to start the journey in the right direction; otherwise, a thousand-mile journey can turn into two thousand miles. Or in the worse case scenario, you never reach your destination. This chapter will give you some "nuts and bolts" advice to get you going. It will help you organize your vision, set goals, and outline the best way to use this book.

# GOALS

## GETTING STARTED: WHEN AND WHERE

An important step in getting started is deciding when and where you will train. If you aren't specific about this, you'll keep finding a way to put it off.

**WHEN.** You need to set a specific time each day to work out. One time is not necessarily better than another. It depends on your schedule. It could be in the morning or before you go to bed. Just don't work out right after you've eaten a substantial meal; give yourself a couple of hours to digest.

**WHERE.** Know where you are going to train. If it's at home, choose a spot where can you spread out your mat and limit interruptions. Create your own home gym. If you train at a health club, then the answer is obvious.

When and where you train are important steps in creating the habit, the ritual.

## CREATING A VISION

What are your workout goals? In other words, how much time can you realistically devote to a workout program? The most important element in answering this question is to be brutally honest. We want everything. A beautiful and healthy body, a satisfying love life, a fulfilling career, loyal friends, a good relationship with our family, a creative outlet, and an enriching spiritual practice. Be patient; you can't have everything all at once. You want a great body and you want it now. Just don't take on a workout schedule that's an unrealistic commitment. This is just setting yourself up for failure.

For the Complete Core Program, you need to start out by setting aside approximately three hours a week. This translates into three workouts that take about an hour each. The Complete Core Program combines core training with strength training, cardio, and a stretching routine. This is a foundation for a lifetime of fitness.

Your ultimate vision for fitness and wellness must be a lifelong process. Being fit and healthy is not like winning the Lotto, where you take the millions and never work again. Working out does not have to be something that is dreaded; it can become a natural part of the day. You and your body are together for life. In many cultures a physical practice is integrated into daily life. This is the case with yoga in India, tai chi in China, and tae kwon do in Korea.

Although America is health conscious, we still don't think of exercise and wellness as an integrated part of our lifestyle. The goal of the Complete Core Program is to give you a physical practice that you can integrate into your life. Core training is uniquely American. It is a melting pot, taking the best of all from many exercise systems and customizing them to our cultural needs.

### CONSISTENCY

Timewise, when it comes to working out, it's best to be conservative. It's better to underdo it and stay on the program than to be overambitious and quit. The key to getting started and to achieving your ultimate fitness goals is to choose a program that enables you to exercise consistently for the long haul. By the long haul, we mean for the rest of your life. It does no good to think "I'll work out this year and take next year off." You want to look and feel good every year. There will come a day when working out is something you want to do, not something you dread. Then it all gets easier.

### BE SAFE

The last question is, "Do you have any specific medical problems or limitations?" Before doing any of the exercises in this book, you should be 100 percent sure that you're not putting yourself at risk of injury or other health concerns. If done correctly and safely, exercise will improve your body and mind. But you should always check with your doctor before beginning a program. If you are recovering from an injury or have chronic problems, make sure you get clearance from your specialist.

## THE "GET STARTED NOW" PHILOSOPHY, OR HOW TO USE THIS BOOK

### START HERE NOW

This book is a comprehensive guide to training your core. You don't have to read the whole book before you start exercising. In fact, we recommend you don't. We recommend the "Get Started Now" strategy. This chapter will give you a plan to get going. Regardless of how advanced your fitness level is, Level One: Get Started Now is an excellent way to initiate yourself into the world of core training. The plan is simple. Go to Part Three: The Core Workout System (page 39) and follow the plan.

### CHAPTERS AT A GLANCE

To give you a feel for the book and to help you create a reading strategy, the following chapter thumbnails will give you a quick tour of the book:

## PART ONE: INTRODUCING THE CORE

**CHAPTER 1: CORE CONSULTATION** offers strategies for using the book and getting off to a good start.

**CHAPTER 2: CORE AT A GLANCE** introduces you to the history, development, and basic philosophy of core training.

**CHAPTER 3: FITNESS LEVEL: KNOW THYSELF** identifies your fitness level and your fitness personality. It will help you avoid common pitfalls and increase your chances of staying on the program.

## PART TWO: THE CORE MIND

**CHAPTER 4: CORE GOALS** offers you tips for setting effective workout goals.

**CHAPTER 5: CORE MIND SKILLS** teaches techniques to help you harness the power of your mind, utilizing basic relaxation, visualization, and meditation skills.

**CHAPTER 6: CORE MOTIVATION** introduces you to basic motivation concepts and theories.

## PART THREE: THE CORE WORKOUT SYSTEM

**CHAPTER 7: INTRODUCTION TO THE COMPLETE CORE WORKOUT** gives you the information you need to get started on the Core Workout System.

**CHAPTER 8: LEVEL ONE: GET STARTED NOW.** This is the first phase of the program. Its goal is to initiate you into the Core Workout System philosophy and build a foundation of core strength.

**CHAPTER 9: LEVEL TWO: CREATING STRENGTH AND ENDURANCE.** This level increases your strength and helps to create muscular balance in your core.

**CHAPTER 10: LEVEL THREE: CORE POWER** builds on Levels One and Two by introducing more challenging moves and putting you on the path of core mastery.

## PART FOUR: THE CORE BODY

**CHAPTER 11: CORE BASICS: THE INNER CORE** teaches you how to activate and integrate your inner core into exercise and daily activities.

**CHAPTER 12: A TRAINING PRIMER: BASIC PRINCIPLES AND TECHNIQUES** gives you the basic knowledge you need to train safely and effectively.

**CHAPTER 13: CORE POSTURE AND MOTION** teaches alignment and movement basics for exercise and for life.

**CHAPTER 14: CORE ANATOMY** outlines basic anatomy and movement principles that will improve the quality of your workouts.

**CHAPTER 15: CORE EATING** gives you basic eating strategies for improved performance, optimal health, and increased energy.

## PART FIVE: THE COMPLETE CORE PROGRAM

**CHAPTER 16: WELLNESS: THE BIG PICTURE** introduces you to basic wellness concepts and the elements of a complete fitness program.

**CHAPTER 17: CORE CARDIO** initiates you into a progressive cardio training program.

**CHAPTER 18: CORE STRENGTH TRAINING** introduces you to a basic strength routine and gives you challenging core moves.

**CHAPTER 19: CORE STRETCHING: BASIC MOVES** provides you with a basic stretching routine.

**CHAPTER 20: CREATING YOUR OWN ROUTINE** guides you through the principles and methods needed to customize your own routine.

## PART SIX: THE ROUTINES

**CHAPTER 21: INTRODUCTION TO THE ROUTINES** gives you a brief overview of the section.

**CHAPTER 22: CORE ROUTINES** contains a variety of core routines. You can find a detailed list in the Contents.

## PART SEVEN: THE EXERCISES

**CHAPTER 23: INTRODUCTION TO THE EXERCISES** guides you through the basics of this section.

**CHAPTER 24: FLEXION MOVES** contains all the flexion exercises.

**CHAPTER 25. EXTENSION MOVES** contains all the extension exercises.

**CHAPTER 26: ROTATION AND CROSSING MOVES** contains all the rotation and crossing moves.

**CHAPTER 27: BUTT AND HIP MOVES** contains all the hip and glute exercises.

**CHAPTER 28: COMBO CORE MOVES** contains all the moves that use more than one movement direction or pattern and work more than one muscle group.

## READING STRATEGIES: HOW TO USE THIS BOOK

Like we said in the opening, the easiest way is to begin with "Level One: Get Started Now" (page 43). Then you can pick up the readings as you go. A simple way to proceed with the readings is to go through the book in order. It was put together logically for this purpose.

But there is always a little bit of conflict between book order and the information you need right away to get started. Here are some alternative readings:

- **If you are unsure about your fitness level or the best place to start, read Chapter 3 to discover your fitness level. This chapter will give you useful advice whether you're a beginner or a gym rat. But we stress, even if you are an advanced exerciser, start with Level One of the Complete Core Workout. This will give you a clear introduction to the components of core training. It will also make it easier to integrate these ideas into your own workout vision.**
- **Other key information chapters that relate directly to your workout are Chapter 11 on the inner core and Chapter 14 on anatomy and movement.**
- **If you have no workout experience, Chapter 12 will teach you basic workout essentials.**

# 2

# CORE AT A GLANCE

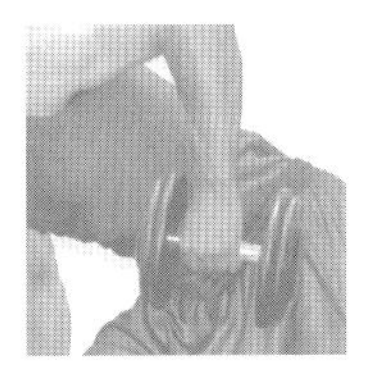

## LIFE IS AN ATHLETIC EVENT

Like an athlete who must be able to withstand the physical challenges of his sport and still thrive, you must be an athlete in the game of life. Daily life's physical challenges may be less dramatic, but the cumulative effects can lead to chronic pain and decreased levels of performance. Sitting, standing, carrying a heavy bag, driving, and working at a computer day after day take a major toll on the body. *The Complete Book of Core Training* will improve how you function and minimize long-term wear and tear on your body, helping you to thrive. It will improve your performance in life and in your favorite recreational activities. It will also give you a great body.

Increasing core strength and stability will help you move through life's challenges with more ease and grace. Core training is sometimes called functional training. It is designed to make you function more efficiently, effectively, and safely. Core training will make your life easier. It will make daily tasks like picking up your baby or loading groceries in and out of the car effortless. It will turn you into an athlete prepared to excel in the game of life. It will also give you a foundation on which to build higher levels of fitness, strength, energy, and endurance.

## THE CORE CONNECTION

As you prepare to embark on your core training program, you will be engaging in both a cutting-edge fitness trend and one of the oldest known training philosophies. Although it has had different names, developing a strong core dates back to ancient civilizations in both the East and the West. The core has roots in the training systems of yoga, martial arts, Greek Olympiads, and classic and modern dance. Core training is not a fad; it is a proven, time-tested, universal training principle.

**YOGA AND PILATES.** Yoga and Pilates have led the way in making core training mainstream. Both of these systems promote a healthy spine, demand that you focus your mind on the process of exercising, and initiate all movements from your center. If you are familiar with yoga and Pilates, you will recognize some of the exercises in this book.

**MARTIAL ARTS.** The popularity of tai chi has introduced the concepts of "chi energy" and being centered into our contemporary vocabulary. Most martial arts emphasize moving from one's center when punching and kicking. The power behind these strikes comes from the core. Martial arts has always made the core the focal point of both physical and mental training. In the Core Routines section you will learn basic principles as practiced in martial arts. You don't need to be a black belt to do them or to apply them to your daily activities.

**THE OLYMPIADS.** Core training was also utilized by the first Olympiads when the participants practiced the discus throw, shot put, javelin, high jump, and wrestling. Joseph Pilates studied the drawings and texts of ancient Greece when he developed his system. Core training and sports training have remained closely linked. Most professional strength coaches who train the world's elite athletes make core training a key element in their strength and conditioning programs. Elite trainers know that the core is your power center and almost all movements are transferred through the core.

For an athlete to be powerful and explosive, he or she must have a strong core. This is true for both an efficient and powerful golf swing and an explosive dunk. In this book, you will learn techniques to improve your performance in your favorite sport.

**DANCE.** Core training is also key in the world of dance. Ballet and modern dance stress the center. All movement, from classical arm extensions and pliés to explosive leaps, begins from the dancer's center. When you move gracefully, you are moving from your center. The pelvic floor and the transverse abdominis, two important core muscles, have always been emphasized in dance. We will talk in detail about these often neglected muscles.

## WHAT IS THE CORE?

How do all these ideas come together to create what has now been defined as core training?

Leading experts define the core differently. Some experts define the core as the entire spine and integrate many yoga moves into their workouts.

Joseph Pilates talked about the power center: the area that encircles your body from your lower ribs to the bottom of your butt (the gluteal fold).

Many physical therapists, following the latest research, focus "core work" on the smaller inner muscles: the transverse abdominis and the multifidus muscles (small lower back muscles that help keep the vertebrae aligned).

Professional strength and conditioning coaches (trainers who work with professional and elite athletes) focus on all of the above areas, along with the muscles that stabilize the scapulae (shoulder blades). This stabilization is important for throwing, swinging, and striking.

Core work also involves training the body through basic movement patterns instead of isolating single muscles in an exercise, like biceps curls or a crunch. This places an emphasis on how your body functions and moves, not just how it looks. Leading strength coaches have been using ideas in this book for years; the core philosophy is now going mainstream.

All of these definitions are accurate. Leaders in the field use all the above techniques, depending on their target audience. The goal of this book is to consolidate the best information in these areas and make it accessible and user friendly, so that both the beginner and the most advanced athlete can benefit from this book. We will talk more about these concepts throughout the book.

## THE COMPLETE CORE WORKOUT

The central component of the Complete Core Program is the Complete Core Workout. The exercises in this workout focus on the area from your breastbone (sternum) to just below your butt, wrapping 360 degrees around your body. The Complete Core Workout trains:

- **the deep muscles of the inner core transverse abdominis, internal obliques, and multifidus.**

- **The famous external ab muscles: rectus abdominis (the six-pack) and external obliques (the love handles).**
- **The lower back muscles: the erector spinae and lumbar groups.**
- **The glute muscles and the muscles that surround and stabilize your hips. This means your inner and outer thighs will also get a workout.**

## THE COMPLETE CORE PROGRAM

The Complete Core Program combines all the above elements, plus integral wellness components, to give you a comprehensive fitness program that will make you look good, feel good, and move with grace and power. The program also works three other key areas:

- **Cardio**
- **Stretching**
- **Strength and stabilization training**

These additional three elements help you function with optimum efficiency, allowing the body to work as an integrated system, as a team that plays well together. The Complete Core Program treats your body as an organic whole, not as parts and muscles functioning separately.

If your body is out of balance, unnecessary tension is created, and your core and other areas have to compensate. If your core is weak, other areas outside the core have to compensate and do its work. These compensations create wear and tear on the body. When your body works against its master design, its efficiency and grace decrease. This inefficiency saps you of vital energy and causes fatigue. A weak link in this organic system forces other links to compensate and move in ways they aren't designed to move. The Complete Core Program is designed to balance, align, strengthen, and stabilize your body so you can handle the demands of life with grace and energy.

## THE COMPLETE CORE PROGRAM WILL:

- **Train and strengthen your body to move in all directions (just like in life).**
- **Stabilize key joints and important structural areas for efficient, safe, and enhanced speed and power.**
- **Work the smaller, inner muscles to help support you and prevent lower back injury.**
- **Develop core support strength 360 degrees around your body.**

# HEALTH AND FITNESS BENEFITS OF THE COMPLETE CORE PROGRAM

- Helps you achieve and maintain your optimum weight.
- Increases overall body strength.
- Decreases chances of injury.
- Enables you to function with ease and power in your daily life and in your favorite recreational activities.
- Builds athletic and aesthetic muscles.
- Strengthens your heart and improves the efficiency of your cardiovascular system at a variety of energy levels.
- Increases muscle tone, strength, and flexibility.
- Helps correct imbalances and weaknesses that cause wear and tear on your body.
- Helps you sleep better.
- Improves your sex life.
- Increases energy levels.
- Slows down the effects of aging, keeping your body functioning at a high level as you reach your senior years.

# 3

# FITNESS LEVEL: KNOW THYSELF

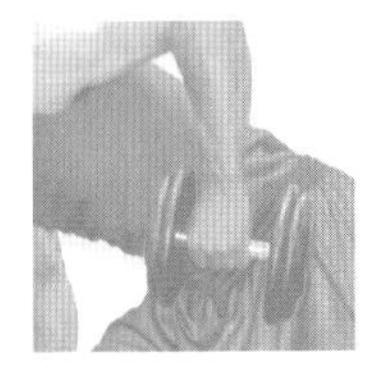

## TO THE CORE

How would you describe your fitness level? Beginner? Intermediate? Advanced? Are you currently working out? Do you get in the start-and-stop syndrome? How long has it been since you worked out? Is this your first time on a program? Have you been working out consistently for more than a year? Are you a gym rat? Are you a perfectionist? Do you get into the compare-and despair-syndrome?

# GETTING TO KNOW YOUR FITNESS LEVEL

In the beginning, along with setting goals, it is important to know your fitness level and your fitness personality. Usually, this is done with a personal trainer. It's kind of like fitness therapy.

The following guidelines will help you discover your fitness level. See where you fit in.

### THE BEGINNER CORE

The beginner falls into two basic categories:

**THE TRUE BEGINNER.** Someone who is just starting out for the very first time.

**REPEAT BEGINNER.** Someone who has started a fitness program and stayed consistent for less than six weeks, then stopped working out for at least six weeks. You're a repeat beginner because you never really got past Stage One. The important thing is you're still trying.

Be clear about what is motivating you. State it in a simple sentence. Here are some examples:

- **You just had a baby and want to get back in shape.**
- **You want to stay competitive at your favorite sport.**
- **You want to slow down the aging process and stay functional and vital as you age.**
- **You want to get in great shape for the beach.**

### STRATEGIES FOR THE BEGINNER

1. For you, the goal is simple. Just follow the Complete Core Workout. If you just had a baby, start the program with the Postpartum Core (page 212). If Level One of the Complete Core Program seems too difficult, then begin with the Pre-Core Routine (page 159).
2. Be patient. It takes at least six weeks before you start to see results.
3. Don't push yourself too hard, for that will lead to excessive soreness and possible injury. Your goal is to train consistently and establish a healthy exercise habit, not to overdo it and quit.
4. As you progress, add the elements of the Complete Core Program (cardio, strength training, stretching.)

### GUIDELINES

1. When learning a new movement, practice it while you are fresh, not when you're exhausted. This can lead to unnecessary frustration. A good strategy is to set aside a little extra time at the beginning of your workout.
2. In the beginning, your main focus should be on mastering proper technique.

## THE INTERMEDIATE CORE

The intermediate falls into two basic categories:

**THE BIG LAYOFF.** Someone who is coming back after a long layoff, at least six months. This layoff could have been because of an injury, a baby, or just laziness. Whatever the reason, you're back!

**START-AND-STOP SYNDROME.** You want to be fit and healthy, but you struggle to stay on a consistent program. You're stuck in the hellish limbo of the start-and-stop syndrome. You've done workout tapes, taken classes, joined a gym, probably bought a piece of fitness equipment (that is now in the closet), you've read health and fitness magazines (or browsed through them on the stands), and you've purchased an exercise book.

You stay with a workout for a while, then quit exercising for a few weeks or a couple of months. You need to get to the next level and make fitness and wellness a natural and consistent part of your life.

## STRATEGIES FOR THE INTERMEDIATE LEVEL

1. Start with the Complete Core Program and work your way through all the levels. If you just had a baby, start the program with postpartum Core.
2. Unlike the beginner, you are going to have some muscle memory and you will have done some of the exercises before. But don't let your ego get in the way and try to get back to your old form too quickly. Although your mind will want to jump ahead, your body needs to move at the pace of a beginner. So go slow and work your way through Level One of the program. Patience and consistency is your path to the next level.

## GUIDELINES

1. Stick with the pace of the program; don't be impatient and try to move forward too fast.
2. Even if you think you know the exercise, review the instructions and trainer's tips before you jump into it.
3. Set realistic goals. Even if you'd like to do more, under-promise. Starting and stopping often boils down to trying to do too much. Then "I don't have enough time" becomes an excuse to quit.
4. Find ways to motivate and challenge yourself when you feel like quitting. Hire a personal trainer for a month, or train with a friend. Do whatever it takes.
5. After you've trained for three months straight, give yourself a break and take a few days off. The important thing is that you consciously choose the break. You're not giving up. Taking these breaks will be the very thing that allows you to come back and train at a higher level.

### ADVANCED LEVEL: THE ELITE CORE

If you're in the Elite Core you've made fitness an important and integral part of your lifestyle. You've been working out consistently for at least two years.

### STRATEGIES FOR THE ELITE CORE

1. There are many ways this book can challenge you. You can go through the Complete Core Program but add weight to the movements so your repetitions stay in the prescribed range. This would be our recommendation.
2. You could start with Level Three of the Workout.
3. You could start with the Advanced Core System.
4. You could do any of the specialized routines to challenge your core, adding variety and excitement to your training.

### GUIDELINES

1. At this level your challenge is to harness the power of the mind, using the mind-muscle link. Focusing your mind on the muscles/area you're training will take your training to new heights.
2. Continually find new ways to motivate and challenge yourself with a complete program that includes weight training, cardio, and stretching.
3. This is key for you: Don't overtrain and/or become too self-critical. This takes the joy and pleasure out of the process. If you miss a workout, don't beat yourself up.
4. Look at Creating Your Own Routine (page 145) to incorporate advanced principles into your program.

### DISCOVERING YOUR CORE PERSONALITY

Part of being a personal trainer is like being a therapist, so now it's lie-down-on-the-couch time. This section gives you some pointers to start a dialogue between your personality and your workout goals.

Before we get into the personality types, let's go over some basics. First of all, each type is just a simple outline of dominant characteristics. Everyone is a combination of different types. Each of us has a social side and a reclusive side; a single trait is not a valid representation of your complete character. These categories give you a way of thinking about yourself and your tendencies. It is also important to understand that one personality type is not better than any other—each type has its own virtues and paths to achieving a goal.

## BASIC TYPES

**SOLO OR SOCIAL:** These two types explore how you relate to the world. Ask yourself this question: What do I do to relax and recharge?

**SOLO:** Likes to be alone or with a close friend to recharge.

**SOCIAL:** Likes to go to parties or other social situations to relax and recharge.

**WORKOUT STRATEGY:** If you're the social type, take classes. If you're the solo type, train alone or with a close friend. Get a book or tape instead of taking a class. This is common sense, but so many people choose a workout plan that goes against their personality.

It's also fine to mix it up. Sometimes you want to be alone, other times you want to be around people. Listen to your needs.

## STEP-BY-STEP, OR THE BIG PICTURE

These two types explore your learning style. Ask yourself this question: How do I best learn things?

**STEP-BY-STEP:** Likes to learn things one step at a time and understand the reasons that connect each step. Likes concrete facts, details, and specific instructions.

**THE BIG PICTURE:** Likes to see the whole first, to understand the larger concepts and general patterns before filling in the details.

**WORKOUT STRATEGY:** A lot of information we give you in this book is practical, detailed, and step-by-step. This organized structure is an inherent part of a "how-to" book. The step-by-stepper should feel comfortable with this structure.

But this type of detail work and specificity might drive the big-picture type insane. It may grind against your nature, making you want to quit the program. Not to worry: This book can also work for the big-picture person. That's why we recommend the Get Started Now approach. So jump right in and fill in the important details as you go.

Know your learning style and let it work for you, not against you.

## THE PLANNER, OR GO WITH THE FLOW

These two types explore how you structure your life and make decisions. Ask yourself this question: How do I like to organize my day?

**THE PLANNER:** Likes things clearly ordered and mapped out for the day.

**GO WITH THE FLOW:** Likes to take things as they come instead of having a firm plan.

**WORKOUT STRATEGY:** Okay, we know what the planner needs. We know the virtues of being well organized and having a clear vision. This is a skill we all need to move ahead in the world, and we all have it in different degrees.

This book follows that philosophy. To have a plan is not that much different than having a dream. We all have dreams. To the planner I say keep it up, but also be careful. Don't let your planning turn into a rigid compulsion. Be open to taking a detour. Listen to your body, for it may need a break. Being too rigid can lead to burnout and injury.

If you're the type that needs to go with the flow, a strict routine is a surefire recipe for getting discouraged and quitting the program. However, variety and change are important training principles. But as I did with the planner, I will give you a word of warning: Learn the basic techniques and build a foundation. The single most important reason for this is safety. Proper technique and a base of strength are key for preventing injury. This means you must stay with the plan, learn the basics, and build a foundation on a schedule. So the early stages, when it is essential to stay on track, may be your biggest challenge. You need to keep some consistency and structure to get results, especially in the beginning. Don't worry, this isn't forever; once you have this foundation, you can be an exercise improv artist, creating from a repertoire of exercises and routines.

# PART TWO

# THE CORE MIND

# 4
# CORE GOALS

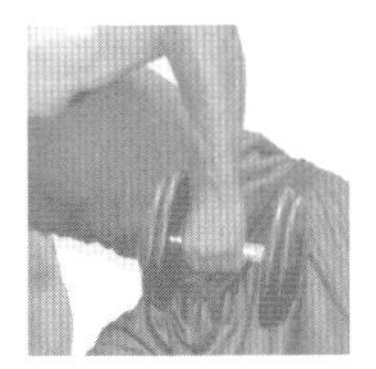

## GOALS: KEEPING YOUR EYE ON THE PRIZE

**This chapter gives you strategies to create goals. Having a clear vision will help you stay on the path. Setting goals will:**

- Focus your attention
- Give you a way to measure your progress
- Mobilize your effort in a consistent and specific way
- Keep you focused on the big picture and daily goals
- Allow you to evaluate and adjust your strategy

## ENDS AND MEANS

There are two basic ways of thinking about goals: the ends and the means. These two ideas are interlocked in the journey of making your vision a reality. You need to be clear about how these concepts work together.

End goals are centered around a specific result and are clear-cut, such as:

- **Lower my body fat by 5 percent**
- **Complete Level Three of the Complete Core Workout**
- **Do cardio three times a week**

The means is the process or the strategy you execute to achieve your goals. This process, or means, is the day-to-day struggle to reach your goal. It is about "walking the walk." Goal setting is a combination of a long-term plan and short-term goals that focus on this process.

## THE LONG AND SHORT OF GOAL SETTING

You need to set long-term, intermediate, short-term, and daily goals. Change doesn't happen overnight. You need a long-term vision and practical daily steps to help you achieve your goal. You also need intermediate goals to help you evaluate your progress and process. These are like quarters and halves in a basketball game.

**LONG-TERM GOAL.** This is your dream, your grand vision.

**INTERMEDIATE GOAL.** This is the midpoint of the process. If you had a six-month exercise plan, this would be your three-month benchmark.

**SHORT-TERM GOAL.** On a six-month plan this could range from one month to a week, depending on how detailed you need to be.

**DAILY GOAL.** These are your bread-and-butter goals. These little steps will take you to your dream. If it's a technique goal, make it as specific as possible. For example, "I'm going to focus on activating my inner core before I start each exercise."

## MAKING ADJUSTMENTS

You will not achieve every goal like clockwork. An important goal-setting skill is the ability to adjust and fine-tune your goals. From time to time you need to honestly evaluate your end goal and your means. You have to be willing to adjust your goals up or down. It can be a difficult proposition to adjust them down, because this can make you feel like a failure. You need to be open and adaptable. Don't let your ego get in the way. If you push yourself too hard, this will lead to injury or burnout. Either one of these outcomes will leave you much farther from your goal than the adjustment.

Circumstances that you can't control can also make an adjustment necessary. Don't push yourself if you have the flu or a cold, an exhausting project at work, or any other type of crisis. Adjust to the situation. The key is not to stop completely. In almost any situation, you can find fifteen minutes a few times a week to maintain your gains and relieve stress. Remember, the ultimate goal is consistency over the long haul. A goal is a way of making your dream more specific. It is a fundamental first step in getting the results you want.

## SETTING GOALS: RULES OF THUMB

1. Make your goals specific. There's no reality in generalities. Your goals need to be stated in measurable terms. "I want to get in shape" is too general. A more specific plan would be to complete all three levels of the Complete Core Program.
2. Make your goals challenging but doable. In the beginning, it is better to err on the side of the doable, gaining confidence and momentum.
3. Write down your goals. It's not a goal if it's not written down. Writing it down is an action, a commitment. We make our clients sign a contract. Once you've written your goals down, you need to read them daily. Read them on days when you're excited about working out; read them on days when you're dreading working out. On both days, this will give you an extra boost.
4. Have a support system. Whenever you're trying to achieve a goal, it's good to have help. This can get tricky. Your friends and lover may actually try to lure you away from your workouts, urging you to have dessert and another drink. Family and friends with similar goals can be effective. Tune out the naysayers.

# 5

# CORE MIND SKILLS

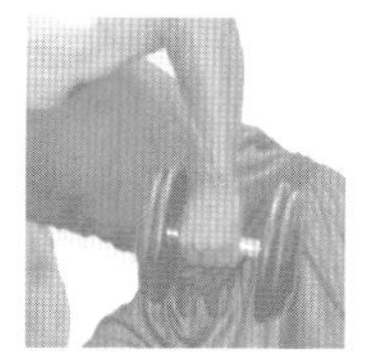

## INTRODUCTION

In this section you will learn basic mind skills to help you improve your performance and manage stress. Your mind responds like a muscle; you need to train it to make it strong. If you don't use it, it will become weak.

## RELAXATION

Relaxation is the foundation for performance. You need to be able to quiet your mind and bring it to a point of concentration before you can concentrate on a challenging activity. Remember, just like any other skill, the more you practice these techniques, the better you will get. These techniques are simple and powerful. We'll begin with a breathing technique.

## CONTROLLED BREATHING

One way to achieve a relaxed state is to concentrate on your breathing. To begin, get into a comfortable position, lying down or sitting, and focus on your breathing; inhale and exhale for approximately one minute.

Then begin to inhale through your nose for a count of five and exhale through your mouth for a count of five. Keep repeating this smooth, regular pattern. Make sure you breathe deeply, letting the breath drop low into your body.

Focus on feeling the air coming into your lungs and imagine it being transported to every cell of your body. Every time you exhale, release any muscular stress or negative thoughts on the breath. Each time you breathe in, imagine the breath purifying your body. Continue this process until you feel relaxed and centered.

This steady, counted deep breathing will calm your nerves. When you're nervous, your breath is shallow and fast. In fact, if you start to take shallow, fast breaths, you'll begin to feel a little nervous. It's a classic example of the mind-body connection. Deep, steady breaths change this pattern and give your body and mind the message to relax. So, whenever you need to feel calm and centered, use this technique.

## HEAD TO TOE: PROGRESSIVE RELAXATION

This technique gives you a tool to consciously program your body to relax. The process is simple. You start from your feet and relax all of your major muscles, from your feet up to the top of your head. You can do this two ways. As you move through your body you can tense and relax each muscle, or you can just give the muscle the mental command to relax. In the following example we will be using just the verbal command. In the beginning, it is helpful to tense and relax, so you can clearly feel the difference between tension and relaxation.

To begin, settle into a comfortable position, either lying down or sitting, and take a couple of deep breaths. Feel where your body is making contact with the floor or the chair.

Now move your focus down to your feet and give them the message to relax, telling all the little muscles on the soles and across the top of your feet to let go. Move up to your calves, and give them the message to relax. Move up to your thighs and hamstrings, telling them to relax. Go to the muscles of your buttocks and tell them to relax.

Then move to your back one section at a time. Give your lower back, middle back, and upper back the message to relax. Then, one area at a time, tell your abdominals, chest, shoulders, arms, and hands to relax.

Finish with your neck, head, and face. Give your neck muscles the message to relax. Tell all the little muscles around your eyes, cheeks, and jaws to relax. Tell your forehead and scalp to relax.

After you have given your entire body, part by part, the message to relax, allow yourself to sink deeper into relaxation with each breath, giving in to gravity and melting into the floor or chair.

You can end the relaxation session anytime you wish by simply saying, "On a count of three, I will open my eyes and feel relaxed and energized, ready to go on with my day." This technique is also good to do with a partner. Have them talk you through each part of your body.

After you have gone through this process a few times, give yourself a relaxation cue word or phrase that will bring you back to this relaxed state. It could be something as simple as the phrase "Let it go," or the name of your pet.

The initial session goes like this: Say your cue word to yourself, followed by a relaxed breath. Then tell yourself, "Whenever I say this word three times, I will return to this relaxed state."

With practice, this verbal reminder, backed up by the breath, will bring your body into a deeper state of relaxation and help reduce the stress of the moment. Your key word is like your password on your computer, but instead of letting you into your hard drive, it is your password to relaxation.

### A BREATHING MEDITATION

The goal of meditation is simple yet difficult. You want to keep your mind focused in the moment and on one task. When your mind resists or wanders, you gently bring it back to the moment and the point of concentration. Over time, this allows you to be in control of your mind, instead of your mind controlling you.

The rules for this meditation are simple. Sit with your spine long, your head floating up and on top of your neck, and your shoulder blades dropped down and together. Then focus on your breathing. Feel the breath come in through your nose and out through your nose. Also, become aware of the natural pause between each cycle of inhalation and exhalation. Keep your mind tuned and focused on your breathing process; when your mind wanders, bring it back. This is different from controlled breathing, in which your breath is controlled in a strict count. In this technique, you allow each breath to be organically what it is. Let your breath mirror what is happening in your body and mind.

## THE PERFORMANCE EDGE

The following techniques—self-talk, visualization, and focusing—are designed to improve your workouts and help you in the process of reaching your goals.

## POSITIVE SELF-TALK

Self-talk is what you are saying to yourself or thinking in the moment. Positive self-talk involves three steps:

- **Slowing down and becoming aware of the negative tape that is playing in your head**
- **Pushing the pause button**
- **Making a new, positive recording**

Taking these three steps puts you in control of your world. It allows you to choose how you are going to respond to life's events. You can't control life's events, but you can control how you respond to them.

Self-talk has two basic forms: positive and negative. Positive self-talk keeps you optimistic and focused in the moment. Phrases like *I feel energized and committed.* Or in a sport it might be a simple cue like *Keep my head down and follow through*.

Negative self-talk prevents you from taking a new action. It keeps you dwelling on the past moment. *I'll never get in shape.* Or in sport you might say something like *I can't hit my nine iron.* Negative self-talk will hold you back in life.

## APPLY SELF-TALK TO EXERCISE

Use self-talk:

1. **For motivation.** *I'll feel so much better after I work out.*
2. **As a reminder.** *Activate my inner core.*
3. **To maintain good habits.** *Stay focused and breathe.*

## SELF-TALK STRATEGIES: TURN NEGATIVES INTO POSITIVES

Just because you know about practicing positive self-talk, the negative self-talk isn't going to just magically stop. You need to become a skilled self-talker, to turn negative self-talk into positive self-talk. It takes consistent and repetitive self-talk to replace the negative tape with a new one.

## EXAMPLES

Negative: I hate warming up.

Positive: Warming up makes the rest of my workout so much better.

## SELF-TALK BASICS

1. **Keep your statements positive:** I will succeed. Negative phrasing: I will not fail.
2. **Keep phrases in the present moment:** I am strong. Not: I will be strong.

3. **Keep it simple:** I feel energized. Wordy: I feel energized because I finally got eight hours of sleep.

## VISUALIZATION

Visualization is the creation of mental pictures. At an unconscious level, you create images all day and all night. These pictures affect your behavior and influence your actions. The goal of a conscious visualization is to create positive images to replace negative images, helping you achieve your goals.

## ELEMENTS OF EFFECTIVE VISUALIZATION

1. Ideally, find a quiet place where you won't be disturbed.
2. Start the visualization with a relaxation technique or controlled breathing to center your body and mind.
3. Set the scene in your visualization, using all your senses to fuel your imagination.
4. Create a scene in your visualization: who, what, where, and when.
5. See in specific details, not in generalities.
6. Let the scene affect you emotionally. Feel the emotions run through your body.
7. See how you affect others in your visualization, and how they react to the new you.
8. Practice the visualization process consistently.

## GETTING FOCUSED AND STAYING FOCUSED

Focus means paying attention to what is important in the moment and disregarding what is unimportant.

When you're working out, you want to focus on the muscles you are training and maintain proper technique. You also want to tune out irrelevant thoughts like *I think I'll have Italian tonight.*

This is the drama of concentrating: struggling to keep your focus on what's important and not letting your mind drift. It's very important when you are working out to keep your mind focused on the exercise and the area you are working. This creates a mind-muscle link, helping you achieve the best results in the least amount of time.

## FOUR TYPES OF FOCUS

Sports psychologist R. M. Nideffer defined four different types of focus; his breakdown can be applied to both sports and exercise. We will define each type, then give you an example of how each focus can be applied to exercising.

1. **Broad focus** happens when you take in the whole scene instead of focusing on a specific spot. It is a wide-angle shot, as opposed to zooming in tight.
2. **Narrow focus** happens when you zoom in on a single element or a small part of a scene or exercise.
3. **External focus** happens when you focus on something outside yourself.
4. **Internal focus** happens when you focus on your thoughts and feelings.

### EXERCISE APPLICATIONS

Let's take a set of Supermans as an example:

1. Broad external focus: Check out your space, then situate yourself on the floor where you have space to do the exercise.
2. Broad internal focus: Get yourself psyched up with a little pep talk. *Come on, let's push hard.* This is a general self-talk psych-up.
3. External narrow focus: Do a specific scan of your body—head, hips, legs—to make sure you are in the proper starting position.
4. Internal narrow focus: Consciously activate your inner core before you start the exercise, and focus on feeling your muscles work—the mind-muscle link in action.

### TO SUM UP

These focus types give you a systematic way to use concentration when you're training and in real life situations. During a set of 12 reps your focus may cycle through these four different types several times. Becoming aware of these focus types will help you effectively apply them during your workout.

### DEVELOP A TRAINING RITUAL

The following is a sample preparation ritual:

**Step 1:** Take a deep breath and get centered, bringing your concentration to the moment and the task at hand.

**Step 2:** Visualize the exercise you are going to perform in perfect form.

**Step 3:** Activate your inner core.

**Step 4:** Keep your mind focused on the movement and muscles.

**Step 5:** After completing the exercise, evaluate your performance. Make a note of any adjustments or things you want to work on. Give yourself a little positive self-talk for doing the exercise and move on.

# 6 CORE MOTIVATION

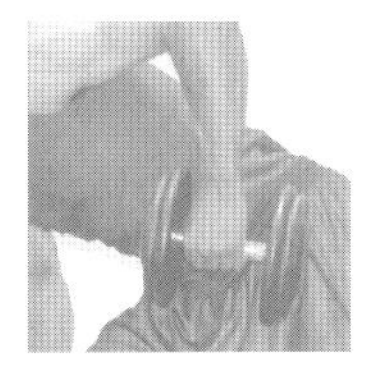

## INTRODUCTION: THE MOTIVATIONAL CHALLENGE

The challenge of motivation begs the underlying existential question: Why do I get out of bed in the morning? Why don't I just give in to a life of sloth, watch TV, and eat junk food? What makes me push for that promotion at work? To be or not to be? Why do anything when in the end we're all food for worms? Staying motivated and consistently striving to achieve one's goals on a daily basis is one of the great challenges of life. Our goal is to give you some motivational strategies to help you achieve your goals.

Motivation is also about choice. Do you really want to stay where you are? Or do you want to create a better life, one in which you look and feel better, get more enjoyment doing things you love, and still be able to do those things as you age? In order to be someone you've never been, you have to do things you've never done.

Here's our motivational argument for working out, in a nutshell: A life in which you don't have a regular exercise routine is less enjoyable than a life in which you have a consistent workout program. Believe us when we say "Life does get better when you work out." It makes everything better. Food tastes better, because every cell in your body is hungry. Sleep is better, because your body is a "good tired" instead of just a "stressed tired." You have more energy, because your body has become more efficient and stronger. Sure, more energy is a good thing, but how can you say "No" to anything that makes eating and sleeping better. And, as you've read in so many places, being in shape improves your sex life. Okay, now you're excited.

Ultimately, motivation is like a muscle: You have to use it consistently, so it is strong and ready when you need it the most, in moments of weakness. You are going to need it. So you need to keep your motivation muscle strong and ready to face the challenges and the obstacles in front of you. Henry James said, "The most important thing to have in life is a mighty will." Let's take a closer look at motivation in theory and in practice.

## OBSTACLES

### HOMEOSTASIS

Homeostasis is a powerful obstacle to motivation. Whereas motivation is about inspiring change and growth, homeostasis is about resisting change and growth. Understanding how homeostasis works is the best way to beat it. Homeostasis is like a computer program installed in your body to resist change—it fights to keep all your systems stable. Without this homeostasis program regulating your body, you wouldn't survive. For example, if our body temperature goes up by just a few degrees, there will be major problems. This system of stabilization is essential for survival.

The problem with homeostasis's vigilant guard against change is that it doesn't distinguish between positive and negative change. Its objective is to protect the norm. A person's normal behavior can evolve into patterns that are not healthy for the body. Homeostasis will protect this unhealthy pattern as ardently as a healthy pattern.

For example, if a person eats processed fast foods high in salt, sugar, and chemical flavoring, homeostasis will protect this pattern. When this person tries to eat healthy whole food, like steamed broccoli and brown rice, it will taste bland, the body will even struggle to digest it, and the stomach will get upset. The taste buds have become deadened by the overseasoned and processed food, so the more subtle tastes of natural foods seem bland. At first, your body will reject the good food in favor of bad food.

The same thing can happen when you begin to work out. Your body is likely to rebel. You may get dizzy or sick during the workout. When workout time rolls around, you may become extra tired. Homeostasis will say, "Hey, this is supposed to be nachos, couch, and TV time."

Homeostasis also has a social aspect. When you pass on going back for a second helping on the free wings at happy hour, your friends may tease and taunt you, calling you "Mr. Healthy." Change is not easy. Each change is a little revolution that will create reverberations in your world.

The purpose of telling you all this, as you start the core program, is to warn you. Beware. When homeostasis kicks in, know what is happening. Your body and your world will resist change at first. There will be a battle before you break through and achieve a healthier new pattern of homeostasis. Know that it is not a lack of character when resistance kicks in. It's natural. It's actually good. It means you are on the path to change. But you have to fight for this healthy change.

Be smart about fighting for change. Negotiate with your friend homeostasis on small changes. These little changes will add up to big changes.

## IMMEDIATE GRATIFICATION

One of the motivational obstacles of our current age is the need for immediate gratification: *"I want it and I want it now."* Because of limited range of attention, we seem to be losing the ability to create a long-term vision and stick to it. This is what we call Cultural Attention Deficit Disorder (CADD for short). CADD is not a pretty word. We can't keep our eye on the ball long term. Over and over we choose short-term gratification over long-term happiness.

The search for instant gratification means we're never happy for long. We have one climatic moment, then land in the void and begin our search for another quasi climax. Instant gratification is like sex without love. It fills a physical need, but something is missing. Our long-term vision muscles have atrophied from disuse; our immediate gratification muscles have grown disproportionately dominant. The two muscles are out of balance. We want everything and we want it now. And we are even proud of this bravado.

We want results without having to go through the struggle of achieving them. We take diet pills and undergo liposuction instead of eating healthy and exercising. We take pills to help us sleep, to keep us up, to cure our anxieties, fears, grief, moods, and sex lives. We treat symptoms, not the underlying causes. We become symptoms.

We lose touch with what is deeper. We don't want to wrestle in the messy middle of things, where the battle of life is fought. We want to skip the day-to-day grind of life. The irony is, this is where all the beauty of life resides. We are, of course, generalizing. This is not true of everyone. By just buying this book and aspiring to get on a fitness program, you have taken a positive step. But this need for instant gratification is something most of us struggle against.

The process, the means, the road traveled determines the beauty of the end result. Here are two different experiences of reaching the top of the mountain. In experience one you climb to the top of a mountain, where the trail is filled with challenges and beautiful vistas. Then, when you reach the top, you savor the breathtaking view. In experience number two you take a helicopter to the top of the mountain, get out and look at the view, then hop back in the helicopter. Which experience would be deeper, more satisfying? What do we lose when we skip the difficult process that would give us the chance of long-term transformation and go for the easy quick fix?

Pushing hard every day with a goal out there in the distance is the opposite of immediate satisfaction. Ultimately you need to have a long-term vision and learn to love the struggle.

## MOTIVATION THEORY

Now let's look at two basic motivational strategies, ways of thinking holistically and long-term, and techniques to stay motivated in the moment, to get into the flow. To do this, we will take a quick look at three different motivational psychologists: Edward Denci, Abraham Maslow, and Mihaly Csikszentmihalyi.

### THE DENCI STUDY: TWO TYPES OF MOTIVATION

Edward Denci, a social scientist, did a classic study in the 1960s that illustrates two basic types of motivation. He gave two groups of college students a Parker Brothers puzzle game. The goal was to put the puzzles together in their proper formation. One group received a dollar for each puzzle they completed in the allotted time; the other group worked on the puzzle without any mention of reward.

After a prescribed amount of time, the students were given a scheduled break. On the table in front of them Denci left a pile of current magazines. The participants were observed through a one-way mirror during this break. The amount of time the players worked on the puzzle during the break was the way Denci measured personal versus external motivation. The participants who received the dollar reward spent significantly less time working on puzzles during the break. They read the magazines. The other group continued to work on the puzzles during the break. This illustrated the importance of personal motivation.

You need to discover the pleasure in the doing of things for their own sake. You need to find deep and satisfying personal reasons. You also need to mix in external rewards. When you reach a goal, treat yourself to something you want. Over the course of a lifetime, you will need both techniques in your motivational tool kit.

## MASLOW AND PEAK EXPERIENCE

A good model for long-term and holistic thinking is Abraham Maslow and his theory of the Hierarchy of Needs. Maslow was a humanistic psychologist who believed in free will and human potential. The end goal of his philosophy was peak experience, or self-actualization. His hierarchical system is based on five levels of basic needs. Maslow believed that each level had to be fulfilled before you could move to the next level. Maslow saw the big picture and how each level was connected and related to every other level. To get motivated and stay motivated, you have to keep an eye on all your basic needs. Maslow's five levels are the following.

**PHYSIOLOGICAL NEEDS.** These are biological needs, which include food, water, clean air, shelter, sleep, sex, and so forth.

**SAFETY NEEDS.** These needs include protection, security, law, structure, stability, and so forth.

**LOVE AND BELONGINGNESS NEEDS.** These needs include relationships, family, community, and so forth.

**ESTEEM NEEDS.** These needs include respect, status, responsibility, social achievement, and so forth.

**SELF-ACTUALIZATION NEEDS.** These needs include personal development, growth, creativity, self-expression, maximizing potential, and so forth.

For a sustained commitment you must be motivated by more than your immediate desires. To stay motivated, you must take into consideration all your basic needs and your environment.

## FLOW AND BEING IN THE MOMENT

In his book *Flow*, Mihaly Csikszentmihalyi, a psychology professor at the University of Chicago, studied the elements that make up optimal experience. There are many names for this state: *being in the zone, playing your "A" game, peak experience, in the groove*, and so forth. These are periods when you are totally engrossed in what you are doing and you forget all your troubles and worries.

Csikszentmihalyi discovered that these experiences happen when you are actively involved in tasks that challenge your mental and physical capabilities, not during laid-back leisure time. Flow can happen at your job, when you are teaching your son to hit a baseball, rock climbing, working out, and so forth. Optimal experience lifts you out of the everydayness of life to a heightened state of enjoyment and productivity.

This, of course, leads to the big question: What are the basic elements of flow and how do you incorporate these elements into your life and your workout? The following are some of the key elements that Csikszentmihalyi says are present during flow:

- **You need complete focus and engagement in your activity.**
- **You need immediate feedback to judge your progress and success.**

- **Your task needs to challenge your skill level, but not be too difficult or too easy.**
- **Your task needs a clear objective and a reasonable chance of completing it.**
- **You need to have control over your actions.**
- **You need to surrender to the process. Don't strive, stress, or strain to reach your goal—enjoy the process.**

Csikszentmihalyi said, "People who learn to control their inner experience will be able to determine the quality of their lives, which is as close as any of us can come to being happy." In short, our intention, what we choose to focus on, and how we respond to the circumstances of our life will determine the quality of our lives, how happy and productive we are. Try to apply these elements to your workouts and the fitness goals you set. This type of active engagement can bring flow into your workouts. These concepts will give you a framework to get motivated and stay motivated.

After all this theory, here are some practical tips to keep you going:

- **Make sure your long-term, intermediate, short-term, and daily goals are clear. Motivation is directly linked to a plan of action. It's hard to get motivated and stay motivated if you don't know how and why you're doing something.**
- **Maintain variety. Keep your schedule flexible so you don't get stuck in a rut.**
- **Change your workout when you get bored with it.**
- **Create rewards for each small goal you achieve. Don't just think of one big reward at the end. If you never get a pat on the back, you lose motivation. These rewards can be as simple as going to a movie, buying a CD, or taking a nap.**
- **Take time off—don't overtrain. Listen to your body; that's how you build a relationship with it. When you reach a point of diminishing returns, take a break. A little rest and relaxation is a great attitude adjuster.**
- **Don't put unnecessary pressure on yourself. Don't connect your entire self-worth with any single project. Keep things in perspective and make it fun.**
- **The goal is to stay active and healthy for a lifetime.**

PART THREE

# THE CORE WORKOUT SYSTEM

# 7
# INTRODUCTION TO THE COMPLETE CORE WORKOUT

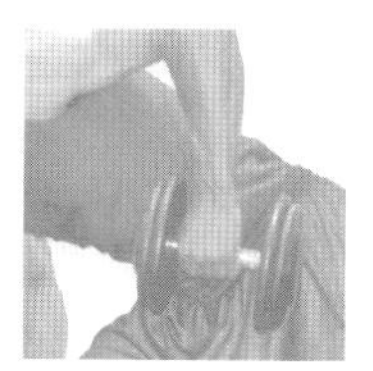

## INTRODUCTION

The Complete Core Workout is a twelve-week core routine that incorporates the latest training techniques to strengthen and define your core.

It has three levels: Beginning, Intermediate, and Advanced. It is designed to fit into your current fitness program or it can be integrated with the Complete Core Program, which includes cardio, strength training, and stretching. Once you initiate yourself into the core workout, you can begin to gradually add the other fitness elements from the Complete Core Program.

Before you begin, you need to warm up to prepare your body to train. You can do either five minutes of light cardio activity or the Dynamic Warm-Up routine (page 157). We highly recommend the Dynamic Warm-Up. It will prepare your core and also improve your agility. If you're already on a fitness program, you can also do this routine at the end of your workout.

## THE COMPLETE CORE WORKOUT DESIGN

The Complete Core Workout exercises all the major muscles of the core:

- **The abdominal muscles**
- **The lower back muscles**
- **The glute (butt) muscles**
- **The muscles that surround and stabilize the hips**
- **The deep inner muscles that support the spine**

The workout is also designed to train major movement patterns. To put it simply, it is designed to train and strengthen your body in all directions, in the way it is naturally designed to move, and the way you use your body in life. It works your body through the following movement patterns:

- **Flexion (forward bending movements, including leg flexion)**
- **Extension (backward extending movements, including leg extension)**
- **Rotational movements**
- **Crossing and side-to-side movements**
- **Adduction (bringing your legs together)**
- **Abduction (spreading your legs apart)**

At each level the Complete Core Workout includes exercises that work these muscles and movements.

## PACE

Each level is designed for a four-week duration. You may reach the prescribed goal in less time or it may take you more time—everyone is different. If it takes you more time to fulfill the requirements, then that's the perfect pace for you. If you reach the goals in less time, you need to hit the prescribed goal at least three times in a row before you go to the next level. These guidelines hold for all three levels.

# 8

# LEVEL ONE: GET STARTED NOW

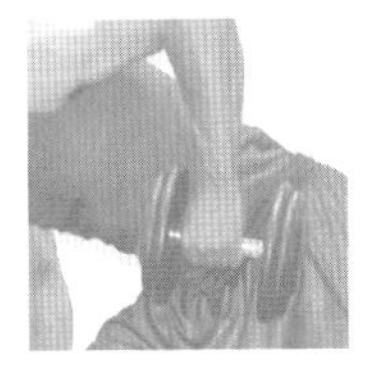

## LEVEL ONE: GET STARTED NOW

Okay, it's time for your first workout. In the beginning, the most important thing is to focus on learning how to do the exercises properly. Don't get frustrated if the movements feel awkward at first. The goal is to just make a little progress each workout. The objective of Level One is simply to get to Level Two.

## GOALS

The fitness goal of Level One is to begin to build a foundation of balanced strength in your core. You will be working many new muscles; some muscles will be weaker than others. Creating a balance helps prevent injuries. This level will also give you a base of strength and endurance that is necessary for good posture and efficient movement.

## GETTING MOTIVATED

It's important at this stage of your training to be patient. You're not going to see immediate results. Consistency is key. If you do a little bit every day, it will add up. Think of it as making deposits in your fitness bank account. Start to use ideas from the core mind section: Clarify your personal reasons, visualize the results you want, give yourself external rewards each week.

## TRAINING GUIDELINES

**SETS:** Do one set of each exercise.

**REST TIME:** The goal is to be able is go through the entire workout without resting between exercises. If you need to rest between exercises, this is okay; don't push too hard. But keep your eye on the ultimate goal, so keep decreasing your rest time, until you can go from exercise to exercise without resting.

**REPS:**

**WEEK ONE:** 10 repetitions for each exercise; if you have to alternate sides, do 5 reps on each side.

**WEEK TWO:** 14 repetitions for each exercise; if you have to alternate sides, do 7 reps on each side.

**WEEK THREE:** 20 repetitions for each exercise; if you have to alternate sides, do 10 reps on each side.

**WEEK FOUR:** Maintain 20 repetitions for three workouts; if you have to alternate sides, do 10 reps on each side.

**LEVEL ONE: GET STARTED NOW**

1. Standing Knee Flexion, p. 243
2. Ball Reach: Knee Level, p. 325
3. Toe Touch 1, p. 228
4. Heel Touch 1, p. 257
5. Glute Bridge, p. 277
6. Prone Crossover, p. 263
7. Back Extension, p. 252
8. Lying Side Leg Raise, p. 290
9. Lying Inside Leg Raise, p. 291
10. Plank: Down Plank, Up Plank, Side Plank: Each Side, p. 314

# 9

# LEVEL TWO: CREATING STRENGTH AND ENDURANCE

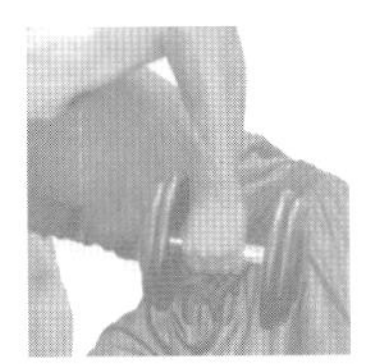

## LEVEL TWO: COMPLETING THE FOUNDATION

Congratulations, you've made it to Level Two. Now that you've mastered the moves in Level One, challenge yourself not only to learn the new moves but to perform these familiar exercises with precision.

### GOALS

The goal of this level is to complete the foundation, cementing the exercise habit and creating an increased base of strength and endurance.

## STAYING MOTIVATED

The middle is a dangerous place. It's too early to see significant results and the excitement of getting started has faded. Focus on the health benefits—how you feel, not how you look.

You might experience the feeling of not wanting to work out, and of not being able to do what you did the last workout. These setbacks aren't what they appear to be. A setback is often preparation for a leap forward. Persevering through these tough days is part of the journey to the next level. So stick with it and believe in the great leap forward. Keep applying the ideas from the Core Mind chapters: read your goals, see your goals, reward yourself. Put these ideas into practice, don't just think about them as an intellectual concept.

## TRAINING GUIDELINES

**SETS:** Do one set of each exercise.

**REST TIME:** The goal is to be able is go through the entire workout without resting between exercises. If you need to rest between exercises, this is okay; don't overdo it. Keep your eye on the prize by decreasing your rest time until you can move between exercises without resting.

**REPS:**

**WEEK ONE:** 10 repetitions for each exercise; if you have to alternate sides, do 5 reps on each side.

**WEEK TWO:** 14 repetitions for each exercise; if you have to alternate sides, do 7 reps on each side.

**WEEK THREE:** 20 repetitions for each exercise; if you have to alternate sides, do 10 reps on each side.

**WEEK FOUR:** Maintain 20 repetitions for three workouts; if you have to alternate sides, do 10 reps on each side.

## CORE SYSTEM LEVEL TWO: COMPLETING THE FOUNDATION LEVEL TWO

1. Standing Knee Flexion with Arms, p. 244
2. Ball Reach: Toe, p. 328
3. Toe Touch 2, p. 229
4. Modified V-Up, p. 224
5. Heel Touch 2, p. 258
6. Leg Over: Single Leg, p. 261
7. Glute Bridge, p. 277
8. Glute Bridge: Single Leg, p. 294
9. Prone Crossover, p. 263
10. Opposite Arm/Opposite Leg, p. 247
11. Back Extension, p. 252
12. Prone Single-Leg Raises, p. 281
13. Lying Hip Rotation, p. 292
14. Plank Series: all positions—30-second holds, p. 314

# 10

# LEVEL THREE: CORE POWER

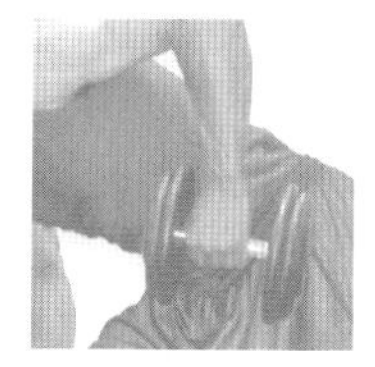

## LEVEL THREE: CORE POWER

Congratulations, you've made it to Level Three. Keep challenging yourself to bring your mind and your body together during your workouts. This level asks more of you by adding new intense exercises.

### GOALS

As you approach these last four weeks, it is important to start adding other fitness elements to your program (if you haven't already). This week, start with the cardio program (page 101).

Next week, add the weight-training program (page 107). The following week, add the stretching routine (page 127). The programs in this book will ease you in gradually, so don't be intimidated.

## STAYING MOTIVATED

Consistency of effort is the key. You will *not* always have consistent results, but you can give each workout a solid effort. In fact, that's all you can do. Even if the workouts seem like drudgery, they are releasing stress, combating anxiety, burning calories, and helping you sleep better. As you approach your goal in this final month, go deeper into your personal reasons for wanting to get in shape. Give yourself rewards at the end of each week, and think of a big reward for finishing the whole program. You are now on the road to making fitness a part of your lifestyle.

## TRAINING GUIDELINES

**SETS:** Do one set of each exercise.

**REST TIME:** The goal is to be able to go through the entire workout without resting between exercises. If you need to rest between exercises, this is okay. But remember your ultimate goal, so keep decreasing your rest time until you can move between exercises without resting.

**REPS:**

**WEEK ONE:** 10 repetitions for each exercise; if you have to alternate sides, do 5 reps on each side.

**WEEK TWO:** 14 repetitions for each exercise; if you have to alternate sides, do 7 reps on each side.

**WEEK THREE:** 20 repetitions for each exercise; if you have to alternate sides, do 10 reps on each side.

**WEEK FOUR:** Maintain 20 repetitions for three workouts; if you have to alternate sides, do 10 reps on each side.

**LEVEL THREE: CORE POWER**

1. Standing Knee Flexion with Arms, p. 244
2. Ball Reach: Heel, p. 330
3. Balance T-Bend, p. 327
4. Toe Touch 3, p. 230
5. V-Up, p. 225
6. Heel Touch 3, p. 259
7. Glute Bridge, p. 277
8. Glute Bridge: Single Leg, p. 294
9. Glute Bridge with Hip Rotation: 45 degree, p. 274
10. Side Superman, p. 238
11. Leg Over: Double Leg, p. 262
12. Prone Double Leg Crossover, p. 264
13. Superman, p. 249
14. Opposite Arm/Opposite Leg, p. 247
15. Back Extension with Rotation, p. 335
16. Prone Single-Leg Raises, p. 281
17. Bent-Leg Kickbacks, p. 279
18. Lying Hip Rotation, p. 292
19. Plank Series: 60-second holds, p. 314

PART FOUR

# THE CORE BODY

# 11
# CORE BASICS: THE INNER CORE

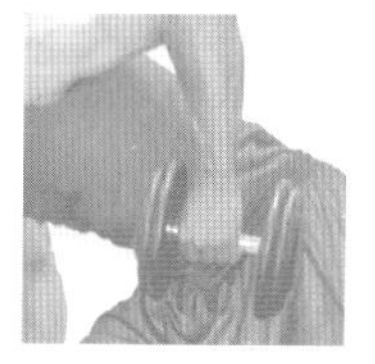

## INTRODUCTION

This chapter introduces you to your inner core. Your inner core is a group of deep muscles that support your spine and give stability to the center of your body. We will focus primarily on the activation of two inner core muscles:

- the transverse abdominis
- the pelvic floor group

# GETTING TO KNOW YOUR INNER CORE

You've probably spent more time training the muscles you want to show off, like the rectus abdominis (the ab six-pack muscle). As a result, you neglect your deep inner muscles, like the transverse abdominis and the pelvic floor. These muscles support your center like a natural girdle or a weight belt. If these inner muscles are weak, regardless of how strong your big external muscles are, you will still be vulnerable to injury and your body will not function at peak efficiency. It is essential that you train your inner and outer muscles. Let's take a closer look at these deep muscles that stabilize and support your spine.

## THE TRANSVERSE ABDOMINIS

The transverse abdominis has become a minor celebrity. The muscle's rise to fame is directly connected to the work of Joseph Pilates. Recent research has shown that strengthening the transverse abdominis is key for alleviating back pain. The transverse abdominis, in a perfect world, is the first muscle to fire when you move, giving your body support. But if you have suffered from back pain, this normal firing pattern can go out of sync and these inner muscles get weak from disuse. So, no matter how hard you train the big outer muscles, you will still be vulnerable to lower back pain. You need to strengthen your inner muscles and restore the natural firing order.

## ENGAGING YOUR TRANSVERSE ABDOMINIS

Your transverse abdominis, the deepest abdominal muscle, runs horizontally across your midsection. It wraps around your waist like a corset and pulls your abdominal wall in, also stabilizing your spine. When your abdomen bulges out, you've lost the support of your transverse abdominis (p. 79).

You activate your transverse abdominis by drawing your belly button toward your spine. It is important to initiate this engagement down low. It helps to think of a spot an inch or two below your belly button. Otherwise, you will be using your rectus abdominis (six-pack muscle) to help execute the movement. The goal is to isolate the transverse abdominis from the rectus abdominis.

You want to gently pull or draw your belly button toward your spine, activating your transverse abdominis. If the activation scale was 1 to 10 (10 being the hardest pulling in), you want to activate your transverse abdominis at an intensity level of about 3.

## YOUR PELVIC FLOOR

The second part of this support system is the pelvic floor. The pelvic floor is the area you work out when you do the famous Kegel exercise. It is a web, or sling, of fascia extending from the front of your pelvis to your lower spine. It surrounds the rectal opening, and in women the vaginal and urethral openings. It is like a thin hammock of support. If your upper body was a barrel, the bottom of the barrel that keeps all the contents in place would be like the pelvic floor.

Before you start to exercise, activate your pelvic floor for support. You don't want to give it a hard squeeze, just a little squeeze to firm up. If the squeeze scale was 1 to 10 (10 being the hardest), you'd want to squeeze at an intensity level of about 3. Keeping this muscle toned, for both men and women, also increases sexual pleasure. For men, it has the added benefit of ejaculatory control.

## KEGELS: THE ESSENTIAL EXERCISE

**THE KEGEL CONNECTION.** Named after Dr. Arnold Kegel, Kegels strengthen the pubococcygeus (PC) muscle. This is the main muscle of the pelvic floor and the major muscle of contraction during orgasm. A strong PC muscle:

- **Improves core support**
- **Improves bladder control**
- **Increases sexual fulfillment**

By increasing blood supply to your pelvis, Kegels can also increase your resistance to urinary tract infections.

## GETTING IN TOUCH WITH YOUR PC MUSCLE

Another function of the PC is to control the flow of urination. When you contract the muscle, it cuts off the flow of urine. There are two simple ways to get in touch with your PC muscle. One is to imagine that you're urinating and then stop the flow; the second is to actually stop the flow when you're urinating, then release the muscle. But it's not recommended to actually do a series of Kegels then, because it can promote, rather than prevent, urinary tract infections. Stopping the flow is just a tangible way to get in touch with the muscle.

**THE KEGEL EXERCISE.** Contract the PC muscle with a moderate, firm squeeze (about a 7 on a scale of 10). Hold the squeeze for five seconds and then release. Do this 10 times in a row, eventually working up to 25 in a row. For optimal results experts recommend working up to 75 squeezes a day, three sets of 25.

Make sure you are not contracting your ab, thigh, and butt muscles at the same time. This will only increase intra-abdominal pressure, aggravating any existing urinary incontinence problem.

**THE KEGEL HABIT.** To be effective, Kegels must be done correctly and regularly for at least three months before results can be expected. So take your time, be patient, and focus. To make Kegels a habit, try doing them:

- **While you watch TV**
- **Before or after working out**
- **Riding in a car or commuting to work**
- **At the movies**
- **At your desk at work**
- **Right now**

## CHOICE OF ENGAGEMENT

When activating your inner core, experiment to find out what works best for you. Research shows that if you activate either your pelvic floor muscles or your transverse abdominis, the other one will also engage. For some people it is easier to activate the pelvic floor and then the transverse abdominis. You will need to experiment. In the beginning it can be helpful to contract your inner thigh muscles by squeezing a towel between your legs.

If you were going to activate the inner core by contracting the pelvic floor, the scenario would work like this. First contract your pelvic floor, then bring your belly button toward your spine. For some people, starting with the pelvic floor helps to keep the focus in the lower ab area, keeping the rectus abdominis from getting involved. For others it is easier to directly activate the transverse abdominis. To do this, bring your lower abdomen toward your spine. There are different mental and verbal cues to help you achieve this goal.

- **Imagine you are tightening a belt around your lower abdominal area.**
- **Hollow or scoop out your lower belly.**
- **Imagine you are zipping up a really tight pair of pants.**

Remember, you don't want to give these muscles the death squeeze, as though you were doing an isometric exercise. That would be like buckling a belt too tight. They are support muscles, so you need them for your entire workout, not just a set or two. A strong inner core will help support your entire body when you exercise and in your daily activities.

## ACTIVATING YOUR INNER CORE: CINCH AND SYNCH

It's a challenge to get a feel for all of this. I like to think of the words "cinch" and "synch." The word cinch has two meanings: It means to draw in or tighten; it also means a thing done with ease, like the phrase "It's a cinch." Tightening with ease is a key element in activating your inner core. This cinching movement is not simply sucking in your gut, which activates your rectus abdominis and causes your pelvis to rotate forward, but rather a tightening and drawing in of the transverse abdominis.

The ultimate goal behind cinching up the inner core is to enable it to work independently and in synch with your bigger external muscles like the rectus abdominis. The inner core supports your body in everyday activities, as well as complicated athletic movements. So think, cinch, and synch.

## BREATHING AND INNER CORE ACTIVATION

### THE DIAPHRAGM

Before we look at breathing, let's take a quick tour of the diaphragm. The diaphragm is a dome-shaped sheath of muscle fiber that arches up inside your rib cage. It is like a mushroom-shaped tent. It is attached or staked out like a tent around the circumference of your lower six ribs, creating an airtight seal. Besides attaching to the ribs, it also attaches to the lower spine and the sternum. In this transverse plane, it creates the floor for your lungs and heart and the ceiling for your stomach, liver, and spleen.

The diaphragm is your breathing muscle. As you inhale, the mushroom dome of the diaphragm lowers and flattens out. As you exhale, the diaphragm rises, re-creating the dome shape.

### BREATHING

Now let's take a closer look at what is supposed to happen when you breathe. As you inhale air, the diaphragm descends and flattens toward the bottom of your ribs where it is anchored. At the same time, the intercostal muscles cause your rib cage to fan out, creating even more space and a vacuum so the lungs expand and fill with air. Then, after a slight pause, the diaphragm releases, rising back to its dome shape, and the ribs move back in. As the diaphragm returns to its dome shape, it helps the lungs expel all their air.

### THE ENEMIES OF BREATH

Breath is life. You can go for weeks without food, days without water, but only minutes without breathing. But breathing has a lot of potential enemies.

**TENSION.** Tension can inhibit the ribs from opening up and allowing a full breath to enter your body.

**SHALLOW BREATHING.** Most people go through the entire day without filling their lungs to full capacity. So the diaphragm and the other breathing muscles become weak from disuse, just like any other muscle.

**HOLDING THE BREATH.** Many people hold their breath and breathe irregularly in little spasms. This causes fatigue and inefficiency. The natural rhythm and power of the breathing cycle gets short-circuited.

**NOT FULLY EXHALING.** Some people breathe in fully, but then have a shallow exhale. That is, they don't fully expel all the air. A full exhalation is what cleanses the body of all the toxins it needs to release. If you don't fully exhale, stagnant air remains in the bottom of the lungs, like a stagnant pool of water.

What does all this have to do with exercise? Working out is your opportunity for full and complete breaths that both energize and cleanse your body.

## BREATHING AND EXERCISE

Proper breathing can be confusing. Part of the confusion is created because there's no one correct way of breathing that fits every situation. Breathing is specific—it matches the task at hand. You wouldn't breathe the same way to pick up a heavy weight as you would to lift a cup of hot coffee to your lips.

Another reason for the confusion is the variety of ways breathing is taught. The following two techniques represent two common, but opposite, ways of teaching breathing.

**THE YOGA BELLY BREATH.** In some yoga classes the instructor tells you to completely relax your belly and let the breath drop deep into your belly. The belly expands in front of the body on the inhalation. Then, on the exhalation, the belly contracts back inward. This way of breathing is good for relaxation but not for sports and working out. It is not three dimensional; it is just frontal.

**THE JOSEPH PILATES BREATH.** This style of breathing is called diaphragmatic breathing, or lateral rib breathing. In this breath the movement takes place primarily in the lateral outward movement of the lower ribs. The belly does not balloon out as significantly as on the above yoga breath. The lateral movement make it easier to keep your inner core activated. It is good for exercise and sports.

These two examples represent two common ways people are taught to breathe, one frontal and the other lateral.

The key thing is to breathe three-dimensionally. This means breath fills the front, back, and sides of your body. And remember, breathing is specific and should fit the task at hand.

Here are some important breathing tips to keep in mind when working out and in life.

1. Don't hold your breath; breathe.
2. Exhale during the working phase of a movement, which means when you're moving against the most force or resistance. For example, if you're doing a glute bridge, exhale as you raise your hips and inhale as you lower them. When you're jumping, inhale as you bend your knees and exhale as you leap.
3. When in doubt, breathe rhythmically in a way that supports the movement.
4. When you have your inner core activated, just squeeze it down low at level 3 intensity and

breathe above your belly button. Even though you are activating an abdominal muscle, your diaphragm should still be able to expand to its full range of motion.

5. Breathing needs to be specific, and the wisdom of your body (for the most part) should take over. It is a balancing act between support and freedom. In the beginning, practicing full, deep breaths (do at least 10 a day) will give your body the power to support its wisdom. Like any muscle, your breathing muscles can become weak and lazy if you don't train them.

6. Your lungs are three-dimensional, so breathe three-dimensionally. Breathe in the entire circumference of your diaphragm. That means into the back of your ribs, into the sides of your ribs, and into the front of your ribs. If you're really winded and your body is recovering, you will notice how your inhalations fill your entire body, 360 degrees around, not just the front or sides of your body.

7. To sum up: When in doubt, breathe. During your core workout, work at having your inner core activated while you breathe freely and powerfully above that inner support. It is like learning to juggle; soon it will be second nature.

## IN SUM: THE INNER CORE

The inner core is made up of the deeper muscles that are closer to your spine. These aren't as famous as the six-pack muscle or your love handles, but they are every bit as important. The two deep muscles that we are most concerned with are the transverse abdominis and the pelvic floor muscles. For a more extensive step-by-step process, see the Inner Core Program (page 163). You don't have to be an inner-core master to start the program, and you don't have to be an inner-core master to begin and receive all the benefits of the Complete Core Workout. But it is something you should concentrate on at each workout. Before you start each exercise, remind yourself to activate your inner core. Be patient and persistent; eventually it will become second nature.

# 12
# A TRAINING PRIMER: BASIC PRINCIPLES AND TECHNIQUES

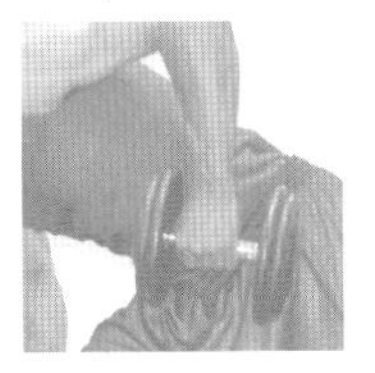

## CORE TRAINING PRINCIPLES

### INTRODUCTION

The following questions cover important workout principles and techniques, and address some of the most frequently asked workout questions. These basics are essential for a safe, productive, and positive workout experience.

## BASIC DEFINITIONS

### *Could you explain to me what a rep and a set are?*

A repetition, also referred to as a rep, is the completion of one entire movement cycle in an exercise. One rep of a Superman (pg. 249) would be raising your upper and lower body off the floor and then lowering them back to the floor. If you did that movement 10 times, that would be 10 repetitions. You probably knew that.

A set is the completion of one or more repetitions. If your goal is to do 10 repetitions of Supermans and you do 10, then you have completed one set of 10 reps. If you just did 9 reps, you still did a set, even though you didn't quite reach your goal. It would just mean you did one set of 9 reps.

## WARMING UP

### *Why do I need to warm up?*

Warming up prepares your body to exercise by:

- **Increasing blood flow to the muscles, allowing them to work more efficiently.**
- **Increasing muscle temperature, allowing the muscles to contract more forcefully and with more speed.**
- **Preparing your body to move in all directions.**
- **Reducing your chance of injury.**

### *What's the best way to warm up?*

In Part Six, The Routines, you will be introduced to the Dynamic Warm-Up, a unique way of warming up your body for core work. The typical warm-up is five minutes of any type of light cardio work. The dynamic warm-up is a series of moves that takes you through your major movement patterns.

## MASTERING TECHNIQUE

### *What's the best way to learn a new exercise?*

It's best to learn a new exercise when you're fresh and focused. You need to give yourself a little extra time to study the photos and read the instructions. You need to get a grasp of the overall movement and the finer points of the exercise. Don't get frustrated if the movements feel awkward or you struggle with some of these finer technical points. In every new endeavor there is a learning curve. Just be patient and stick with it. Here are a few tips:

- **Carefully study the examples.**
- **Break the movement into doable segments: a beginning, middle, and end.**
- **Give special attention to elements of the exercise that you might find are difficult.**

In the beginning, it is essential to master the proper technique for each exercise. This is the first step; everything else takes a backseat. Don't worry about the recommended reps for each exercise, these are just recommendations. It doesn't matter how many reps you do, if you're doing them wrong.

## ADDING INTENSITY

### *How do I know when to add weight to an exercise?*

Adding weight increases the intensity and difficulty of the exercise. You can start to add weight once you've mastered proper technique and reached your repetition goal. If you haven't mastered the technique and try to push it, you increase the risk of injury.

Your repetition goals tell you when you should add weight. A common example is the 8-to-12 repetition scheme. In this scheme, you choose a weight that will allow you to do 8 reps. As you get stronger, the number of reps you can do increases. When you can do 12 repetitions, you add a weight that will allow you to do only 8 reps again. Then work your way back up to 12 reps and add weight again. Exercise is all about positive adaptation. As your body adjusts, adapts, and gets stronger, you progress by adding new challenges, more reps, and increased weight.

Staying in a positive training zone can be a delicate balance. You don't want to push yourself too hard and overtrain. When you work out, especially weight training, you break your muscles down; they need rest to grow back bigger and stronger. That's why you don't weight train every day.

There are other ways to build intensity into a program, besides adding weight. Other intensity builders include:

- **Doing a more difficult exercise for the same body part**
- **Adding an extra set**
- **Increasing the number of repetitions**
- **Decreasing rest times between sets**
- **Doing the exercise in a more challenging form, such as on a core board, on an exercise ball, or standing on one leg instead of two.**

You want to add intensity gradually, usually adding just one intensity builder at a time. This can get complicated. For a more detailed explanation, see Creating Your Own Routine (page 145).

## BREAKDOWN IN TECHNIQUE

***I hear trainers sometimes tell their clients, "One more rep." How do I know when I should stop instead of trying to go for one more repetition?***

The clearest answer is a breakdown in technique. This means you should stop when you can no longer do the exercise properly. For example, a Roll-Up (page 231) requires that your feet stay on the floor through the entire movement. So on your tenth repetition, if you have to bring your feet off the floor to complete the movement, you have suffered a breakdown in technique—it's time to stop. When your technique gets sloppy, you're no longer effectively working the targeted area, and you're increasing your chances of injury.

Another familiar example is swinging your upper body when you're doing biceps curls, using momentum instead of your biceps muscles. Be vigilant in spotting these tendencies.

## FULL RANGE OF MOTION

***What does full range of motion mean?***

A full range of motion means doing the exercise through its entire range of movement. For example, on Knee Touches, you want to be able to touch the tops of your knees, not just your thighs, with your hands.

## THE NEGATIVE TO POSITIVE SIDE OF A REPETITION

***I get confused about the different phases of a repetition.***

You'll often hear fitness trainers say something like this: "Control the weight on the negative phase of the rep." This is a simple concept, but it can be confusing if no one has explained it to you. First, let's look at an exercise example. In a push-up, the positive phase is when you push your body off the floor; the negative phase is when you lower your body back toward the floor. You want to keep the stress on the muscles, so you want to lower your body back toward the floor at a little slower rate than you raised it. You want to fight the forces of gravity by slowing or controlling the negative (lowering) phase of the push-up movement.

Let's look at another exercise. When you are squatting, the negative phase is when you lower your body into the squat position and the positive phase is when you raise back up to the standing position.

Here's a more concise definition of these two concepts that you can apply to almost any exercise. The positive phase of the exercise (pushing your body up away from the floor in a push-up) occurs when you move against the most resistance. During this phase you increase the speed with a controlled, but powerful, movement.

The negative phase of an exercise (lowering your body toward the floor in a push-up) occurs when you move against the least resistance. During this phase you slow the speed down a little.

## SPEED OF MOVEMENT

### *How fast should I do the exercises?*

As a rule, no matter how fast or slow you are exercising, you need to maintain proper technique throughout the full range of motion. This keeps tension on the muscles and doesn't let gravity take over. When you decrease the speed of exercise, it often becomes more difficult to perform. Varying the speed beyond the norm is an advanced technique.

## THE FOUR SPEEDS

We will outline four basic speeds. The following guidelines will give you general parameters.

**STANDARD SPEED.** This is the norm. It's medium, neither fast nor slow. This can be a little tricky, because standard speed is connected to the positive and negative phases of the exercise movement. As we said earlier, normally you execute the positive phase of a movement at a faster rate than the negative phase.

Let's look at a push-up again. A standard speed for a push-up would be approximately one second to raise your body and two seconds to lower it. This makes for a more explosive positive phase and a more controlled and slower negative phase. Now let's look at four speed variations and see how they relate to this standard speed.

**SLOW.** This means you downshift and slow the movement down by a gear. For example, when you downshift, the positive phase of a push-up may take two seconds and the negative phase may take three seconds.

**SUPER SLOW.** This means moving in a very slow and controlled motion. If this speed is prescribed, you will be given an exact count to follow. For example, you might take a ten-second count on both the positive and negative phases of a push-up.

**FAST.** This means you speed up the pace of the movement by one gear while still maintaining proper technique. For example, you might perform the positive phase of a push-up in a half-second and the negative phase in one second.

**SUPER FAST.** This means you do the movement as fast as you can while still maintaining proper form.

As you become more advanced, depending on your reason for doing the exercise, you may choose to vary the speed. There are many ways to do this. You can mix and match speeds during different phases. For example, you could do the exercise with a very fast positive phase, combined with a very slow negative phase. The size of the movement will also determine the ratio. A full squat or dead lift, which covers a bigger range of movement than a push-up, might have a standard speed of a two-second positive and a three-second negative. You may choose to vary the speed:

- to create variety
- to train for sports-specific movements
- to train for explosiveness and speed
- to train a movement utilizing different energy systems (slow, medium, and fast systems)

## RESTING

### *How long do I need to rest between exercises?*

The purpose of rest time is to let your muscles recover for the next exercise. Many variables determine how long you should rest between exercises. In the Complete Core Workout your rest time is set for you. We limit your rest time between exercises, usually moving directly from one exercise to the next. Your goal and your fitness level will determine your rest time. Here are some principles to keep in mind:

- If you're a beginner, you may need more rest time.
- If you're doing athletic explosive movements, you'll also need recovery time.
- If you are trying to build endurance, you want to limit rest time, keeping the muscles working.
- If your goal is strength, you may want to increase the rest time, so you're fresh to handle heavy weights.

## BREATHING

### *How do I know if I'm breathing properly when I exercise?*

Breathing when you're exercising or doing any activity is essential to stay energized and efficient in your movements. That's one of the great things about yoga—the instructor constantly reminds you to breathe in each posture.

During exercise, the rule of thumb is to exhale during the positive phase of the exercise movement and inhale during the negative phase. To review, the positive phase is when you are moving against the most resistance; the negative phase is when you're moving against the least resistance. You should inhale during the negative phase of the exercise to refuel your body, bringing in fresh oxygen and energy for the positive phase of the move. For a push-up this means you would inhale for energy as you lower your body toward the floor and exhale for power as you press up.

If you're doing a lunge, you would exhale as you straighten your legs from the kneeling position to standing and inhale as you lower your knee back toward the floor.

### HOLDING POSITIONS

If you're holding a position for a longer count, such as planks, then you should breathe in a rhythm that supports your body's position. Most important, *don't hold your breath!*

### CASE STUDY: THE ART OF EXERCISING

***Does every repetition count, or are only the last few important?***

Let's look at the big picture when it comes to doing a set. Quality is more important than quantity. This is true when it comes to doing each repetition and when it comes to doing an entire set. Each rep has a beginning, middle, and end. The same is true of a set.

Every set is a cumulative build to failure. Just because your first repetitions are easy doesn't mean you just phone them in. You need to strive for quality in each repetition.

Let's say your goal for a set of Supermans is 12 repetitions. You cruise along 1 quality rep after another. Then around rep 7 you start to feel the fatigue and burn. You stay focused on proper technique, you keep your mind focused, and you work through the good pain on reps 8 and 9. On rep 10 you really struggle to squeeze it out.

Now let's slow things down for that dramatic moment of failure. On rep 11, you let the entire weight of your body give in to the floor, then use the floor to push off, and pull your head up to help raise your torso off the floor. These are all signs that the set is over. You've had a breakdown in technique. You're no longer executing quality repetitions and receiving the benefits of the exercise. By giving your weight into the floor and by pushing off the floor, you're using momentum instead of your lower back and muscles. You also used your head, instead of your lower back muscles, to help raise your torso. This not only takes the tension off the working muscle, it also puts you at risk of injury. So you didn't quite make the goal of 12, but the important thing is quality, not quantity.

### THE EXERCISE ARCHETYPE

***When I take a class, I often feel lost and confused. What can I do?***

In every exercise there is a sequence of steps. They will vary from exercise to exercise, but underneath this difference is a structural pattern that will be true for almost every exercise. Understanding this structure will improve your exercise IQ and help you keep your bearings during a workout. Every exercise has:

- **A beginning, the correct ready position and proper mental focus**
- **A middle, the exercise's movement sequence**
- **The end, the strict return to the beginning position**

All of these phases interconnect. Mastering proper technique is the key to getting the best results in the least amount of time.

## GOOD PAIN VS. BAD PAIN

### *Is "no pain, no gain" really true?*

You don't get to a new and better place without being challenged and pushing yourself. You must always push yourself through some discomfort. How hard you push depends on your goals and fitness level. If you're training for improved health and fitness and not as a competitive athlete, then you don't need to push yourself to the edge. Giving a 70–80 percent effort will give you all the health and wellness benefits of the exercise, plus increase your functional strength, help you lose weight, and build muscle.

No matter what level you're training at, an increased level of fatigue will hit your body as you approach the last repetitions. When you're pushing yourself through the last repetition, you need to be able to tell the difference between good and bad pain. You want to challenge yourself, not injure yourself. Here are some points to keep in mind.

**Good pain** is the feeling of being "pumped," as Arnold Schwarzenegger used to say. It's the positive feeling of knowing you worked your muscles hard. One day you may even start to love this feeling, seek it out, push toward it.

**Bad pain** is a warning sign that says, "Stop! Don't push!" These warning signs are shooting pains, sharp pains, and spasms. Whenever pain moves beyond the area you're working, that is a sign to stop and evaluate. Bad pain is an indication that you've injured yourself or you're putting yourself in danger.

It is also important to gradually increase your workout intensity. You need to build a foundation, a strong base, before pushing to the edge.

## SORENESS

### *Should I train when I'm sore?*

Muscle soreness is common after a workout. Don't worry if you're a little sore (good pain). Soreness is the result of microscopic tears in the muscle; they need time to recuperate and repair so they can come back stronger. Most of the time it is good to train through mild soreness. The increased blood flow in the area will help repair the tissue. If you are too sore to train for your next scheduled session, you've overdone it.

Remember: Train hard, train smart.

# 13

# CORE POSTURE AND MOTION

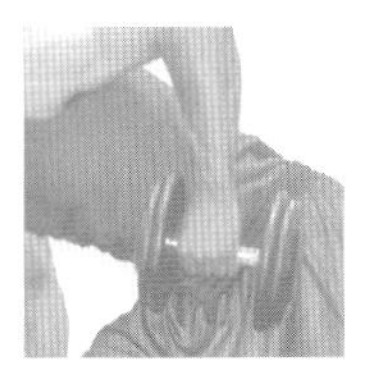

## INTRODUCTION

Proper posture is a major issue even for advanced exercisers. Good posture is important in your daily life, and the correct ready position is critical when you're working out. The following guidelines will give you a set of tools to build good posture and the correct ready position for working out. Good posture will make you taller and take unnecessary stress off your spine and organs, allowing you to function with optimum efficiency.

The second part of this chapter explains how your body moves. This will help you understand core training and help you design your own routines as you become more advanced.

## PART ONE: POSTURE AND READY POSITION

### THE SPINE: TRACING THE CURVES

To understand the concept of proper alignment, you need a basic understanding of the spine's structure. The healthy spine has three natural curves: one in the lower back, one in the middle area of the spine, and one at the neck. The overall shape of the spine is like a gentle, elongated S. The following illustration is of a healthy spine, all of the gentle curves creating a wavelike form.

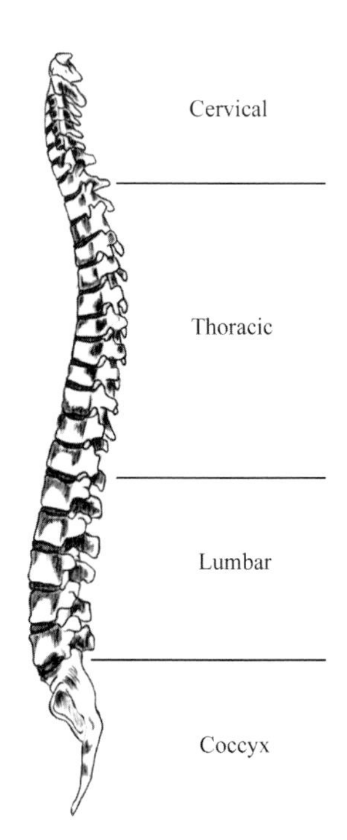


Following these curves, the spine is divided into three parts: the lumbar area, the thoracic area, and the cervical area. These three areas make up the twenty-four movable vertebrae of the spine:

- **The lumbar area makes up the five vertebrae of the lower spine.**
- **The thoracic area makes up the twelve vertebrae of the middle spine.**
- **The cervical area makes up the seven vertebrae of the upper spine.**

### THE SPINE FROM TOP TO BOTTOM

Each part of the spine affects every other part of the spine, and spinal alignment affects your entire body. Any exaggerated curve or diminished curve in your spine negatively stresses the entire length of the spine. It also puts stress on other key areas of your body. These include:

- **Your shoulder blades and stabilization muscles that support your shoulder joint**
- **Your hips and the muscles that help stabilize your hips**
- **Your hamstrings, hip flexors, and psoas muscles**

Postural problems occur when these natural curves are either exaggerated or diminished. The following postures are three common postural pitfalls. Being aware of these common tendencies will help you maintain your spine's natural and healthy curves.

**HUNCHED POSTURE.** Rounded shoulders and a hunched or caved-in chest are signs of this posture. A hunched position pulls the shoulder blades up and away from the spine, decreasing shoulder stabilization and inhibiting proper breathing. It creates an unnaturally large curve in the middle area of your spine (the thoracic area). It also increases the spinal curve in your neck area, causing your head to jut forward.

**SWAYBACK.** An exaggerated curve in the lower back is a sign of this posture. This puts excessive pressure on the lumbar vertebrae. This posture creates an unnatural curve in your lower spine. It also increases the spinal curve in your neck area, causing your head to jut forward.

**FLAT BACK.** A backward tilt or tucking in of your pelvis is a sign of this posture. This diminishes the natural curve in your lower spine, flattening out your lower back. This flattening affects all the curves along your spine, causing neck and back strain.

## THE READY POSITION

For exercising, you need to take proper alignment into a ready position. By ready position we mean a state of readiness where your body is balanced and prepared to move. This ready position has two components: one mental and one physical. The mental component means you are focused, you know what you want to accomplish, and you're motivated to give your best effort. The physical component, which we will concentrate on in this chapter, has to do with your posture and stance. We will focus on five checkpoints of alignment. You can adapt these guidelines to different positions: standing, lying, and all fours.

## PHASE ONE: PROPER ALIGNMENT

**CHECKPOINT ONE: THE FEET.** Evenly distribute your weight on both feet and feel your feet connect to the ground, creating a solid foundation of support. If you need to move to the balls of your feet for an exercise movement, do so after you have grounded yourself by planting your feet firmly and evenly.

**CHECKPOINT TWO: THE KNEES.** Unlock your knees. This means your knees should be slightly bent, an inch or less. If your knees are locked, the first thing you have to do before you can move athletically is unlock your knees. A good way to get a feel for this is to stand and gently lock your knees tight for a couple of seconds, then let them relax. You will feel your knees unlock. This is your natural, unlocked position. A more familiar example is the jaw. You don't want to go through the day tightly clenching your jaw closed; you want to let it relax. It wasn't designed to be held shut tight, nor were your knees designed to be constantly locked.

**CHECKPOINT THREE: YOUR HIPS AND FINDING NEUTRAL.** Okay, now things are going to get a bit more complicated. Now we're at the center of your body, so it's crucial to get this area set in proper alignment. The ready position for your hips is a neutral position. Finding neutral is like finding the balance point in a teeter-totter. When a teeter-totter is balanced, it is level; neither end is pointing up or down. In neutral, your pelvis is balanced level; it is not tucked in backward or tilted forward. Let's try to make this concrete.

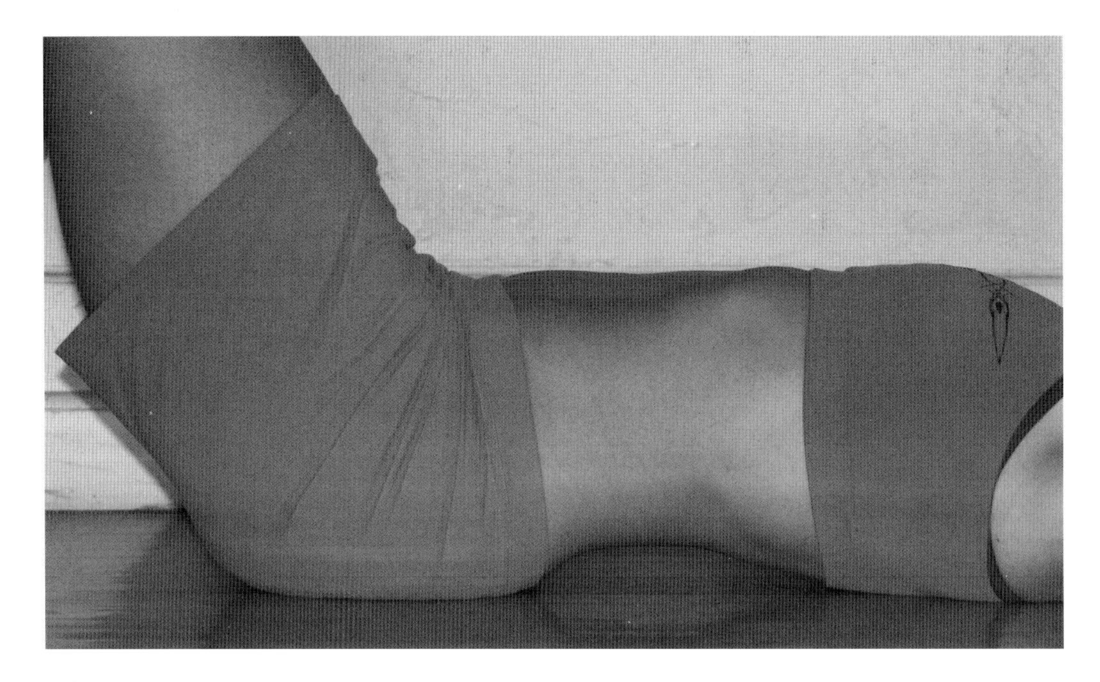

The best way to get a sense of neutral is lying on your back with your feet flat and your knees bent. To understand neutral it is helpful to feel what it is like to be out of neutral. First, tilt your pelvis forward toward your feet, increasing the curve in your back.

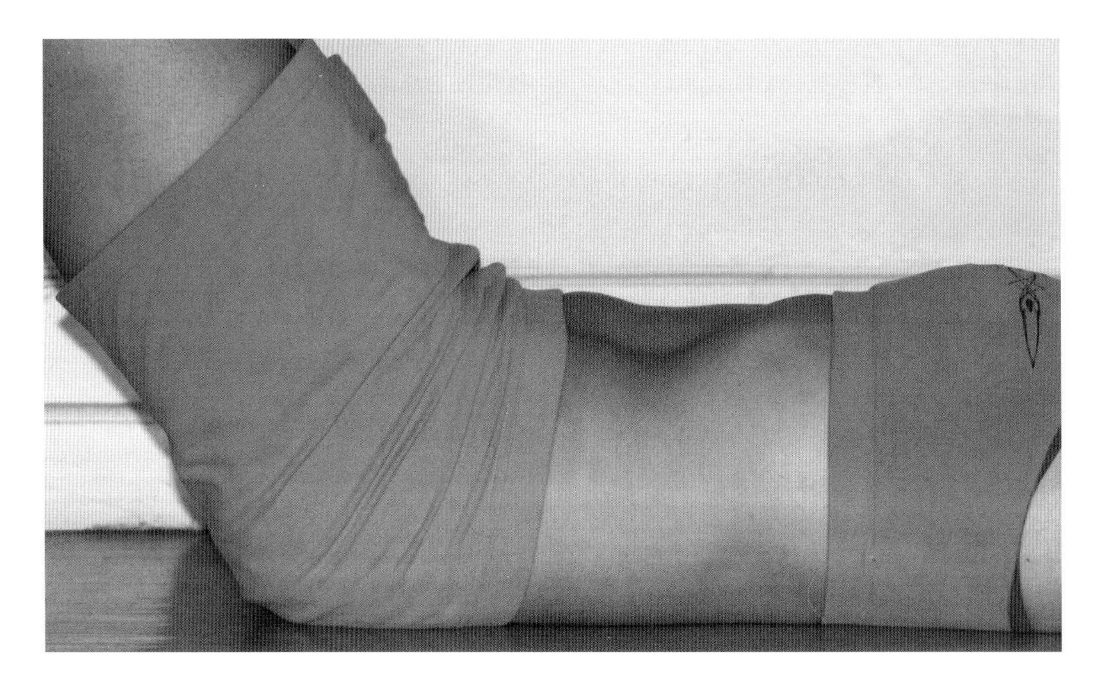

Now tilt your pelvis backward, rounding your lower back against the floor.

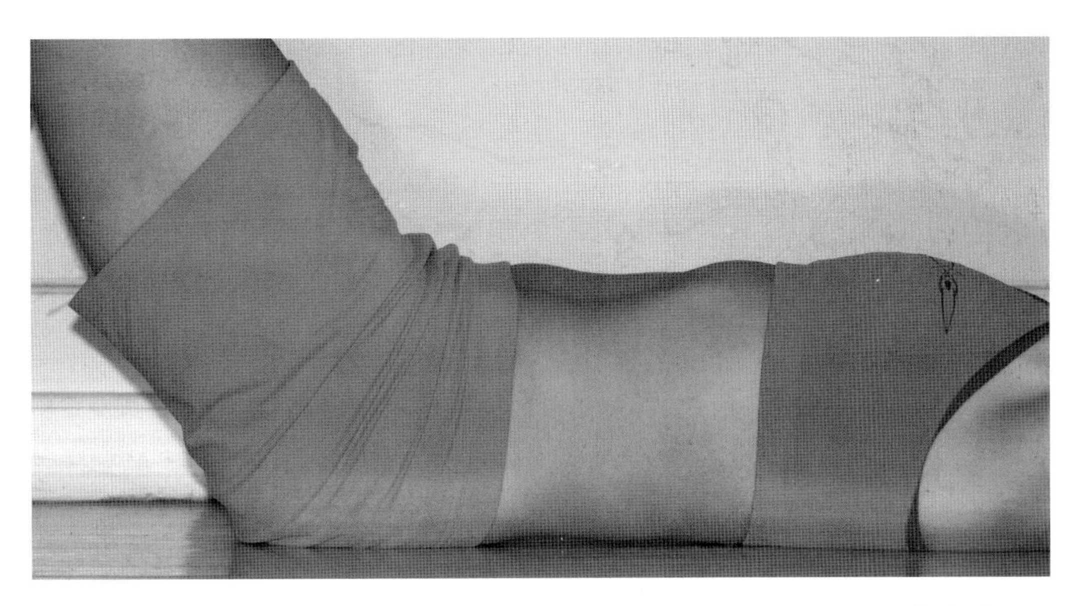

Now let your pelvis rest in the middle, balanced between these two extremes and relaxing toward the floor. This is neutral, like a balanced teeter-totter.

The goal of a neutral pelvis is to set the correct and natural relationship between your pelvis and lower spine and to create a strong bridge between your upper and lower body. If your pelvis is out of neutral, it will affect the rest of your spine. Being neutral will help you move efficiently and powerfully. You want the spine to maintain its natural curves. There will be many times during working out or playing a sport when your hips move out of neutral, but you want to start from the optimal position. When your hips are out of neutral, it puts extra stress on other muscles and joints. The Complete Core Program will strengthen all the key areas, allowing you to handle the extra stress when you're out of neutral, and still perform at your highest level.

***ALL FOURS.*** The same principles apply to the all-fours position. Your hips should be in neutral; your back should not be rounded or arched. Your joints should be lined up: elbows and wrists directly under your shoulders and knees directly under your hips.

***TAKE IT TO STANDING.*** The same principle also applies to standing. You don't want your pelvis rotated forward or backward. Use the same methods of moving through the extreme backward and forward tilt, then find neutral between these two extremes.

**CHECKPOINT FOUR: SHOULDERS.** Release your shoulders down and back, so they are aligned over your hips, knees, and ankles. This means you could draw a line straight down through shoulders, hips, knees, and ankles. You don't want to round your shoulders forward so you're hunched, or force your shoulders back in a military posture. You want to let your shoulder blades release down and together. This puts your shoulders in proper alignment. This position should also be maintained when you're lying on the floor.

**CHECKPOINT FIVE: HEAD AND NECK.** Elongate and release your neck up. It's helpful to think of your head as a helium balloon that effortlessly lengthens your neck and floats up. This will help balance your head on top of your spine with your ears directly over your shoulders. Think of keeping your chin level (parallel to the floor), neither tucked down nor pointed up. Keeping your focus straight ahead at eye level will also help your neck and head to be aligned.

Doing core exercises that emphasize the abdominals, chin position can be a little more confusing. A simple way to check this when you're doing core abdominal work is to imagine you are holding an apple between your chin and chest. Another way is to keep a fist's distance between your chin and chest. There is a tendency to bring the chin to the chest during ab work. You may need to make an extra effort to keep proper head and neck alignment during these exercises.

### STACKING

We'll review by giving you a simple feedback system to check your alignment.

Think of your body as made of building blocks stacked on top of each other. Your body is an interrelated system, each block dependent on every other block for proper alignment. Your blocks should be stacked so your ears, shoulders, hips, knees, and ankles are aligned directly above each other. This body block check gives you a quick feedback system to place your body in proper alignment.

### STANDING TALL

Besides stacking, you want to stand straight, not lean in one direction. Here's a simple way to get straight. Lean your body forward, then backward; decrease the lean each time until you feel balanced between these forward and backward points. Then do the same thing from side to side, decreasing the lean until you feel balanced between these two side-to-side points.

Correct posture takes practice and awareness. If you get in the habit of going through these basic checkpoints, over time, proper alignment will become second nature.

Now that you understand the basics of the ready position and alignment, the next step is understanding the way your body moves.

## CORE MOTION: THE MOVING BODY

Core training is about movement. Movement is life. We often take our natural movements for granted, until something goes wrong. Behind even the most mundane everyday tasks is a complex system of thousands of motor units communicating with dozens of different muscles. Just picking up a glass of water involves a chain of interrelated events that happens with such speed and seamless harmony that it's easy to forget the wonder of what is happening. When you pick up a glass of water, almost simultaneously with thought, the body chooses the best path of travel, negotiates the angle of the reach, the speed of the movement, when to accelerate, slow down, and how tightly to grasp the glass, and the proper contraction of all the primary and secondary muscles. Then on the way up it has to hit the target, your mouth, without spilling any of the contents.

The goal of core training is to train the body so it can move with power, efficiency, and grace for a lifetime. A natural side benefit of this is a trim, muscular, and athletic body.

**CORE MOTION: THREE-DIMENSIONAL MOVEMENT**

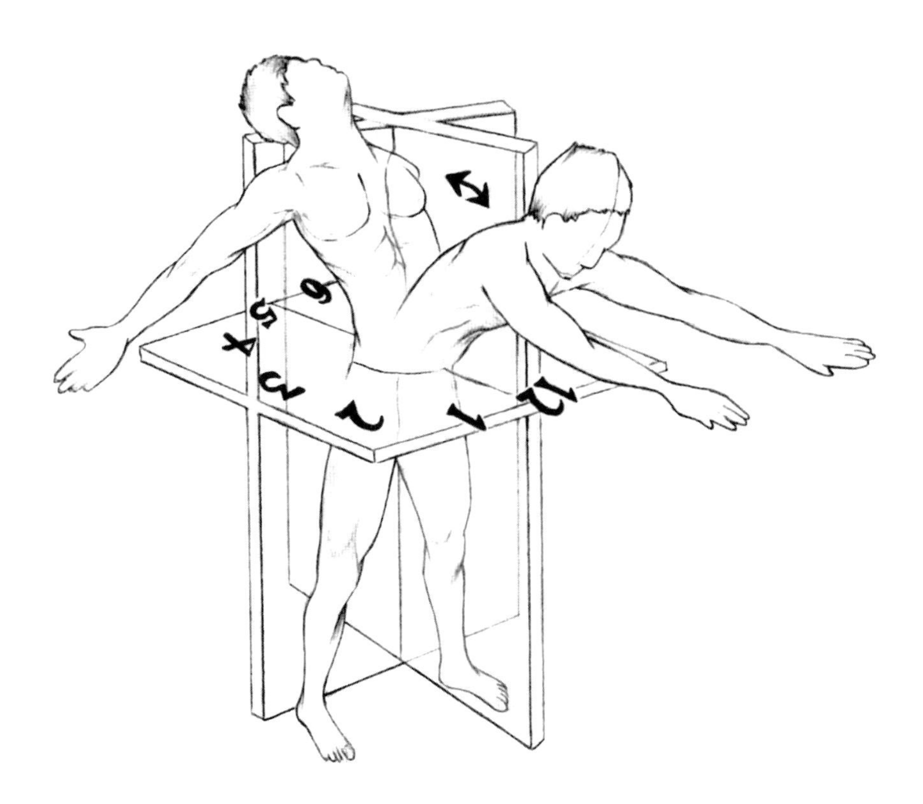


The Complete Core Workout will train your body in all directions. Your body moves in space in three basic ways. To help you understand these movement directions, we'll refer to the core clock.

**FORWARD AND BACKWARD MOVEMENT.** On the core clock this would mean bending forward and backward along the line that runs through 12 and 6 on the core clock. This is also called flexion and extension. A movement in this direction could be as small as a crunch or as big as a dead lift.

**EXERCISE EXAMPLES:** Dead Lift, Superman, Roll-Up

**FLEXION:**
Flexion occurs when the body bends at the joint, much like a hinge that opens and closes. When you flex a joint, the open angle of the joint decreases.

**MOVEMENT EXAMPLES:**

- **Torso flexion—bending at the hips to touch your toes**
- **Arm flexion—bringing your hand to your shoulder**

Both of these movements decrease the angle of the joint.

**EXTENSION:** Extension means to extend or straighten the joint so the angle of the joint increases.

**MOVEMENT EXAMPLES:** the opposite of the above flexion movements:

- **Raising up from a forward-bend-toe-touch position**
- **Extending your arm away from your shoulder**

Both movements increase the angle of the joint.

**SIDE-TO-SIDE MOVEMENT.** On the Core Clock this would mean bending from side to side or raising or lowering legs along the line that runs through 3 and 9. This is also called lateral flexion and extension. When you bend at the waist and straighten you increase and decrease the angle.

**EXERCISE EXAMPLES:** Side Bend, Jackknife

**ROTATIONAL AND CROSSING MOVEMENTS.** These include all twisting and rotational movements of the upper and lower body. On the Core Clock, twisting movements and rotational movements can run either clockwise or counterclockwise.

**EXERCISE EXAMPLE:** Russian Twist

Crossing movements travel at an angle. They can travel at an angle: from 5 to 11, 7 to 1, 8 to 2, 4 to 10, and any crossing variation in between.

**EXERCISE EXAMPLE:** Catches

## MOVEMENT PATTERNS

Movements represent basic ways the body is designed to move. This is based on our body's musculoskeletal system. These movement patterns work in combination with the movement directions outlined above. Different movement patterns also combine to create an almost infinite number of movement possibilities.

## THE BASIC PATTERNS

1. A Squat
2. A Lunge
3. Leg Flexion and Extension (moving your legs forward and backward in running and jumping motions)

4. Lateral Step (moving from side to side)
5. Leg Crossover (crossing one leg in front of or in back of the other)
6. Arm Articulations (all articulations that involve movement in the shoulder joint)

### ACTIONS

Basic actions are the ways you commonly combine movement patterns and directions into performance events. By performance events, we mean actions that have a specific goal in mind. Most performance events have a primary action at their center.

1. Walking and running
2. Rotational swinging and throwing
3. Striking and kicking
4. Changing direction and turning
5. Jumping

### MOVEMENT QUALITIES

The quality of a movement describes its essential characteristics: speed, force, direction, and tempo. These are common movement qualities you use in life and sports.

- **Sustained and explosive**
- **Acceleration and deceleration**
- **Straight and circular**

These directions, patterns, actions, and qualities represent the basic ways we move. This is not an exhaustive list, and the human body is capable of virtually infinite variations and combinations. It is a basic movement template, a way to think about movement. It is a guide for creating workout routines. Ideally, you want to include all these movement elements in your workout. It also provides a way to evaluate the strengths and weaknesses of your body.

These movement directions, patterns, and actions are behind the design of the Complete Core Program, so all you have to do is follow the program step by step. The program will give your body strength and balance in all directions. It will train your body through the most-used movement patterns and in the basic performance actions of life and sports. This will give you a functional, muscular, and athletic body to meet the challenges of life.

# 14
# CORE ANATOMY

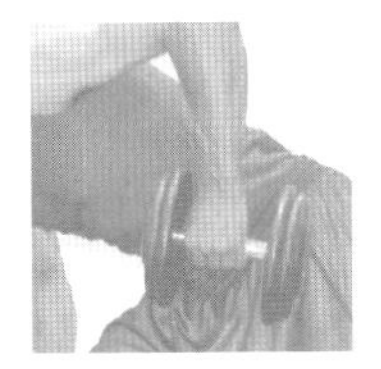

## INTRODUCTION

Workout books usually talk about just the famous muscles: the ab six-pack, the perfect butt, toned and trim thighs, rippling biceps, "pecs," and "lats." This makes sense. After all, these are the muscles we look at in the mirror. However, in this chapter we are also going to look at the little-known deep muscles below the surface. These deep muscles are essential for core stabilization, body wellness, and performance—for example, the multifidus muscle which is essential for keeping your vertebrae aligned. Maybe one day the multifidus muscle will be a household name.

# ANATOMY BASICS

This chapter emphasizes knowledge that can be applied to your workouts. First, let's take a look at how the body hangs together.

## BONES

Bones create the framework of your body and also serve as levers that create movement when acted on by muscles. Bones are also alive. It is easy to think of them as dead, because that's the way we usually see them on skeletons or in the food we eat. But they are living and grow just like muscles. Bones respond to exercise by getting thicker and stronger. And when bones are understimulated, they shrink. Strong and thick bones are harder to break. Working out is, obviously, one of the best ways to prevent osteoporosis and decreases your chances of injury.

## JOINTS

Joints are places in the body where bones come together. Some joints, like the sacroiliac joint, are capable of little or no movement. Ball-and-socket joints (hip and shoulder joint) and hinge joints (knee and elbow) move freely. These are called synovial joints, because they contain synovial fluid, which lubricates the joint, allowing it to move without friction.

## CONNECTORS

If you looked at a skeleton, you would notice that it is held together and moves through a series of wires and pins. If you took away these wires and pins, the bones would just form a pile on the floor. Your body does not have wires and pins to keep it together. Instead, your body has ligaments and cartilage to connect and help your bones move.

**LIGAMENTS.** Ligaments hold your joints together. They are made of very strong fibers that act like straps to bind your joints together.

**CARTILAGE.** Cartilage helps your joints move efficiently and without pain. The moving surface of your joints is covered with cartilage. This protective covering absorbs pressure, reduces friction, and increases the movement of the joint.

## SOFT TISSUE

Now let's look at soft tissue: tendons, fascia, and muscles. They also act as connectors, but their primary function is to produce movement.

**TENDONS.** Tendons are a strong tissue that connects to the bone. Muscle then connects to the tendon. Tendons are a secure bind that helps strengthen the muscle connection to bones.

**FASCIA.** Fascia means bandage. Fascia is a thin sheath of connective tissue that binds and surrounds muscles and organs.

**MUSCLES.** Muscles are attached to bones. Their primary function is to produce movement. A muscle is the motor that moves the bones.

## MUSCLES IN ACTION

Muscles come in a variety of sizes and shapes, matching their form to their function. Muscles that act as stabilizers, such as those that support the pelvis, are short. The major muscles of the legs and arms are long and capable of producing large and sweeping motions in these limbs. This is why some exercises, like hip and shoulder blade stabilization exercises, may seem frustrating. The muscles are small and range of motion is only a few inches. This makes the movement hard to feel.

Your body is also made up of layers of muscles. Both the deep and surface muscles are essential for your body to function at an optimum level.

The goal of this chapter is to make you see and feel your body from the inside out, to make you aware of the smaller deeper muscles, as well as the bigger external muscles.

Understanding and being able to visualize these key muscles will deepen your training experience. We will start from the deepest muscles and work our way out to the external muscles.

## THE CORE MUSCLES

This section will examine the major muscles that make up your core area.

## BODY AREA: ABDOMINAL AREA (FRONT AND SIDES OF YOUR UPPER BODY)

This section looks at the muscles of the abdominal area and the pelvic floor. These muscles create support for your core.

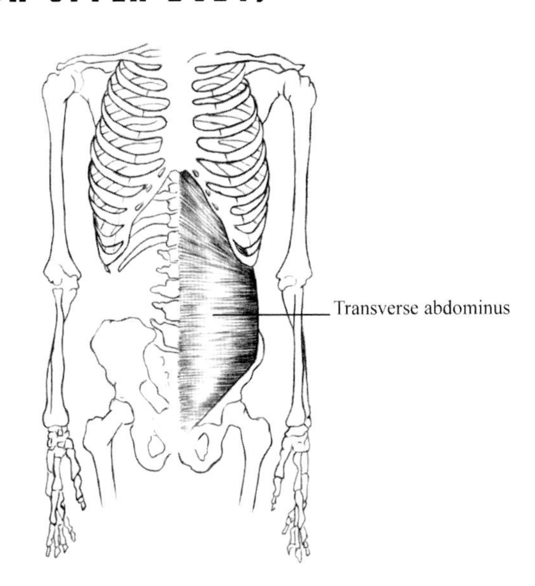


### THE TRANSVERSE ABDOMINIS

**DESCRIPTION:** This is the deepest abdominal muscle. It wraps around the body horizontally like a wide belt or girdle, giving support and protection to the spine. It originates at the top of the hipbone and attaches to the bottom six ribs and the breastbone.

**ACTION:** The transverse abdominis pulls your midsection in toward your spine. This tightening gives core support to the center of your body. Whenever you draw your lower midsection in, you're activating your transverse abdominis. There are many verbal cues for this action: bring your belly button toward your spine, scoop in, hollow in, zip it up (like you're zipping up a really tight pair of pants), and so forth.

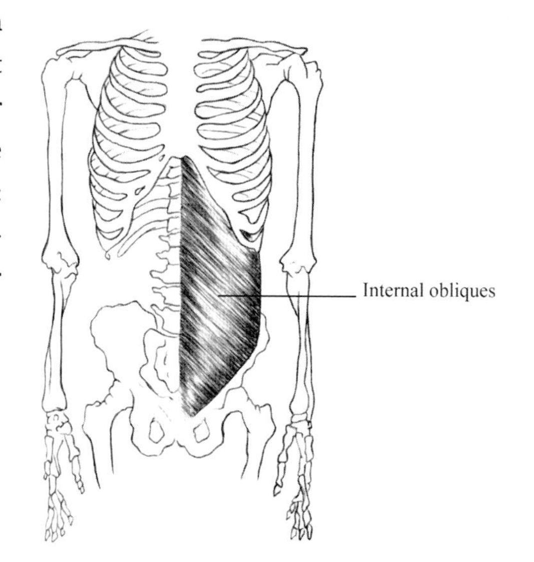


### INTERNAL OBLIQUES

**DESCRIPTION:** The internal obliques are situated underneath your external obliques. They move diagonally upward from the top of your hip and attach to the eighth, ninth, and tenth ribs.

**ACTION:** The internal obliques (along with the external obliques) are prime movers when your body twists or bends sideways. Since they are a deep muscle, they are also an important postural muscle and assist in core stabilization.

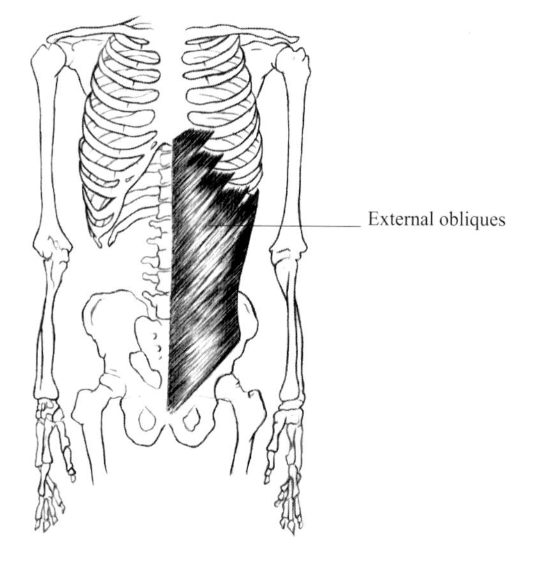


### EXTERNAL OBLIQUES

**DESCRIPTION:** The external obliques originate from the lower eight ribs and run diagonally down, inserting at the front half of the hip. They rest on top of the internal oblique and run in an opposite diagonal direction. The two groups create crisscrossing layers of support.

**ACTION:** The external obliques work in combination with the internal obliques in all twisting, rotating, and side bend movements.

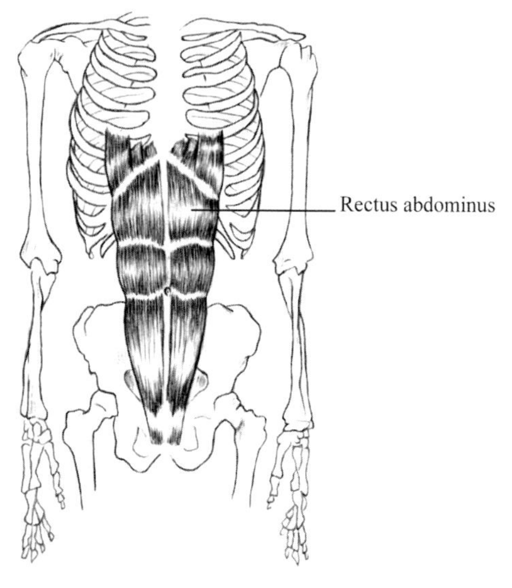


### RECTUS ABDOMINIS

**DESCRIPTION:** The rectus abdominis is one long sheath of muscle that runs from your breastbone (sternum) to your pubic bone.

**ACTION:** The primary function of this muscle is flexion, bending your torso toward your hips and bending your hips toward your torso.

# BODY AREA: LOWER BACK AND SPINE SUPPORT (THE BACK OF YOUR UPPER BODY)

This section looks at the muscles that support and stabilize your spine. The back muscles in general aren't as well known as the muscles on the front of your body. We will focus on two layers of muscles that supply column support for the spine. These muscles connect the vertebrae and run along the spine, protecting and supporting it like tension wire holding up a pole. Both groups use the word "spinalis"; just think of this as being a long word for "spine." The first layer is the inner spinalis group and the second layer is the erector spinalis group.

## THE INNER SPINALIS GROUP

These are the deepest muscles of the spine. They connect each vertebra to stabilize and support the spine.

### MULTIFIDUS

**DESCRIPTION:** This small deep muscle connects vertebra to vertebra.

**ACTION:** The multifidus gives intervertebrate support and stability. It helps keep the individual vertebrae aligned during flexion and extension.

### ROTATORS

**DESCRIPTION:** This small deep muscle connects between each vertebra. It differs from the multifidus in its angle. It swings slightly wider out to the side.

**ACTION:** Besides giving support and stability, this muscle assists the body when it rotates.

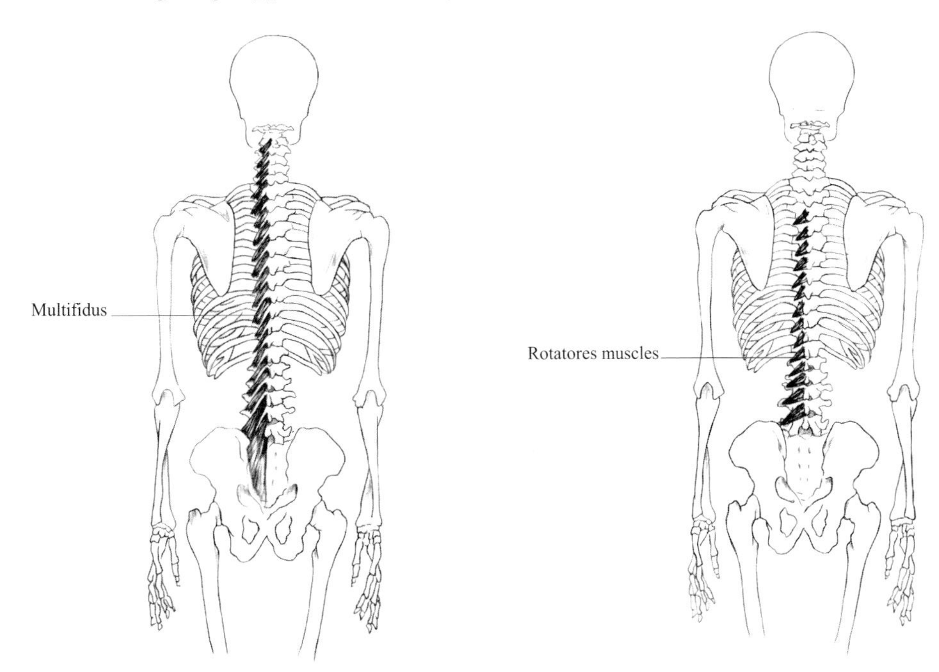

### ERECTOR SPINALIS GROUP: ILIOCOSTALIS, LONGISSIMUS, SPINALIS MUSCLES

This group of muscles, working in combination with your inner spinalis group, is designed to do the heavy work. The inner spinalis muscles stabilize the spine as the bigger erector spinalis muscles do the heavy lifting. If either group is weak, you are a candidate for back pain. Working muscle groups together brings both groups into play.

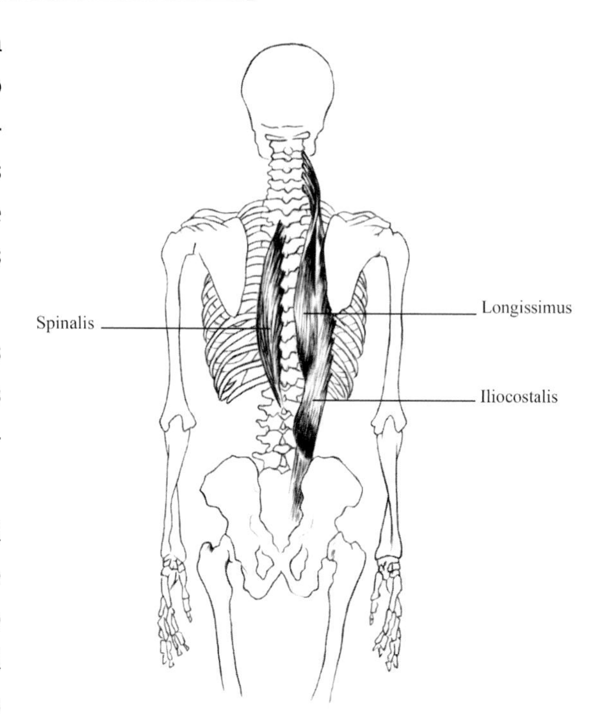


**DESCRIPTION:** The erector spinalis group runs along each side of your spine. These muscles spread out along the spine like tension wires, creating support.

**ACTION:** These muscles allow you to extend and straighten up. When you bend forward at the waist, you use the erector spinalis muscles to straighten up. They also allow you to safely bend backward into hyperextension. These muscles work together with your abdominal group to keep you upright. If you didn't have these back muscles, you would flop forward over at the waist. If you didn't have your abdominal muscles, your torso would flop over backward.

## BODY AREA: THE SHOULDER BLADES

Along with hip stabilization, shoulder blade (scapula) stabilization plays a major role in a healthy spine. It allows you to maintain a healthy and proper curve in your middle spine, the thoracic area. For this to happen, you need to train the muscles that stabilize the shoulder blade, so they can maintain proper position, releasing down and toward each other.

The muscles that allow you to do this get weak when you sit all day and round your shoulders forward. This causes your shoulder blades to float up and move farther apart, which is just the opposite of what you want. The shoulder blades also support and stabilize the shoulder joint, giving you a safe foundation for powerful arm movements such as throwing, swinging, and punching. There are specific exercises for these muscles in the strength routine in the Complete Core Program.

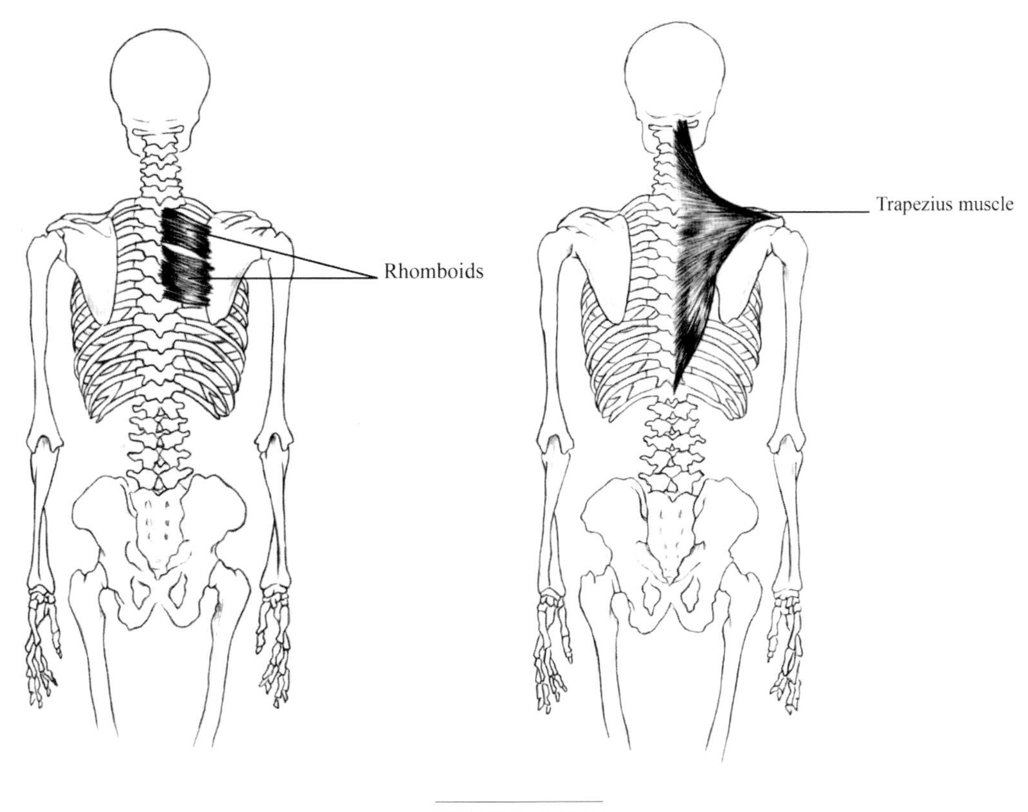


## RHOMBOIDS

**DESCRIPTION:** The rhomboids, located beneath the trapezius muscle, run at a downward angle from the upper part of your middle spine area, attaching to your shoulder blades.

**ACTION:** The rhomboids assist the trapezius in pulling the shoulder blades down and toward the spine.

## TRAPEZIUS

**DESCRIPTION:** The trapezius muscle originates at the base of the skull and along the vertebrae of the neck (cervical) and upper back (thoracic), attaching to the collarbone and shoulder blade.

**ACTION:** The "traps," as they are often called, run in three different directions, giving them three different functions. The upper traps raise your shoulders toward your ears; the middle traps pull your shoulder blades toward your spine; and the lower traps pull your shoulder blades down toward your waist. Most people just do shrugs, which trains only one of the traps functions, raising your shoulders toward your ears. This is not the most important exercise for posture and stabilization. In the Complete Core Program, you will learn how to train all three functions.

# BODY AREA: THE HIPS AND GLUTES

The hips and glutes (buttocks) are a key transition point between the upper and lower body. It is important to have this area strong and stable. This section looks at the glutes and the muscles that surround your hip. You use these muscles whenever you:

**FLEX YOUR LEG**—when you bring your leg forward in a running, jumping, or kicking motion

**EXTEND YOUR LEG**—when you extend your leg backward behind you in a running, kicking, or swinging motion

**SPREAD YOUR LEGS**—when your spread your leg(s) away from the center of your body

**BRING YOUR LEGS TOGETHER**—when you bring your leg(s) toward the center of your body

### HIP FLEXOR GROUP: PSOAS, ILLIACUS, RECTUS FEMORIS, SARTORIUS, TENSOR FASCIA LATAE MUSCLES

**DESCRIPTION:** The hip flexor group originates from the last thoracic vertebrae (which is the lower part of the middle section of your spine) and the lower lumbar vertebrae. It inserts into the upper thighbone.

**ACTION:** The hip flexor muscles are the prime movers when you lift your leg out in front of you. They are also involved in deep squatting motions.

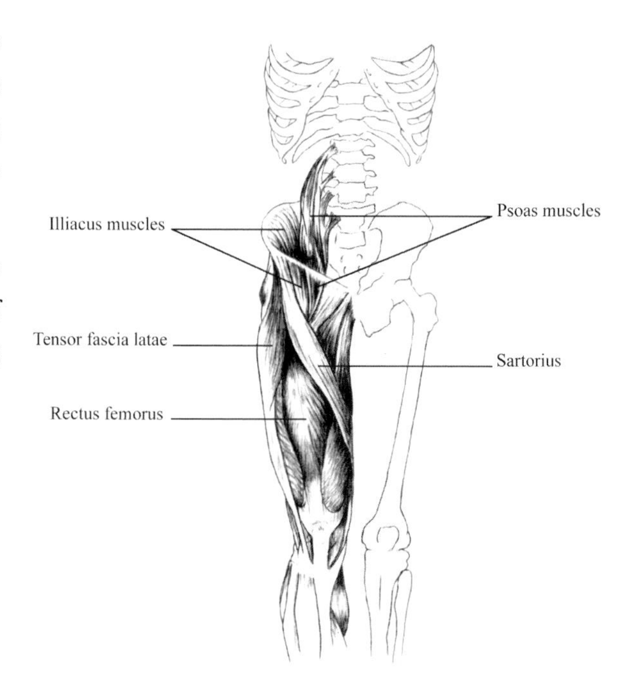

# ABDUCTOR GROUP (OUTSIDE PART OF HIP)

### GLUTEUS MEDIUS AND GLUTEUS MINIMUS

**DESCRIPTION:** The gluteus medius and the gluteus minimus, originating along the hip and attaching to the thighbone, wrap around the outside of your body. The gluteus minimus is located below the gluteus maximus.

**ACTION:** The gluteus medius is the prime mover when you move your leg(s) out from the midline of your body—in other words, when you spread your legs. The gluteus minimus also aids in this movement and acts as a stabilizer when your leg moves backward and forward.

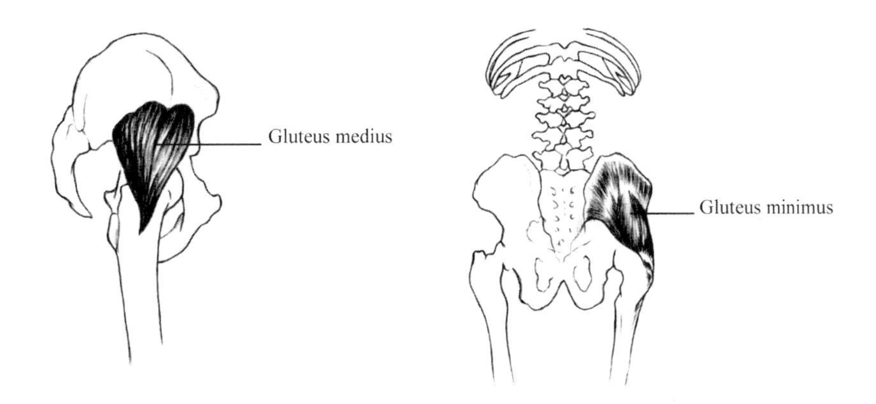


# ADDUCTOR GROUP (INSIDE PART OF YOUR LEG)

### ADDUCTOR MAGNUS, ADDUCTOR LONGUS, ADDUCTOR BREVIS, PECTINEUS, GRACILIS

**DESCRIPTION:** The adductor group originates at the hipbone and attaches to the thighbone.

**ACTION:** This group is the prime mover when you bring your legs inward toward the midline of your body—that is, when you bring your legs together. This muscle group is also key in stabilizing your hips when you move sideways.

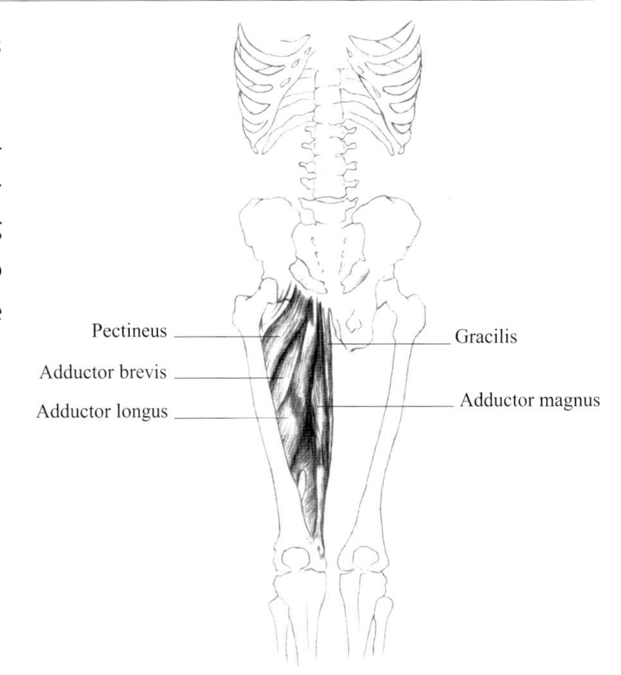

# HIP EXTENSION GROUP: GLUTEUS MAXIMUS

### GLUTEUS MAXIMUS

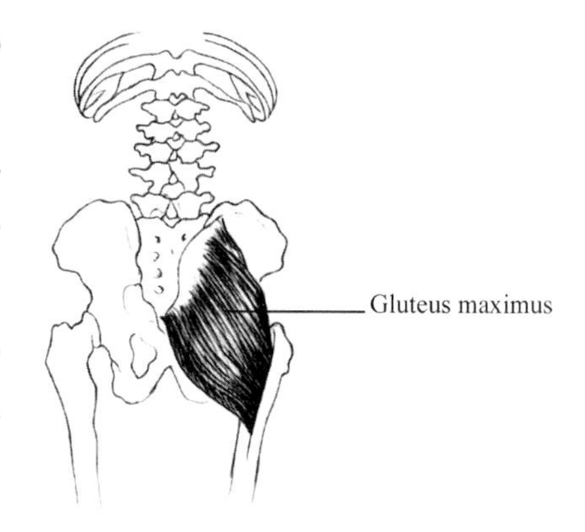


**DESCRIPTION:** The gluteus maximus originates along the hip and lumbar area and attaches to the thighbone.

**ACTION:** The gluteus maximus is a prime mover in hip extension when you extend your leg(s) behind you. It is also activated when you rotate your thigh to the outside.

In summary, the goal of this chapter is to increase your awareness of key areas and to help you visualize and get in touch with your deeper muscles.

# 15

# CORE EATING

BY TRACY MARX

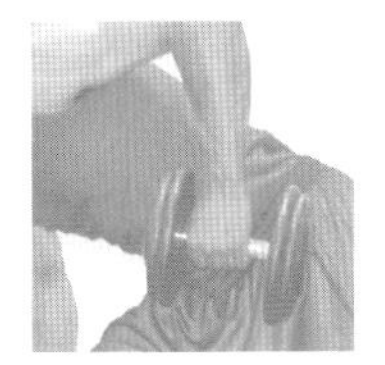

## YOU ARE WHAT YOU EAT

In many ways, we are walking food. On a purely physical level, food becomes the building blocks of our cells, which make up our tissues, which form our organs and blood. On a physiological level, the foods we consume affect our mood, energy, and therefore our future. For example, the more chemically processed and artificial a food is:

- **The less nutritious it is**
- **The more debilitating to the digestive system (note that today's best-selling over-the-counter medications are digestive aids)**
- **The higher in calories it is**

While people in the nutritional world are at war with one another, the truth is that no one way of eating is right for everyone—nor will one way of eating be right throughout an entire lifetime. Dietary needs change from season to season, from year to year; people have varying metabolisms, blood types, genetic inheritance, and energy and stress levels, all of which play a role. For most of us, the point is to stop eating garbage, understand our cravings, and make choices based on our bio-individuality, not on rigid theory. First, you need to get a handle on some nutrition basics.

## NUTRITION PRIMER

### A CARBOHYDRATE IS A CARBOHYDRATE IS A CARBOHYDRATE—*NOT!*

Many of today's most popular diets lead you to believe that entire food groups should be off-limits. While some of these diets will cause you to lose weight in the short term, ultimately their nutritional deficiencies make them impossible to stick to. Your highly intelligent body will eventually demand the nutrients—and the variety—it needs.

Carbohydrates have become particularly demonized, but not all carbs are equal. There's a world of difference between processed carbs and whole, unprocessed carbs from vegetables, whole grains, and fruits. And remember that whole grains are not fattening. People the world over rely on whole grains as their staple food—and most of the world's populations are not overweight. Americans, on the other hand, are overweight, and our diet is very low in whole grains. Whole grains are rich in nutrients, protein, cleansing fiber, vitamins, and minerals. They are a complete food.

### SIMPLE CARBOHYDRATES

These are sugars, primarily table sugar and natural sweeteners like corn syrup and fructose, as well as lactose, found in dairy products. Simple carbs compose the foods many of us commonly eat, most of which are processed, such as white bread, bagels, crackers and pretzels, pasta, pastries, puffed cereals, granola bars, cheese, ice cream, yogurt, and fruit juice.

These carbohydrates are simple in their chemical structure—just two molecules hook them together. They are quickly absorbed into the bloodstream, causing the chain reaction of a rapid energy rise followed by an energy dip and renewed hunger. We will discuss this pattern in more detail later in the chapter.

## COMPLEX CARBOHYDRATES

Complex carbohydrates are composed of long chains of sugars that are bound up with fiber. These sugars must be broken from their chains and the fiber in order to be released into your bloodstream. This process, which first requires chewing, followed by some work on the part of your small intestine, takes many hours—which is the reason complex carbs give you long-lasting energy. A diet that is composed mainly of whole grains, vegetables, beans, fruit, and smaller amounts of animal products keeps blood sugar and insulin levels down, enabling the body to continually burn both sugar and fat. These types of foods are also usually lower in calories and rich in fiber, which encourages healthy elimination.

Some of the best sources of complex carbohydrates include brown rice, oats, buckwheat, millet, quinoa, amaranth, barley, bulgur, and rye. Also, pulpy vegetables—such as squash, carrots, parsnips, rutabaga, and onions—and legumes, such as beans and peas.

## FATS

Like carbs, fats are also misunderstood. Just as there are healthy and unhealthy carbs, there are healthy and unhealthy fats. The fact is, the right kinds of fats are crucial for total body functioning. A proper balance of the essential fatty acids (EFAs)—omega-3 and omega-6—is vital to the integrity of the body's cell membranes and the health of the cardiovascular, immune, reproductive, and central nervous systems. EFAs are the building blocks of prostaglandins—hormone-like substances that regulate every organ, tissue, and cell in the human body. They are also an integral ingredient in the production of sex and adrenal hormones.

Unfortunately, these fats are the ones most likely to be deficient in the diet, especially where women are concerned. The first step in remedying this is to understand how fats are classified so we can make healthy choices. Here again, we come to a question of quality. Like other unrefined foods, unrefined oils contain numerous vital nutrients not found in the refined variety. Regardless of which type of oil you use, it should be labeled as "unrefined."

We can divide fats into four groups:

**GROUP ONE: POLYUNSATURATES (OMEGA-3):** Vegetable sources include flaxseed oil, hazelnut oil, perilla oil, hemp, pumpkin seeds, soybeans, walnuts, wheat germ, wheat sprouts, fresh sea vegetables, leafy greens, and purslane. Animal sources include fortified eggs, oils from salmon, mackerel, herring, cod, sardines, tuna, flounder, anchovies, and cold-water fish such as trout.

**POLYUNSATURATES (OMEGA-6):** Vegetable sources include safflower, sunflower, corn, soy, sesame, hemp, raw nuts and seeds, legumes, spirulina, and leafy greens. Animal sources include mother's milk, organ meats, and lean meats. Additional natural sources include evening primrose oil, black currant oil, and borage oil.

**GROUP TWO: MONOUNSATURATES:** Usually used in cooking, monounsaturated oils exceed both saturated and polyunsaturated fats in one respect: They don't cause cholesterol to accumulate like saturated fats, and they don't turn rancid easily, like polyunsaturates. In addition, monounsaturated oils do not deplete HDL (the good cholesterol) and do reduce LDL (the bad cholesterol). Polyunsaturates also reduce LDL but decrease HDL as well. Vegetable, legume, and seed sources include olive, grapeseed, macadamia, avocado, almond, apricot kernel, peanut, high-oleic safflower and sunflower oils, and rice bran oil.

**GROUP THREE: SATURATES:** These fats are found primarily in animal products, plus a few plant sources. While they have the fewest rancidity problems and work well as cooking oils, in excess they act as roadblocks in the metabolism of the essential fatty acids, preventing the conversion of the good fats into those beneficial prostaglandins (healthy hormones) we mentioned earlier. Overindulgence in saturated fats is also associated with elevated cholesterol levels, which can lead to obstruction of arteries and heart problems. A diet that includes a lot of commercially processed/fast foods makes it especially easy to consume too much. Try to keep your intake of these fats at a minimum and obtain them from quality sources, especially if you regularly eat animal products and/or have cholesterol problems.

Vegetables sources include coconut oil, cocoa butter, peanut oil, palm oil, and palm-kernel oil. Animal sources include pork, lamb, and beef fats (lard, tallow); organ meats; and full-fat dairy products like butter, whole milk, cheeses, and ice cream.

**GROUP FOUR: TRANS-FATTY ACIDS:** Now for the real bad boys—trans fats. These are to be avoided as much as possible. While saturated fats have long been labeled the "bad" fats in the American diet, substantial evidence suggests that today's epidemic of heart disease began when hydrogenated and partially hydrogenated fats (and the foods containing them) were introduced into the mainstream diet. Basically, trans-fatty acids are a synthetic fat created by a chemical process in which hydrogen is added to naturally occurring liquid fat at extremely high temperatures. Consuming trans fatty acids promotes increased total serum cholesterol and blood insulin levels. Cancer, obesity, diabetes, and immune system problems are also now associated with trans fats. The Food and Drug Administration plans to make listing trans fats on foods labels mandatory as of 2006. In the meantime, avoid the following: margarine, vegetable shortening, lard, partially hydrogenated vegetable oils, and the numerous baked goods and fried and processed foods made from them.

## PRACTICAL EATING TIPS

### MOTHER NATURE: SHE GIVES, AND GIVES, AND GIVES . . .

In trying to navigate all the conflicting dietary ideas coming our way, it's important to know alternatives that don't get as much play as "Got milk" ads. This can greatly expand your menu. For example, to most Americans, calcium means dairy products. But on closer examination there are several alternate sources of calcium (have you ever wondered where cows get it?).

This is good news for the many people who are lactose intolerant or suffer other negative effects of consuming dairy, including aggravated allergy symptoms and PMS. For example, one cup of milk contains approximately 300 mg of calcium. Compare this to the one-cup calcium content in the following non-dairy foods:

**VEGETABLES (1 CUP)**

- **cooked collard greens, 360 mg of calcium**
- **cooked kale, 210 mg**
- **cooked bok choy, 250 mg**
- **fresh broccoli, 140 mg**
- **turnip greens, 252 mg**
- **mustard greens, 196 mg**

Here are some other good sources:

**PROTEIN FOODS**

- **one tin sardines, 480 mg**
- **3 oz. salmon, 290 mg**
- **4 oz. tofu, 150 mg**
- **One cup cooked beans, 100 mg**

**SEA VEGETABLES (3 OZ.)**

- **hijiki, 1,400 mg**
- **wakame, 1,300 mg**
- **kombu, 800 mg**
- **kelp, 1,093**

**NUTS AND SEEDS (3 OZ.)**

- **Almonds, 254 mg**
- **Walnuts, roasted, 83 mg**
- **Sesame seeds, 160 mg**
- **Raisins, 62 mg**

When it comes to what to put in your cereal, a variety of non-dairy milks are now widely available, from soy and rice to oat and almond. If you are feeling limited when it comes to eating, do some exploring. Nature has provided literally hundreds upon thousands of nutrition choices.

## TAMING YOUR CRAVINGS: A LOOK AT SUGAR

For many of us, cravings are such a way of life that we take them for granted, constantly fighting them and then indulging them. Sugar is the most common culprit. Countless people suffer from sugar cravings, and a surprising number describe the feeling as "uncontrollable." It may be helpful to understand that although your body is craving sugar, that doesn't mean it's craving donuts, candy, cookies, or ice cream (foods composed of simple carbs as opposed to complex carbs—more on those later). It is craving the quick but temporary rise in energy levels and mood that sugar can produce. But once the levels ebb, a craving arises to reproduce the same wave, and a pattern is created. This is problematic because sugar and processed foods cause rapid and extreme elevations in both blood sugar and insulin. Elevated insulin signals the body to burn the sugar and store the fat—one of the ways people gain weight. High insulin can also result in other serious disorders, including adult-onset diabetes and some types of cancer.

A good way to deal with this craving is to add small doses of sweetness to your foods throughout the day. Add sugar or honey to your tea, use sweet salad dressings, have fruit for dessert or snacks. And believe it or not, eat your vegetables. Consider trying a daily serving of one or more of the following naturally sweet vegetables: sweet potatoes, yams, carrots, onions, the many varieties of squash, and parsnips. These provide gentle elevations in blood sugar, as opposed to extreme highs and lows.

## NEGOTIATING WITH YOUR CRAVINGS

On the other end of the spectrum, consuming an excess of nonnutritious sugary foods will eventually result in a craving for something that feels "nutritious." In this case, you may feel the need to fill up on a steak or other high-protein, high-fat food. Now your body is on the roller coaster of trying to rebalance itself. If you find yourself tossed between extremes, try experimenting with your diet. If you are lacking in one area, like greens, try increasing your intake and see what happens. Whatever your craving is for, sweet or salty, crunchy or spicy, remember that cravings are a symptom of an underlying imbalance—one that you can easily deconstruct if you give some thought to it. We are often really hungry for nutrients, not necessarily more food/calories.

## ADD MORE GOOD FOOD

Think in terms of adding foods to your repertoire, rather than taking them away. As your taste buds awaken to new and forgotten flavors, and you discover a wider variety of foods you enjoy, these new additions may ultimately "crowd out" the less desirable ones. A good diet need not include deprivation and denial.

## GMOS, HORMONES, ANTIOBIOTICS, AND COMMERCIAL MEATS

Today's commercial food supply is more processed, chemicalized, and genetically modified than ever—from pesticides and chemical fertilizers, to dyes and wax, to the antibiotics and hormones injected into farm animals. Studies suggest that nonorganic supermarket produce is sorely lacking in trace minerals as compared to organic produce. Take care of yourself by consuming the highest quality foods you can—you will literally taste the difference.

If you are a meat eater, know that most of the commercial red meat in the United States contains traces of the hormones used to fatten the animals. The fat in red meat, and similarly in poultry, serves as a depository for these and other unhealthy substances, many of which have estrogenic effects that may increase the risk of certain cancers. Fish is a cleaner choice, but be aware of mercury poisoning and environmental toxins—especially if you are pregnant or may become pregnant. Mercury in the bloodstream can be harmful to a developing fetus, as well as to young children. The safest choices are cold-water fish, such as wild Alaskan salmon, sardines, and herring. These also are good sources of health-protective omega-3 fatty acids.

## VARIETY IS THE SPICE OF LIFE

When it comes to eating for optimum health, it's indisputable that a diet high in a variety of fresh foods from the various food groups will cover all the nutritional bases, giving you the immune-boosting phytochemicals, antioxidants, and other micronutrients, vitamins, minerals, and fiber you need to prevent and overcome illness, promote healthy digestion, and achieve your optimum weight and energy level. The lower the percentage of processed foods in the diet, the better. Make the highest quality food choices you can to minimize your intake of any harmful elements. A variety of color can be one good clue to the range of benefits you're getting from your diet.

## FOOD FOR THOUGHT

A balanced diet in terms of food is just one part of a balanced life. Believe it or not, the body also commonly hungers for exercise as a way of releasing tension, but too often we try to satisfy this hunger with food. Exercise is a primary food; so are loving relationships, rewarding work, and a spiritual life, which may include meditation, yoga, prayer, or religious practice. Don't forget about these primary sources of nourishment in your life. Healthy eating habits are related to lifestyle.

PART FIVE

# THE COMPLETE CORE PROGRAM

# 16

# WELLNESS: THE BIG PICTURE

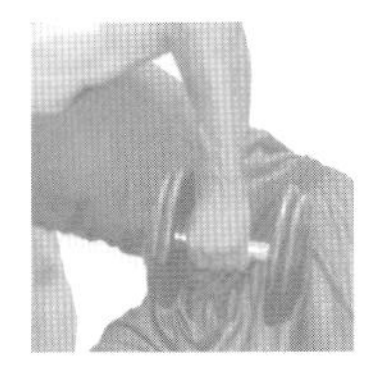

## WHAT IS WELLNESS?

Complete wellness is a lifestyle. It asks you to take responsibility for how you live and the choices you make. Wellness means taking an active role in improving every aspect of your life in order to achieve a productive, healthy lifestyle.

A strong, balanced core workout can be the center of your physical wellness program, but it is not a complete wellness program. This chapter will give you a brief overview of the six dimensions of total wellness.

## THE SIX DIMENSIONS OF WELLNESS

There are six major dimensions of wellness: physical, emotional, intellectual, social, spiritual, and vocational. How you develop these dimensions determines your lifestyle. Becoming proactive in your wellness choices is the first step to a healthy lifestyle. The following are brief descriptions of the wellness dimensions.

**PHYSICAL WELLNESS** encourages all issues concerning your physical body. These include daily exercise, diet, and medical care. They also include the use and abuse of tobacco, drugs, and alcohol.

**EMOTIONAL WELLNESS** emphasizes awareness and acceptance of your feelings. An emotionally well person maintains satisfying relationships with others while feeling positive and enthusiastic about his own life. You also maintain minimal levels of stress, develop healthy feelings, and use nondestructive emotional outlets.

**INTELLECTUAL WELLNESS** encourages creative, stimulating mental activities. Intellectual stimulation and learning are crucial elements in adapting to change and understanding the world we live in.

**SOCIAL WELLNESS** encourages contributing to the human community and physical environment. A socially well person emphasizes interdependence with others, with nature, and within his or her own family. A socially well person has developed healthy ways to interact, react, and live with other people.

**VOCATIONAL WELLNESS** encourages growth and happiness in your work. A vocationally well person seeks jobs that give personal satisfaction and enrichment.

**SPIRITUAL WELLNESS** is the quest for meaning and purpose. A spiritually well person develops, evolves, and practices his religious, political, environmental, and personal beliefs.

## YOU ARE UNIQUE

It's important to understand that everyone's pie chart is different. For instance, a professor may have a larger intellectual dimension than a massage therapist, who works more intuitively and physically. An athlete would have a larger piece of the physical dimension than a church minister, whose religious beliefs are the substance of his life. Your pie chart will be a reflection of your individuality.

## THE PHYSICAL DIMENSION

Since this is a fitness book, we're going to take a close look at physical well-being—specifically, exercise wellness.

Just as you created your overall wellness profile, you can also create a profile of your physical wellness. Within the physical wellness piece of pie, besides the core workout, we will focus on three elements: cardio work, strength training, and stretching. There are many benefits of exercise: stress reduction, weight loss, cardiovascular benefits, muscular strength, endurance, and increased flexibility. To achieve these benefits, however, you need a complete fitness program. This chapter will get you started on the Complete Core Program.

## GETTING STARTED ON THE COMPLETE CORE PROGRAM

It's important that you begin your comprehensive exercise program slowly and increase your exercise levels gradually. Keep in mind, these workouts are in addition to your core workout. The goal of these workouts is to get you started. They are the first step in building a complete program. How you ease into the Complete Core Program will depend on your goals and how much time you can commit. The entire program will take about one hour and you need to do it three times a week. The breakdown looks like this:

- **10 minutes of stretching**
- **30 minutes of cardio**
- **20 minutes of lifting**

Before you start the program, make sure you check with your doctor.

## STRATEGIES

There are a lot of ways to work this program into your life:

- **Start out doing the Complete Core Program twice a week. You will still look and feel better, even if you do it just twice a week. When your schedule gets hectic, doing the program twice a week is a good way to maintain your results.**
- **Break up the program as you integrate it into your core workout. You can alternate days. For example:**

  MONDAY: **core work and cardio**

  TUESDAY: **weight train and stretch**

  WEDNESDAY: **core work and cardio**

  THURSDAY: **weight train and stretch**

  FRIDAY: **core work and cardio**

  SATURDAY: **weight train and stretch**

- **The above is just on example. Adapt it to your own life. Maybe you are already taking a yoga class two or three times a week; then you wouldn't need to do the stretching program. You want to put your focus on weight training and cardio work.**
- **You can also start out by adding just one element of the program at a time. If you start out by working up to 30 minutes of cardio a day, that's big. Then, when you've accomplished your cardio goals, tackle strength training. The main thing is, you need to start thinking about the big picture—a complete fitness plan.**

In the following chapters we will look at each element of the Complete Core Program.

# 17

# CORE CARDIO

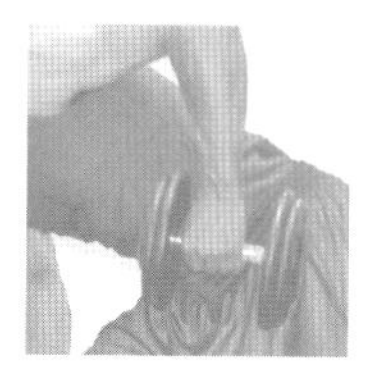

## INTRODUCTION

Cardiovascular fitness is achieved by performing activities that tax the heart, lungs, and circulatory systems. Cardio work puts a demand on the oxygen-exchange systems of your body. Oxygen is taken from the lungs into the circulatory system, then distributed to the muscles that are being used during the exercise. The oxygen is then used to help break down stored fats into energy for the working muscles. This exchange system forces the lungs and heart to become extremely efficient, so that the working muscles can continue their activities.

The American College of Sports Medicine recommends thirty minutes of cardiovascular exercise, at least three times a week, to achieve significant health benefits. During this thirty-minute period you need to maintain your heart rate, 65–85 percent of your maximum heart rate, for at least twenty minutes. Popular cardio exercises are walking, jogging, swimming, bicycling, and various classes (step, tae bo, spinning, and so forth).

## THE CARDIO ZONE: FINDING YOUR TARGET HEART RATE

The following formula will determine your target heart rate. For an example, let's use someone who is thirty years old.

At birth, your maximum heart rate is 220 beats per minute. Each year you age, your maximum heart rate decreases by one beat. So to determine your maximum heart rate, you subtract your age from 220. If you are 30, your maximum heart rate is 190 beats a minute.

## DETERMINING YOUR TEN-SECOND PULSE RATE

As we said earlier, your target training zone is between 65 and 85 percent of your maximum heart rate. The most practical way to test this during a workout is to figure out your ten-second pulse rate. The way to do this is to multiply your maximum heart rate (220 minus your age) by 0.65 and 0.85, and then divide those figures by 6 (because there are 6 ten-second periods in a minute). The two resulting figures are the low and high ends for your target zone.

When working out, you want to keep your heart rate between these parameters. In the example above, the numbers round out to 21 and 27 beats in the ten second count. Here's the math:

**Subtract for maximum heart rate. 220 – 30 = 190 beats per minute**

**Multiply for lower end of target. 190 × 0.65 = 123.5 beats per minute**

**Multiply for upper end of target. 190 × 0.85 = 161.5 beats per minute**

**Divide by 6 for 10 second count for the lower target. 123.5 ÷ 6 = 21**

**Divide by 6 for 10 second count for the upper target. 161.5 ÷ 6 = 27**

These days, this is an old-school method. A good investment is a heart rate monitor. They are fairly inexpensive, especially if you get one without all the bells and whistles, which you don't really need. This way you can get constant feedback.

## CARDIOVASCULAR PROGRAM

The following are guidelines for a progressive cardiovascular program. The program gradually eases you into aerobic training. If you need to take more time at any level, that's fine; move at your own pace. An easy pace means a pace below your target heart rate.

### LEVEL ONE: WEEKS 1 AND 2

5-minute easy pace

5-minute *target* pace

5-*minute easy pace*

15 minutes total time

### LEVEL TWO: WEEKS 3 AND 4

5-minute easy pace

5-minute *target* pace

2-minute easy pace

5-minute *target* pace

5-*minute easy pace*

22 minutes total time

### LEVEL THREE: WEEKS 5 AND 6

5-minute easy pace

10-minute *target* pace

2-minute easy pace

10-minute *target* pace

5-*minute easy pace*

32 minutes total time

### LEVEL FOUR: WEEKS 7 AND 8

5-minute easy pace

15-minute *target* pace

2-minute easy pace

15-minute *target* pace

5-*minute easy pace*

42 minutes total time

### LEVEL FIVE: MAINTENANCE

5-minute easy pace

20-minute *target* pace

5-minute easy pace

When you've reached Level Five, try exercising at the top end of your target rate.

## CORE INTERVAL TRAINING

The Complete Core Program incorporates the latest changes that have become popular in such classes as spinning. The essence of these popular classes is interval training. Interval training isn't a new concept—athletes and serious runners have always utilized it. In a nutshell, interval training combines more intense levels of training with less intense levels, as opposed to one steady level. For example, you might train at an increased level of intensity for a minute, then lower your level for a minute, alternating until you reach the cool-down phase of your workout. During interval training you push to the edge or beyond 85 percent of your maximum heart rate.

This type of training is more like life and sports. You don't move through the day or through a sport at a constant pace like a metronome. In most sports you use a variety of energy systems, from standing at rest to a jog and a sprint. The same is true in life. You often move from standing still or walking to a quicker pace. You run to catch the subway or to stop your child from walking into the street; you dive for a ground ball in a softball tournament or drive in for a layup in a pickup game. Core cardio will train you for your favorite activities and for life.

Core cardio also helps you lose weight. The formula for losing weight is simple: Burn off more calories than you take in. Weight loss is connected to the total number of calories you burn throughout the day. Increasing intensity with interval training burns more calories during your workout, making your cardio time more efficient and effective for losing weight.

## INTERVAL TRAINING BASICS

As we said earlier, interval training alternates high-intensity work with lower intensity recovery work. High intensity is when you push to the edge or beyond your aerobic threshold (85 percent of your maximum heart rate) toward an all-out effort. In the recovery or lower intensity phase you return to the low end of your aerobic training zone (65 percent of maximum). The goal of interval training is to allow your body to gradually adjust to increased levels of exertion. This also increases the total caloric burn in your workout.

## RANGE OF PERCEIVED EXERTION SCALE

Guidelines for interval training are expressed in the Range of Perceived Exertion (RPE) scale. This scale has a range from 1 to 10.

The lower ranges, 1–4, represent your warm-up exertion intensity. Levels 1 and 2 would be a brisk walk. Levels 3 and 4 represent an easy jog. Levels 5, 6, and 7 represent your target cardio range (65–85 percent of your maximum). The target will be different for everyone, depending on your age, fitness level, and genetics. Levels 8, 9, and 10 represent high-intensity exertion. Just like the target zone levels, these high-intensity levels will be different for each person.

## A BEGINNING INTERVAL WORKOUT

The following cardio workout is a simple way to incorporate the RPE scale and interval training into a 30-minute cardio session. In this routine you will do 1 minute of high intensity for blocks 2 through 5.

### THE ROUTINE

**BLOCK ONE: MINUTES 1–5.** During the first couple of minutes, ease into your warm-up phase with an exertion level of 1 and 2. Then move up to an RPE of between 3 and 4 for the next 3 minutes.

**BLOCK TWO: MINUTES 6–10.** Maintain a target zone RPE between the 5–7 range. Gradually increase pace as you reach minute 8, which will be your interval minute. This means push up your exertion level between 8 and 10 for 60 seconds. Recover at the exertion level of 5, the low end of your target zone.

**BLOCK THREE: MINUTES 11–15.** Maintain a target zone RPE between 5 and 7. Gradually increase the pace as you reach minute 13, which will be your interval minute. This means push up your exertion level between 8 and 10 for 60 seconds. Recover at the exertion level of 5, the low end of your target zone.

**BLOCK FOUR: MINUTES 16–20.** Maintain a target zone RPE between 5 and 7. Gradually increase the pace as you reach minute 18, which will be your interval minute. This means push up your exertion level between 8 and 10 for 60 seconds. Recover at the exertion level of 5, the low end of your target zone.

**BLOCK FIVE: MINUTES 21–25.** Maintain a target zone RPE between 5 and 7. Gradually increase pace as you reach minute 23, which will be your interval minute. This means push up your exertion level between 8 and 10 for 60 seconds. Recover at the exertion level of 5, the low end of your target zone.

**BLOCK SIX: MINUTES 26–30.** Cool down by using the first 2 minutes to recover at the low end of your target zone. Then drop down to an RPE between 3 and 4 for the last 2 minutes. During the last minute, slow down to a walk.

## NEXT LEVEL

To progressively build on this model, gradually add another 1 minute high-intensity interval to blocks 2 through 5. Start by adding it to the first block. Continue adding high intensity intervals until each block has 2 high-intensity minutes. Space them out so you always have at least a 1 minute recovery period between each high-intensity period.

# 18

# CORE STRENGTH TRAINING

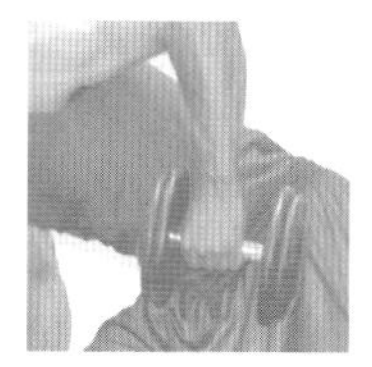

## INTRODUCTION

Weight training provides increased strength gains and increased endurance for your muscles, joints, bones, and ligaments. Strength training benefits include a better posture, stronger bones, increased strength for daily activities, good muscle tone, flexibility, and strength in your joints. The core strength-training program includes exercises designed for all the major muscle groups.

Special emphasis is given to scapula (shoulder blade) stabilization. This is key for sports activities, posture, and overall spinal health. This is accomplished with the alphabet moves Y, W, and M. These moves work the lower and middle trapezius muscles and the rhomboids. These are the muscles that hold your shoulder blades down and together. A problem area for many people is rounding the shoulders forward. This causes the shoulder blades to rise and separate. This, in turn, creates spine and alignment problems. Doing your alphabet will help alleviate this problem.

For each exercise there will be a traditional lift and a core variation. These variations will put you in positions that activate your core stabilization muscles. The following guidelines will help you build a solid and safe foundation on the Basic Eight routine.

## GUIDELINES

- **Build a foundation of strength before you start the core variations. This means at least 6 weeks of the traditional lifts.**
- **Complete this routine 2 or 3 times a week.**
- **For upper body exercises use a 10-to-15 repetition scheme. This means choosing a weight that will allow you to do 10 reps. When you work your way up to 15 repetitions, add weight. Continue this progressive cycle of adding weight.**
- **For lower-body exercises (squats and lunges) use a 15-to-20 repetition scheme. For lunges this would mean 15 to 20 on each side.**
- **For push-ups do your maximum each time.**
- **If you want to devote more time to strength training, after six weeks add an extra set to each exercise.**

BODY AREA: **CHEST** EXERCISE: **PUSH-UP**

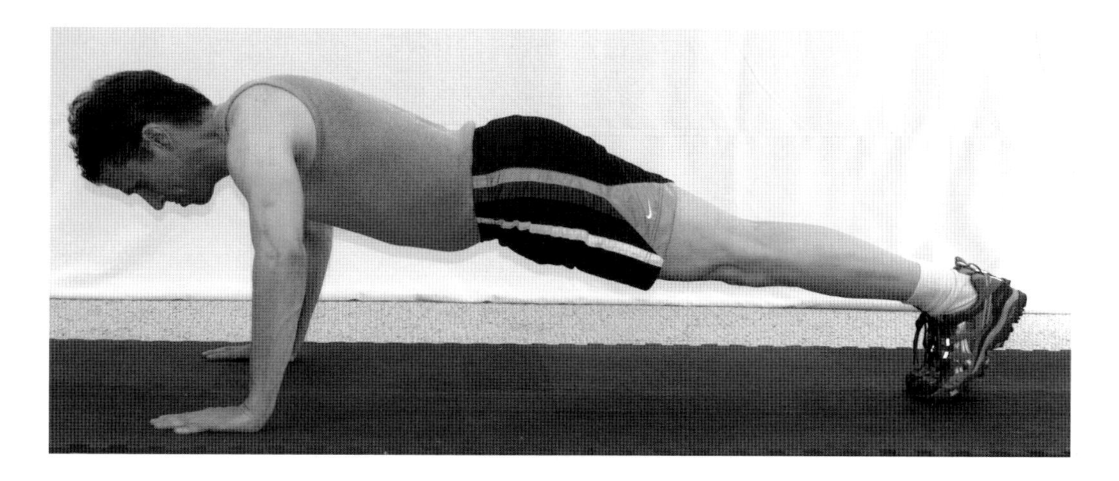

**STARTING POSITION:** Lie on your stomach, legs extended, toes tucked, hands placed outside your shoulders. Straighten your arms, lifting your entire body off the floor, balancing on your hands and toes.

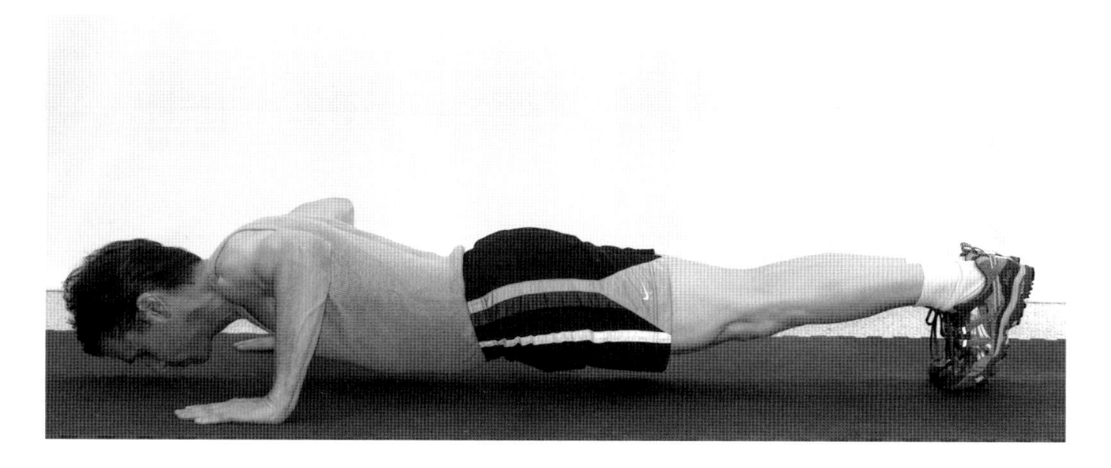

**THE MOVE:** Lower your body, letting your chest lightly make contact with the floor, creating a 90 degree angle in your elbow joint. Then straighten your arms, raising your body back to the starting position. This is one repetition.

## VARIATION

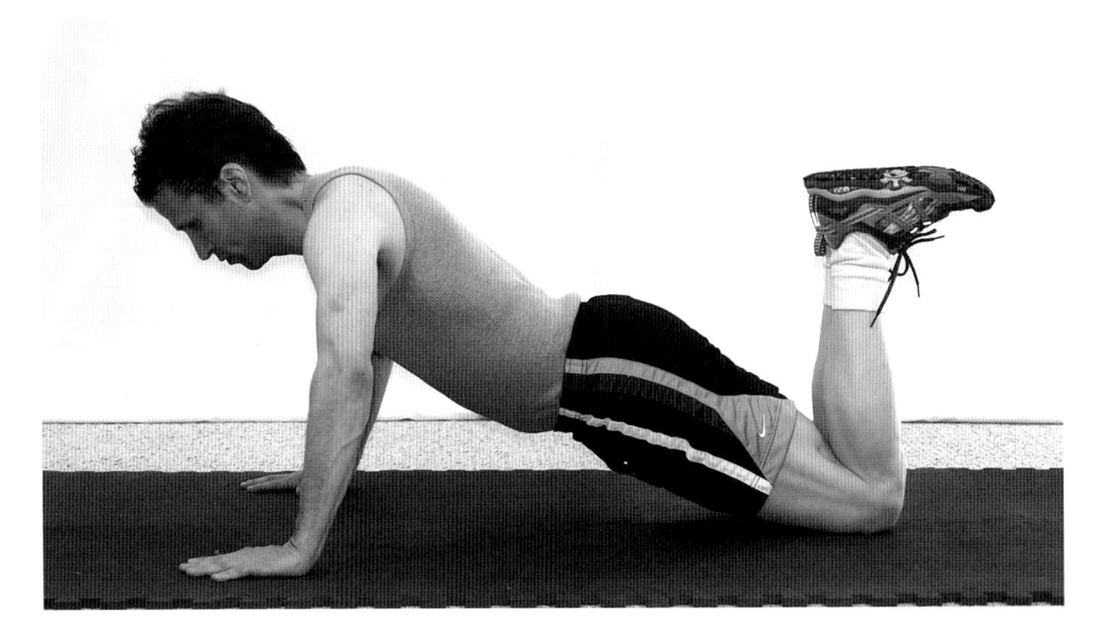

This exercise can also be done from your knees. From the above starting position rest your knees on the floor so your lower legs and feet are up in the air. Balance on your hands and your thigh muscles just above your knees. Then raise your body off the floor.

## TRAINING TIPS

- Think of your body as a solid unit, moving as a whole.
- Keep your head and neck in alignment with your spine, your eyes looking straight down, not up.
- Concentrate on your chest muscles as you go through the entire range of motion.
- Extend your arms just short of locking out.
- Exhale as you push up inhale as you go down.
- Depending on your flexibility, gender, and body type, different parts of your body may be the first to touch the floor. It could be your chest, stomach, or nose. The key is to keep your body aligned and held firm.

## CORE VARIATIONS

### PUSH-UP: SINGLE LEG PUSH-UP

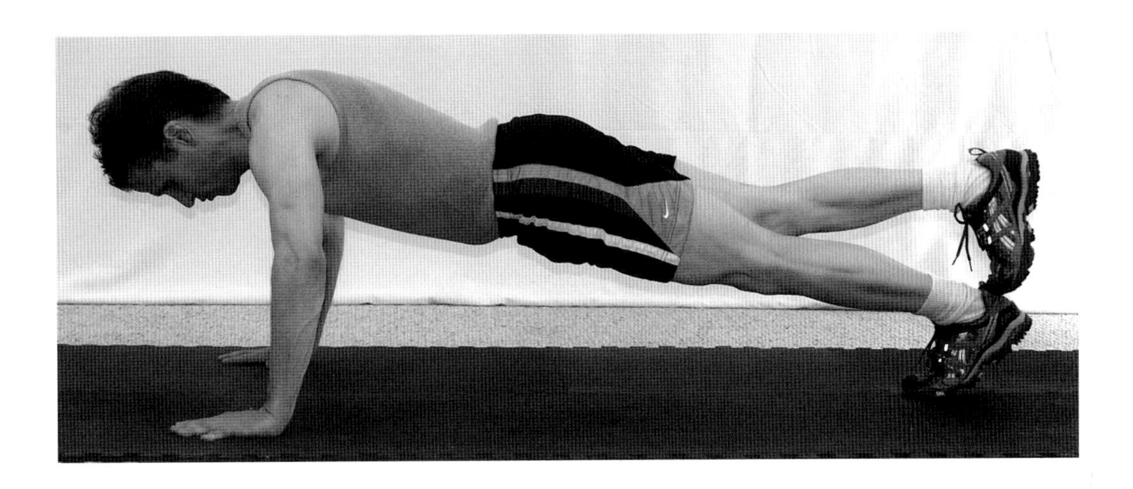

Follow the same procedure as in a normal push-up, but support yourself with just one leg.

### PUSH-UP: PUSH-UP ON THE BALL

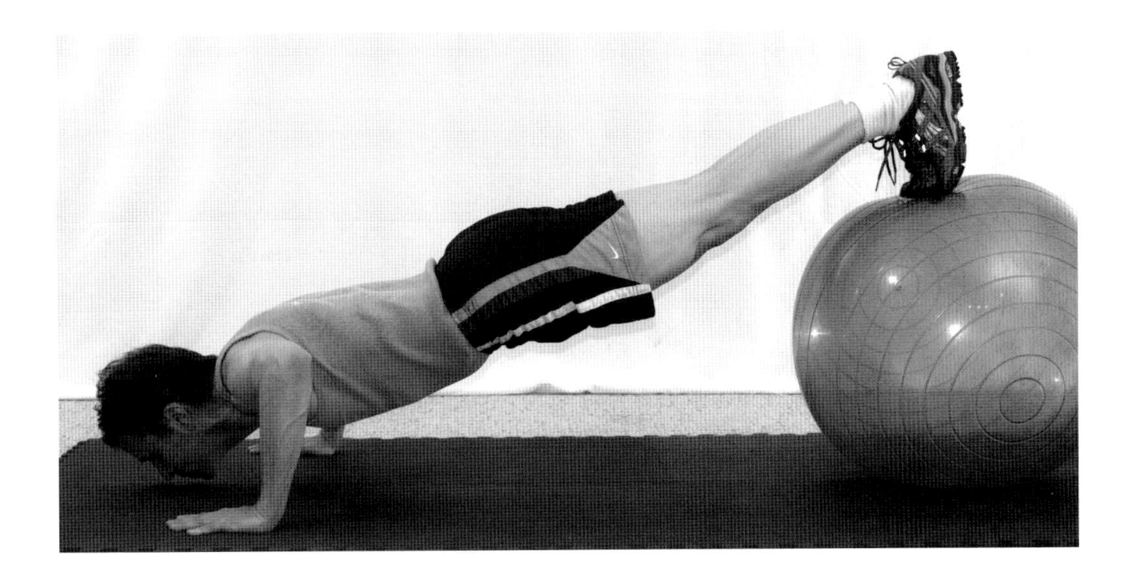

Follow the same procedure as a normal push-up, but rest both feet on top of the exercise ball. You can increase the difficulty by resting the balls of your feet on top of the ball.

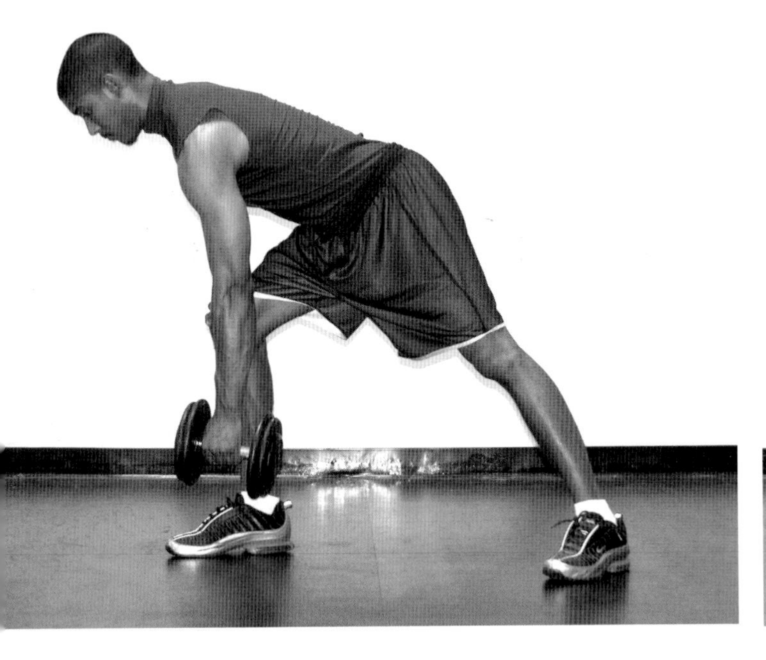

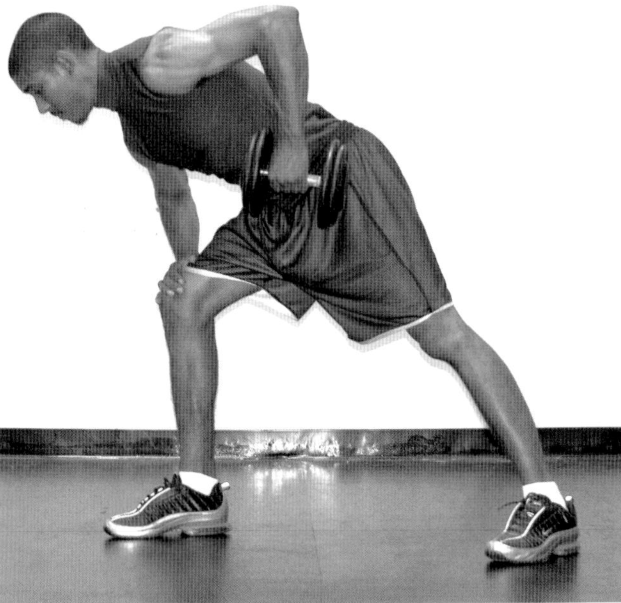

**STARTING POSITION:** Holding a dumbbell with your left hand, step forward with your right leg. Then bend forward at your waist, supporting your torso with your right arm on your right leg. Create between a 45 and 90 degree angle with your upper body. Let your left arm hang down (palm facing in).

**THE MOVE:** Using your back muscles, pull the dumbbell up to your chest. Then lower it back to the starting position in a controlled motion.

### TRAINING TIPS

- Imagine you have a string on your elbows and the movement is initiated from the elbow, instead of your hand pulling.
- Focus on pulling with your back muscles.
- Control the motion on both phases of the movement; don't let gravity take over.
- Exhale as you pull the weight toward your chest; inhale as you lower the weight.

## CORE VARIATION

### BENT ROW: ONE-LEG BENT ROW

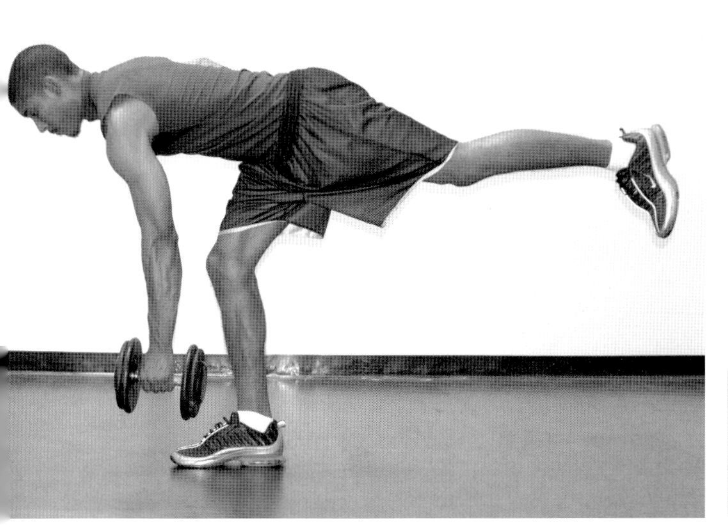

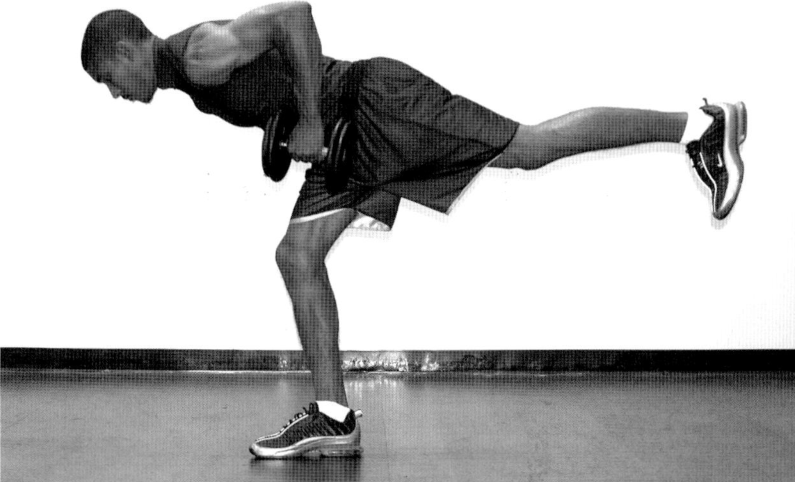

**STARTING POSITION:** Holding a dumbbell with your left hand, step forward with your right leg. Then bend forward, raising your left leg up off the ground and leaning your torso forward, so you are balancing on one leg, making a T-shape. Your left arm is extended at your side. Your right arm hangs down naturally or braces on your right thigh for support.

**THE MOVE:** Using your back muscles, pull the dumbbell up to your chest. Then lower it in a controlled motion while maintaining the balanced T-position.

## TRAINING TIPS

- Activate your inner core to help you maintain balance.
- Feel the movement initiate from your back muscles, initiating the movement from your elbow.
- If you can't make a perfect T-shape, modify it so you can maintain balance.
- Use your free hand for support by hanging on to a chair or wall.

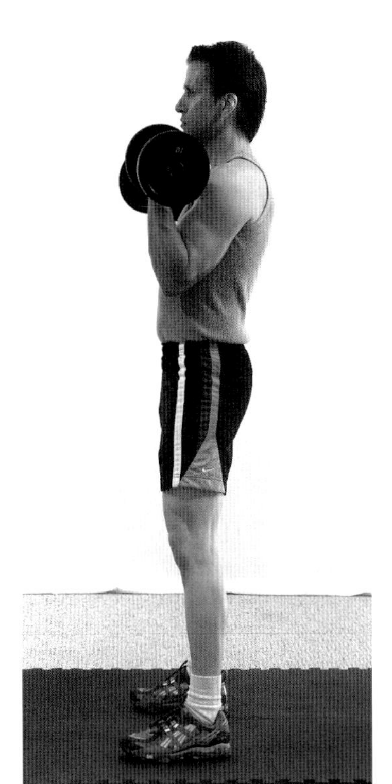

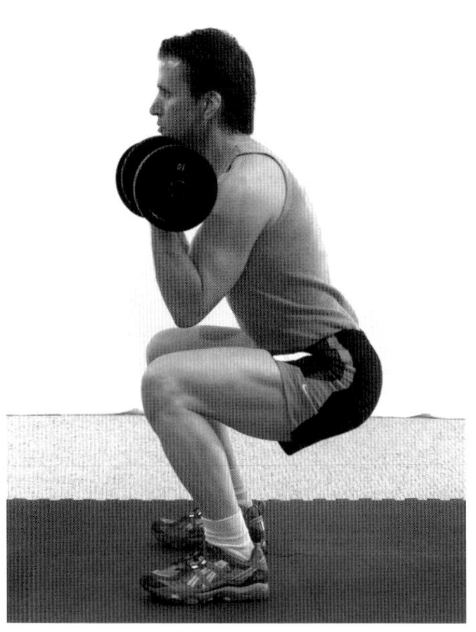

**STARTING POSITION:** Prepare to squat by getting in the Ready Position: feet a little wider than shoulder-width apart, toes pointed slightly out, knees unlocked, weight evenly distributed from the balls of your feet to your heels, shoulders back and down, a neutral spine, head and neck in alignment with your spine, and eyes looking straight ahead.

**THE MOVE:** Descend in a controlled manner (your hips moving backward as if you're sitting and your torso leaning forward to counterbalance) until the tops of your thighs are parallel to the ground. As you lower, don't let your knees come out over your toes. Then return to the starting position.

### TRAINING TIPS

- Add weight by holding dumbbells up at your shoulders.
- Don't bounce at the bottom of the movement.
- Keep heels flat.
- Don't allow your hips to sway backward as you come up.
- Keep your inner core activated for support.

## CORE VARIATION

### THE SQUAT: **OVERHEAD SQUAT**

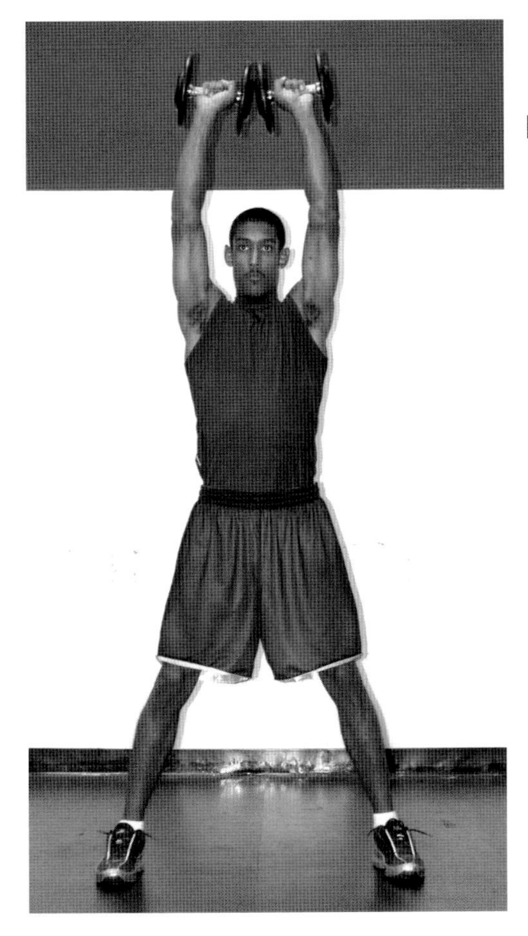

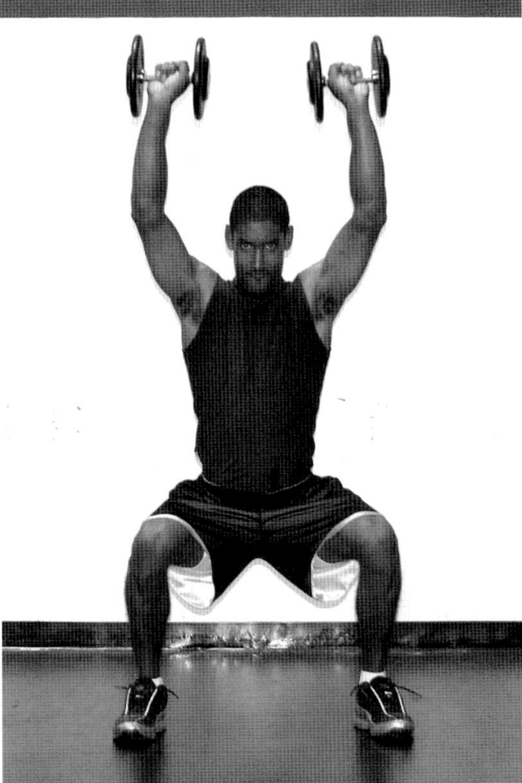

**Follow the same procedure as a squat, but begin with dumbbells or a barbell extended directly over your head. Maintain the overhead position for the entire set. Start out with a light weight.**

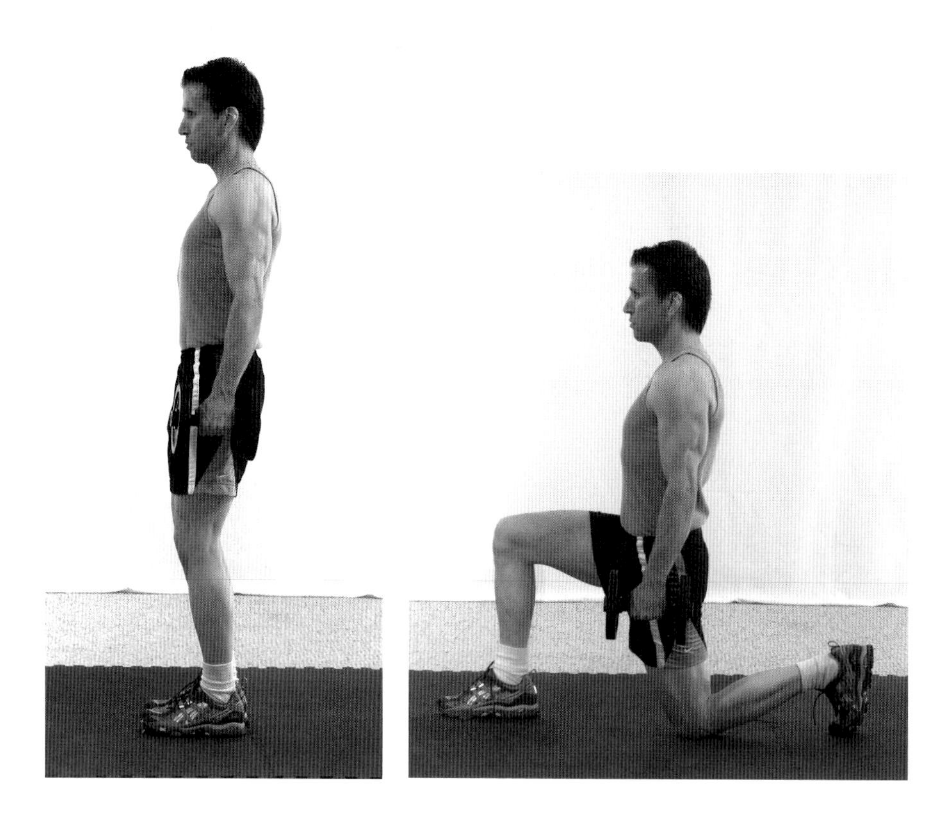

**STARTING POSITION:** Stand in the ready position, feet shoulder width apart.

**THE MOVE:** Lower your body back to kneeling position, keeping your knee an inch above the ground or letting it lightly touch the floor (but don't let your back knee rest on the ground). Maintain proper kneeling position by keeping your front knee behind your toes. Alternate sides.

## CORE VARIATION

### LUNGE: ON THE BALL OR BENCH

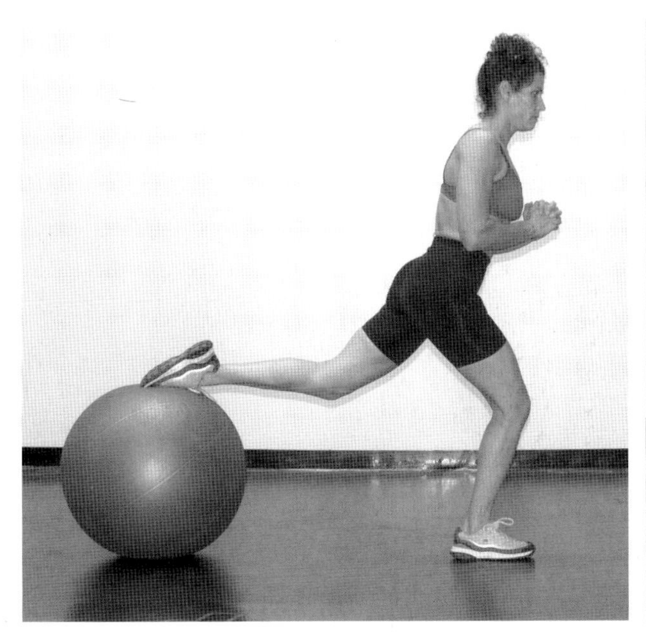

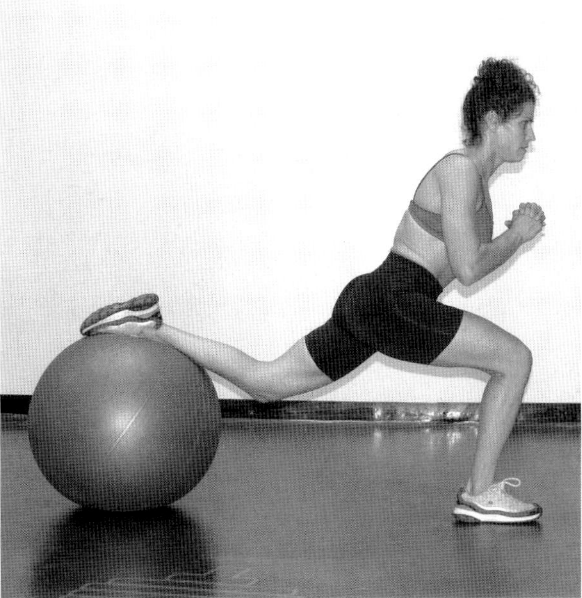

**STARTING POSITION:** Place your back foot on a bench, chair, or exercise ball, then step forward with the other foot. Prepare to lunge by getting your front leg and your upper body in the same ready position as above.

**THE MOVE:** Bend your lead leg, lowering your hips toward the floor, then return to the starting position. Switch sides and repeat.

## TRAINING TIPS

- Step forward so the shin of your lead leg is vertical (perpendicular to the floor).
- Add weight by holding dumbbells at your sides.
- Keep your body upright and your spine in the neutral position.
- Make sure your hips drop straight down, not forward.
- Don't bounce your knee off the ground.
- Look straight ahead throughout the movement.

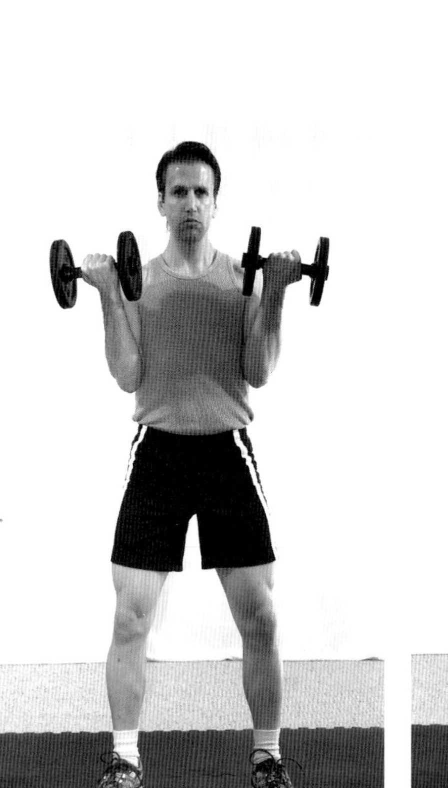

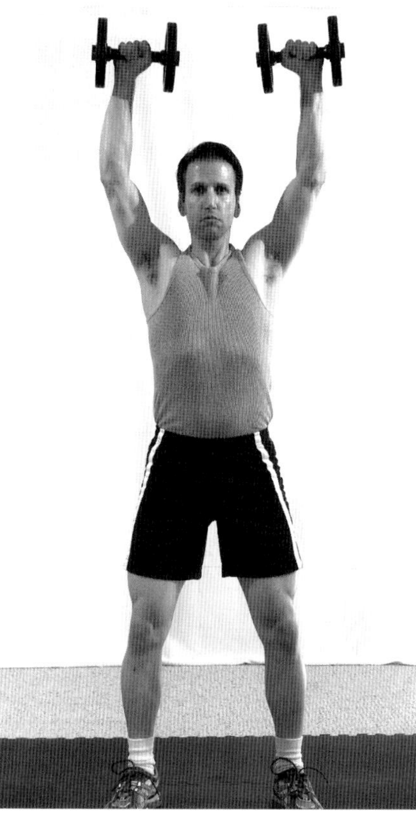

**STARTING POSITION:** Stand with your feet wider than your shoulders, creating a solid base, knees unlocked. Hold both dumbbells at shoulder level with your hands rotated so your palms face your body.

**THE MOVE:** Raise both dumbbells directly over your head as you rotate both hands out so that your palms face away from your body when your arms are extended. Return to starting position under control. Repeat.

### TRAINING TIPS

- Maintain good posture throughout the exercise.
- Avoid arching your lower back as you lift.
- Keep your elbows aligned with your ears.
- Focus your mind on your shoulders throughout the exercise.

## CORE VARIATION

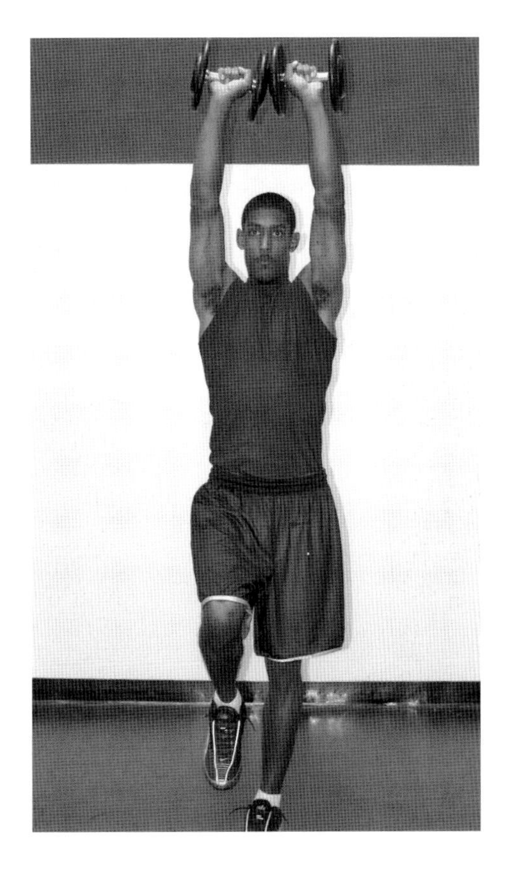

**ON ONE LEG:** Follow the same procedure as the Rotation Press, but balance on one leg. Alternate legs halfway through the set.

**ONE ARM AT A TIME:** Follow the same procedure as the Rotation Press, but press up with one arm at a time. You can use any of the following options:

- Alternate arms.
- Do all the reps on one arm, then switch arms.
- Do the one arm variation, standing on one leg.

**STARTING POSITIONS FOR ALL VARIATIONS:** The starting position can be bending over at the waist, resting over an exercise ball, or resting over a bench.

### Y VARIATION

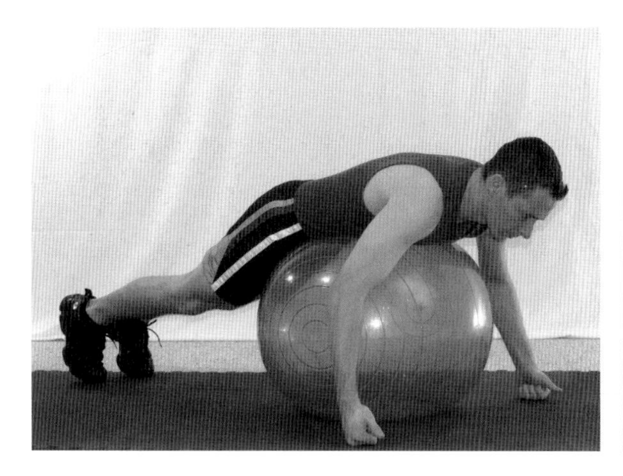

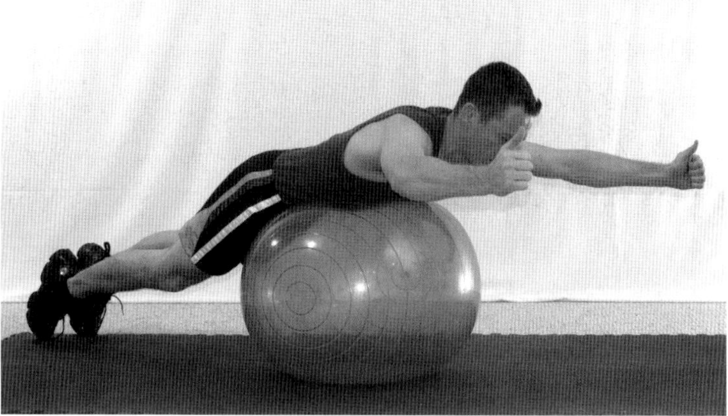

**STARTING POSITION:** Extend your arms out in front of your body, angling your arms into a Y shape. Point your thumbs up. Then lower your arms down to begin.

**THE MOVE:** Raise your arms up to the Y position. Lower and repeat.

### W VARIATION

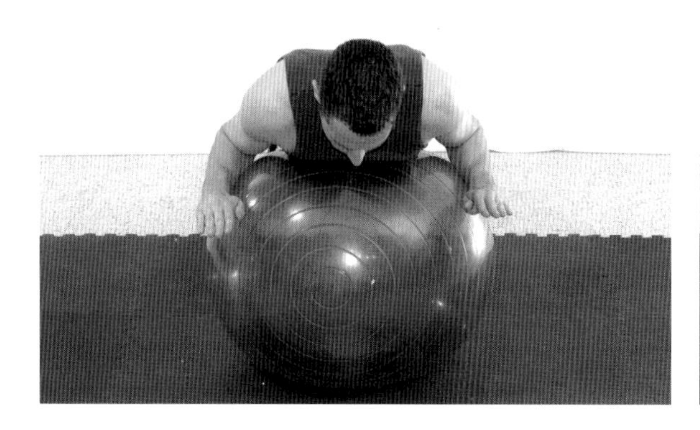

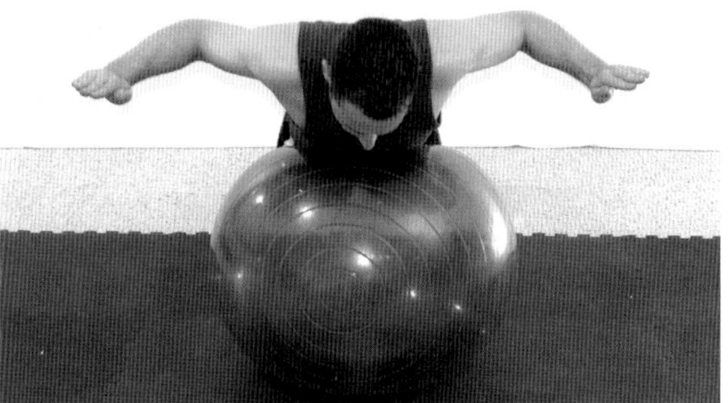

**STARTING POSITION:** Bring your hands toward your shoulders, creating the spacing of a W shape. Then bring your elbows into the sides of your body and let your arms drop at your sides. Point your thumbs up, or keep them neutral.

**THE MOVE:** Bring your shoulder blades together as you raise your arms (like flapping wings in a controlled motion), maintaining the W shape at the top of the movement.

## M-VARIATION

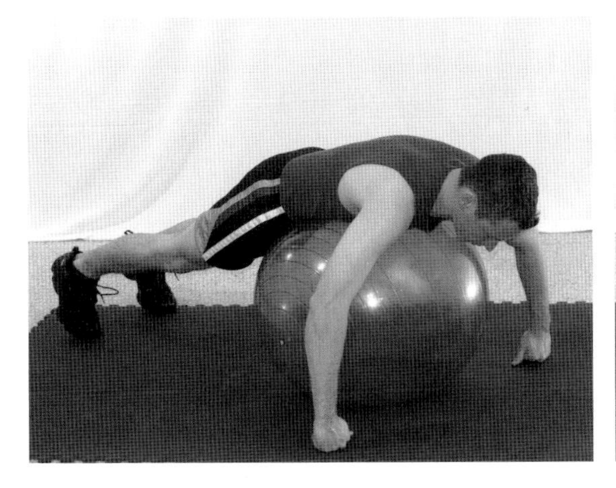

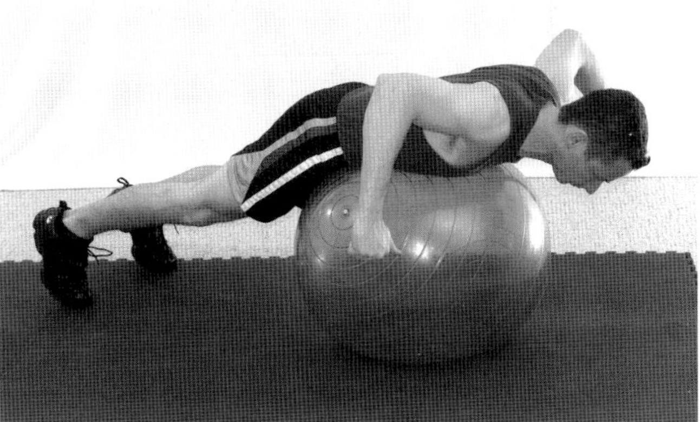

**STARTING POSITION:** Let your arms hang straight down.

**THE MOVE:** Bringing your shoulder blades together, raise your elbows, bringing your arms up and creating an M shape.

## TRAINING TIPS FOR VARIATIONS

- Initiate movements from your shoulder blades.
- Keep the motion controlled; don't try to jerk it up with your arms.
- Keep a neutral spine.
- Keep your head and neck aligned with your spine.
- Keep your shoulder blades back and down throughout the movements.

BODY AREA: **TRICEPS** EXERCISE: **BENCH DIPS**

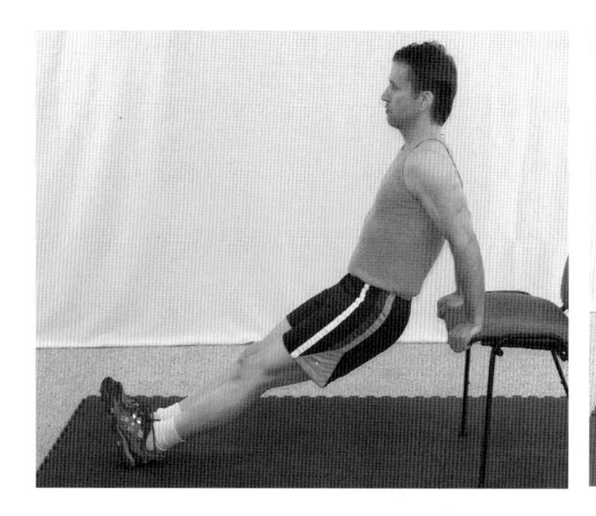

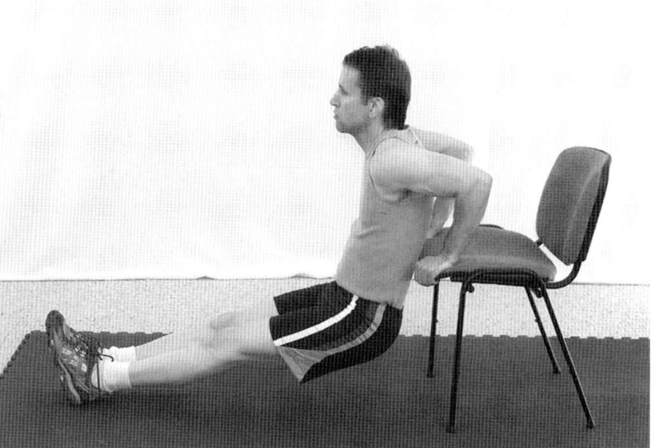

**STARTING POSITION:** To prepare, sit on the edge of a bench or chair and place both hands at the sides of your hips, fingers facing forward. Then extend your arms and scoot forward, sliding your hips off the end of the chair or bench by a couple of inches.

**THE MOVE:** Lower your body until your arms are bent at a 90 degree angle. Return to the starting position and repeat.

### TRAINING TIPS

- Maintain good spine and neck alignment.
- Move your body straight up and down, not out at an angle.
- Focus your mind on your triceps.

## CORE VARIATIONS

### ON THE BALL-1

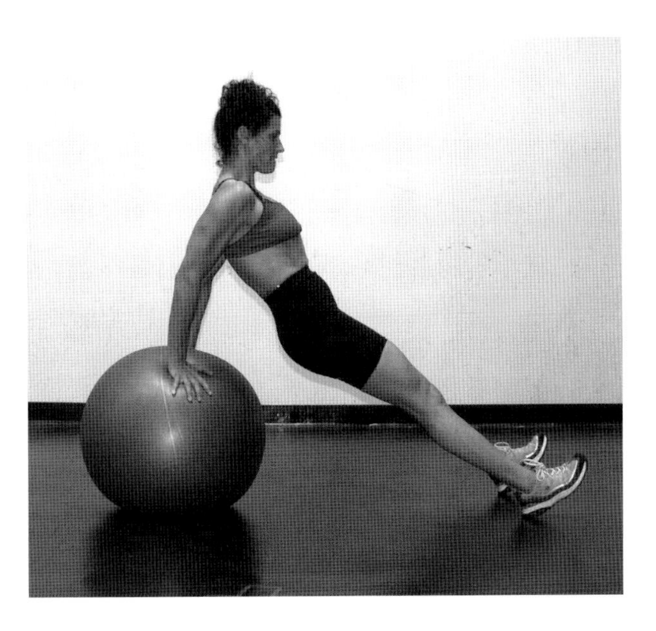

Follow the same procedure using an exercise ball instead of a bench or chair.

### ON THE BALL-2

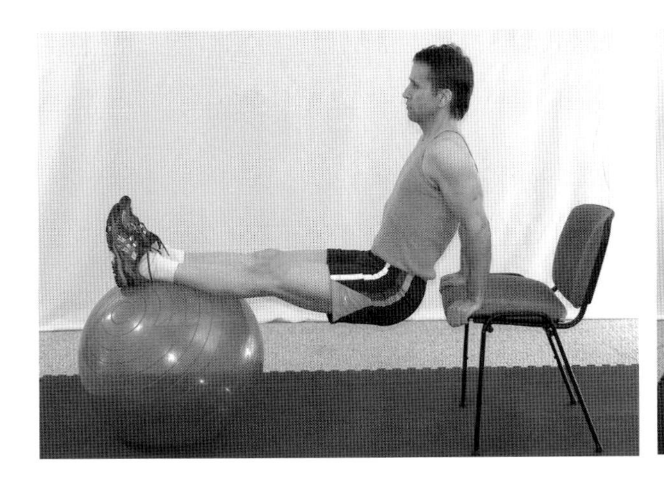

Do the same exercise, but rest your feet on top of an exercise ball. To increase the difficulty, rest just one leg on top of the ball (placing one leg on top of the other).

### ON ONE LEG

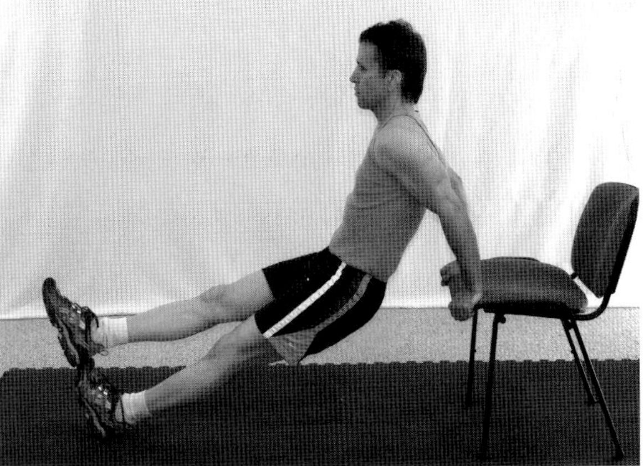

Do the same exercise, but use just one leg for support (placing one leg on top of the other).

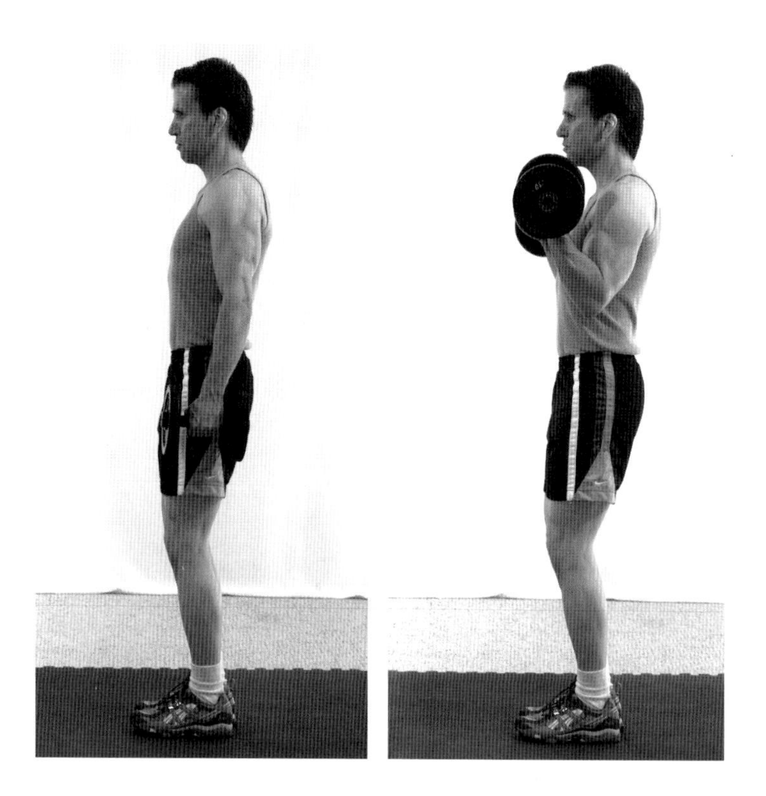

**STARTING POSITION:** Stand with your feet shoulder-width apart, holding two dumbbells at your sides, palms facing in.

**THE MOVE:** Begin to simultaneously curl both dumbbells, rotating your palms up as the weights pass your hips. Continue the smooth arc until the weights reach your shoulders. Then lower the dumbbells back to the starting position.

### TRAINING TIPS

- Keep your upper arms motionless and pressed against your torso throughout the range of motion.
- Aim for a smooth, flowing movement.
- Focus your mind on your biceps.

## CORE VARIATION

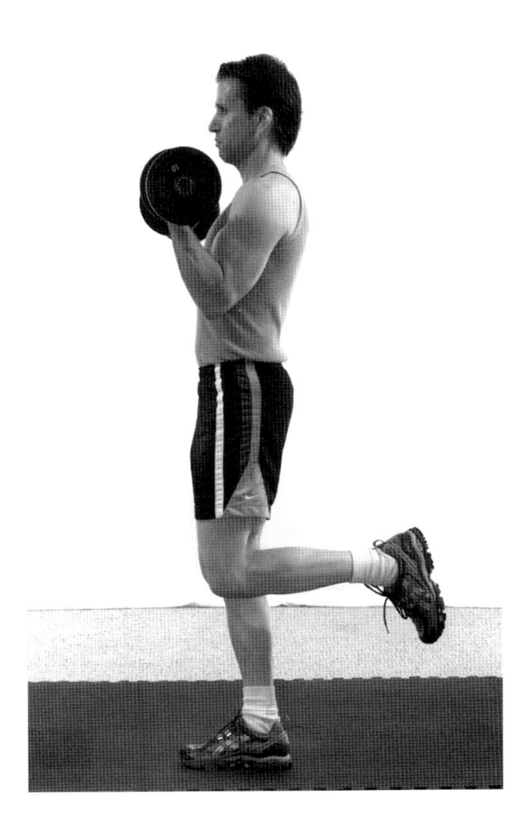

**ON ONE LEG:** Follow the same procedure, but balance on one leg. Alternate legs halfway through the set.

**ONE ARM AT A TIME:** Follow the same procedure as with curls, but curl one arm at a time. Other variations on this theme are:

- Do all the reps on one arm, then switch arms, and complete the prescribed number of reps with your other arm.
- Combine one-arm and one-leg variations.

# 19
# CORE STRETCHING: BASIC MOVES

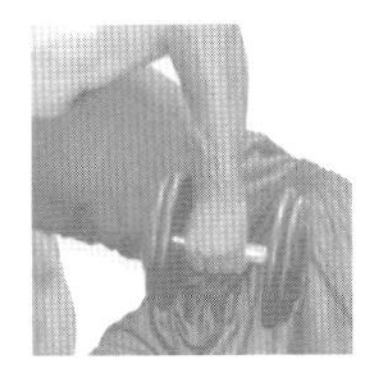

## INTRODUCTION

Stretching works the muscles, ligaments, and joints. Flexibility is important in maintaining posture, joint mobility, and range of motion. You need to stretch all your major muscles at least three times a week. Stretching at the end of a workout is a good way to cool down and safely improve your flexibility when your body is warm.

The goal of core stretching, like all core training, is to increase your body's functionality and flexibility in all directions. The core stretching routine is a combination of forward and backward bends, side bends, and rotation and crossing moves.

This routine is designed so you can hold each stretch for a prescribed time or move from stretch to stretch in fluid motion, creating a dynamic flow to the routine, much like a Sun Salutation in yoga. The stretches are grouped in three positions: standing, on the floor, and on all fours.

## GUIDELINES

- **Start slow and stay within your comfort zone, breathing into the stretch.**
- **Stretch only until you feel slight discomfort (not pain!).**
- **Hold each static stretch for 10–30 seconds, depending on your goals and needs. This means stretch tight areas and tight sides for a longer hold. If you have the time, indulge in longer holds. If you're in a hurry, do 10 second holds.**
- **For dynamic stretch, hold each position for a short pause, then move to the next position.**

### DYNAMIC AND STATIC

These are two fancy terms for when you hold a stretching posture (static) and when you move into a stretching posture and only hold it for a brief pause (dynamic).

## STANDING

### SEQUENCE ONE

# NECK ROLL

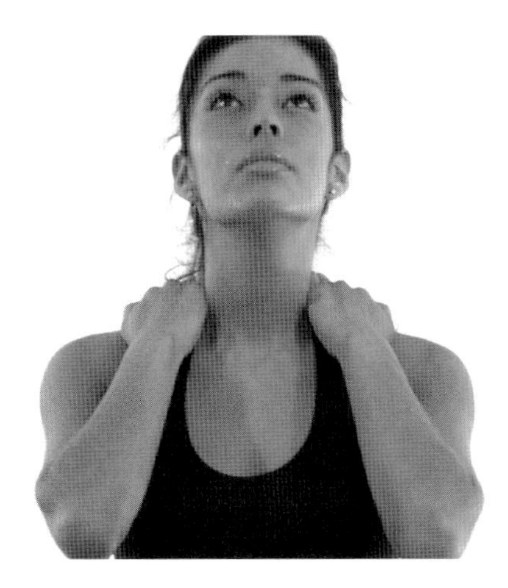
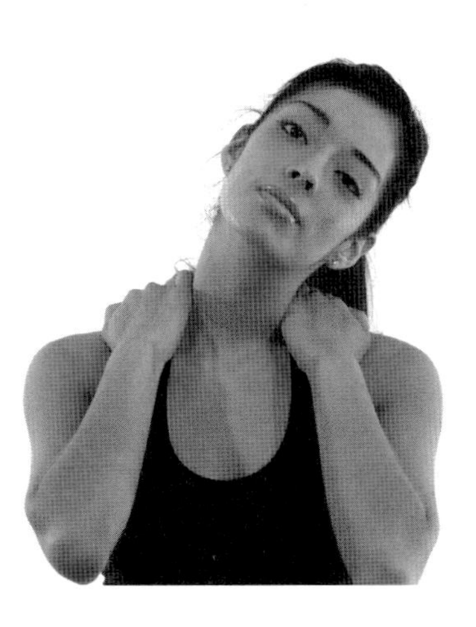
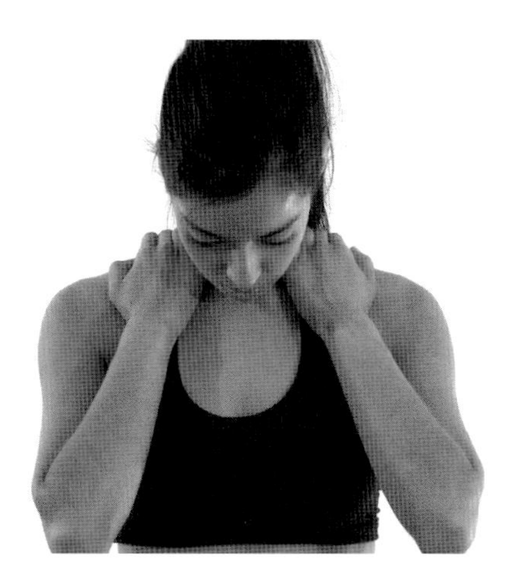

Place one hand on each side of your neck. Draw circles with your nose in a clockwise motion. Draw five circles, then repeat the move in a counterclockwise motion.

- Relax your jaw during the motion.
- Make the circle big enough so you are getting a nice stretch.

# SHOULDER ROLL

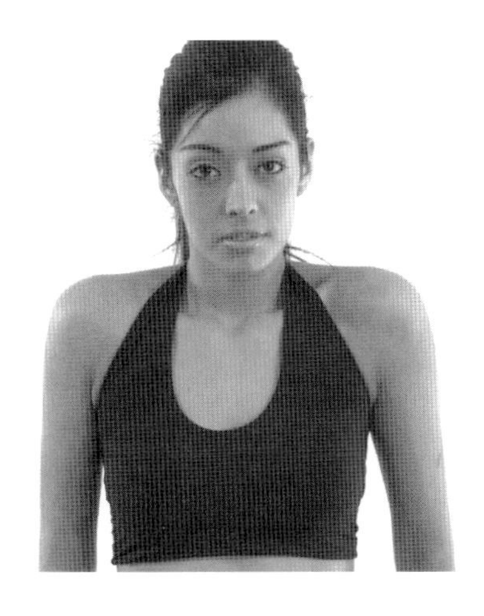
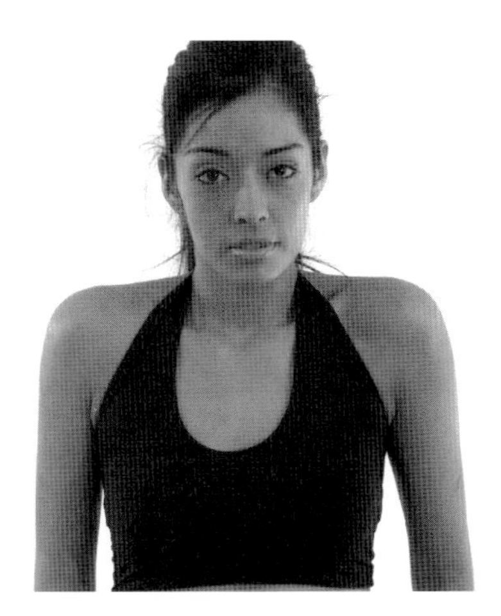
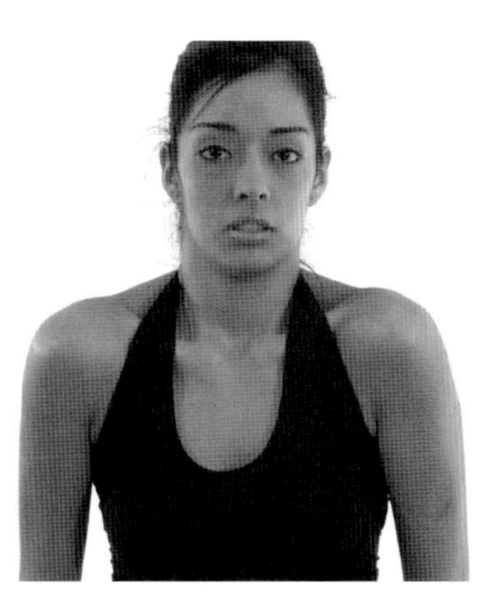

Raise your shoulders toward your ears and then roll them backward. Repeat the movement, but this time roll your shoulders forward. Then bring your shoulders up toward your ears and hold for a count of three and release. Repeat sequence three times.

SEQUENCE TWO

# STANDING BACKWARD BEND

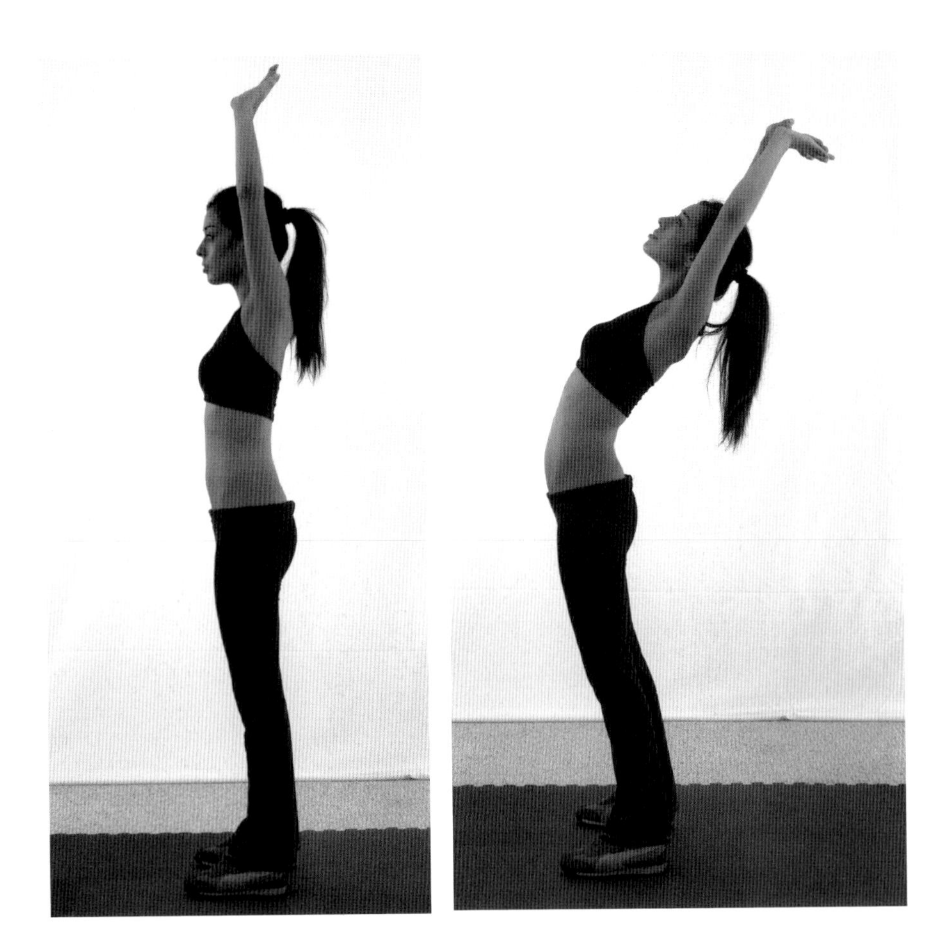

Standing with your feet shoulder-width apart, raise both hands above your head and interlock your thumbs. Then reach up, lengthening your spine but keeping your shoulders down, as you gently bend backward. Hold position and then return to the starting position or move dynamically into the next posture.

## TRAINING TIPS

- Let your neck and head gently follow the curve of your spine.
- Tighten your buttocks to protect your lower back.
- Keep your elbows even with your ears.
- Breath into the stretch.
- Initiate the movement from your center.

# STANDING FORWARD BEND

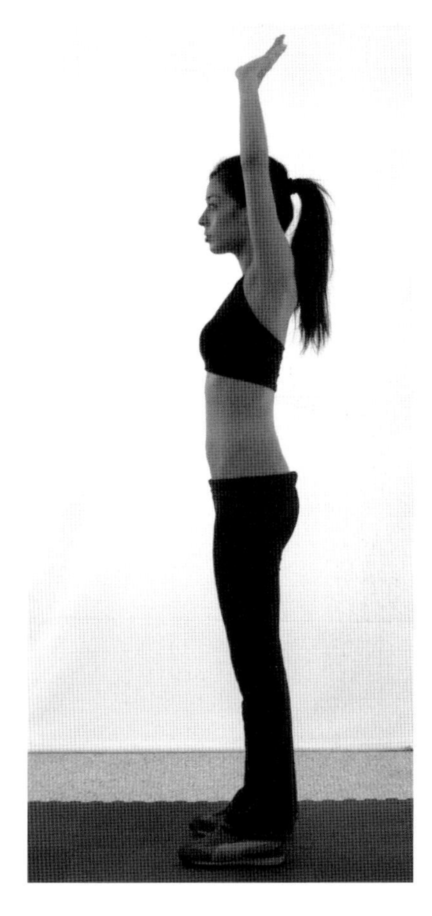

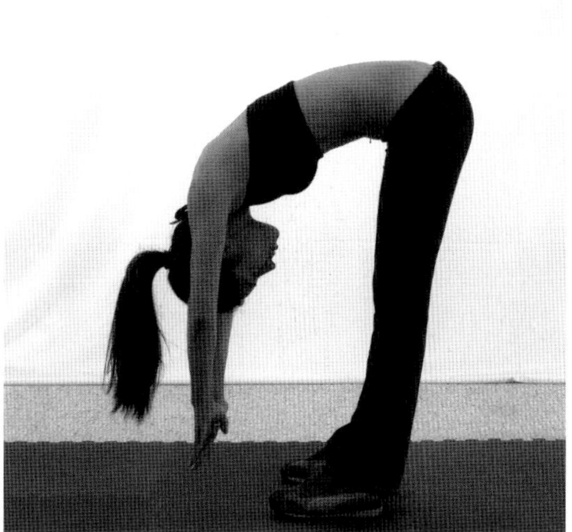

**Keep your feet shoulder-width apart and your hands above your head, thumbs interlocked. Then reach up, lengthening your spine and keeping your shoulders down, as you gently bend forward. Hold position and then return to the starting position or move dynamically into the next posture.**

**TRAINING TIPS**

- **Let your head hang down naturally.**
- **When you return to the starting position, activate your inner core and contract your buttocks as you come up.**
- **Exhale as you straighten to the starting position.**
- **Initiate the movement from your center.**

# STANDING SIDE BEND (NARROW STANCE)

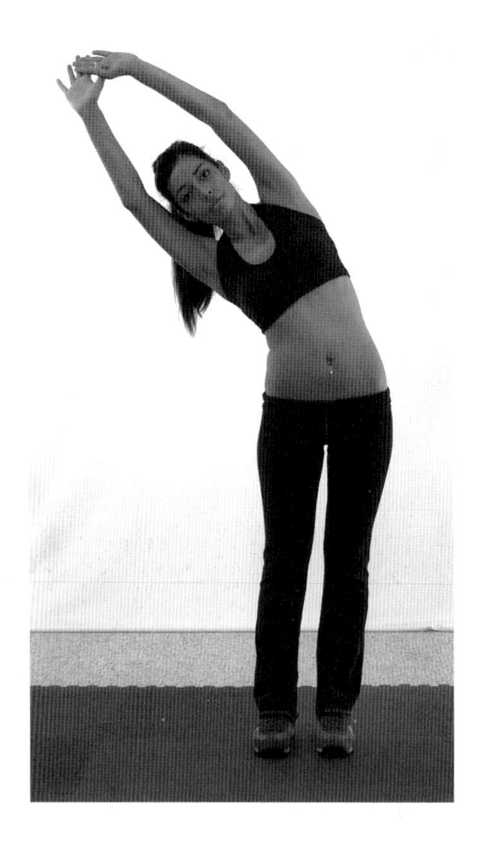

Keeping your feet hip-width apart, raise both hands above your head and interlock your thumbs. Then reach up, lengthening your spine, keeping your shoulders down, as you gently bend to the side, directly over your hip (3 and 9 on the core clock), making a C shape with your body. Hold position and then return to the starting position or move dynamically into the next posture. Repeat on the other side.

**TRAINING TIPS**

- Let your neck, head, and arms gently follow the bend of the stretch.
- Tighten your buttocks to protect your lower back.
- Breathe into the stretch.
- Initiate the movement from your center.

# STANDING SIDE BEND (WIDE STANCE)

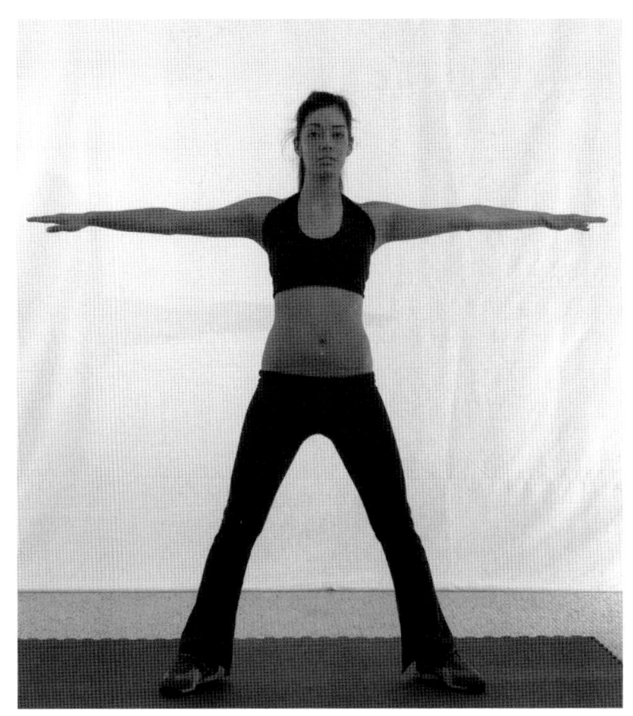

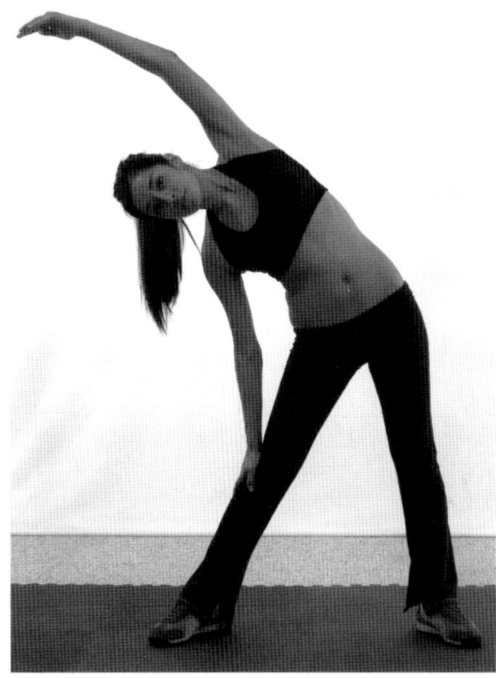

**Spread your feet wide and raise your arms to shoulder level. Then bend directly over your waist, bringing your left arm over your head, as you let your right hand slide down your leg. Hold position and then return to the starting position or move dynamically to the other side. Repeat on the other side.**

### TRAINING TIPS

- **Let your neck, head, and arms gently follow the bend of the stretch.**
- **Breathe into the stretch.**
- **Initiate the movement from your center.**

# STANDING FORWARD BEND WITH ROTATION (WIDE STANCE)

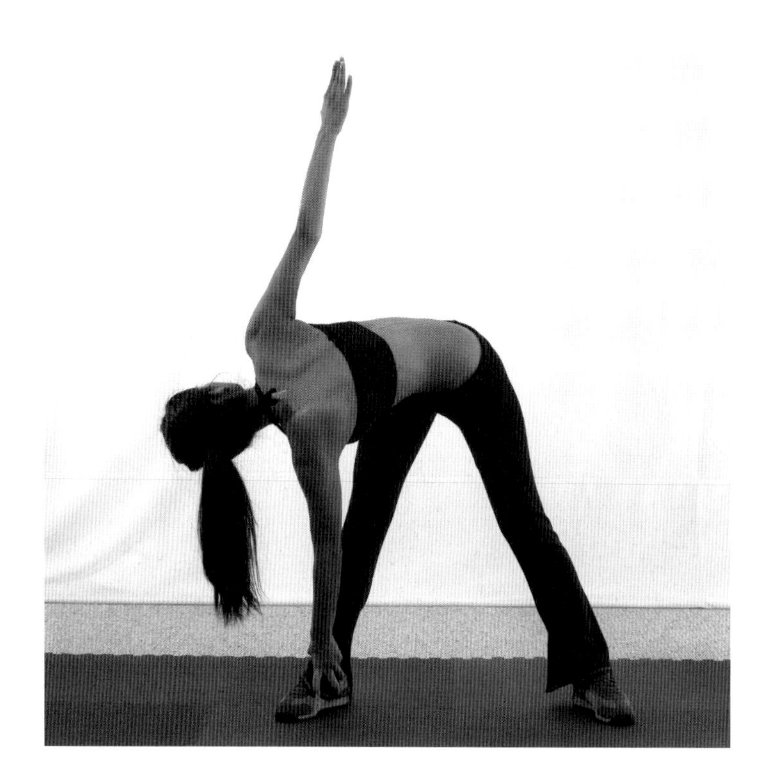

Keeping your feet spread wide and arms at shoulder level, bend forward and at an angle over your right leg, grasping the inside of your right ankle with your left hand as you raise your right arm straight up in the air. Look up at your right arm. Hold the position or move dynamically to the starting position. Repeat to the other side in a fluid motion.

**TRAINING TIPS**

- Gently rotate your spine into the twisting motion.
- Breathe into the stretch.
- Initiate the movement from your center.

SEQUENCE THREE

# KNEES-TO-CHEST HUG

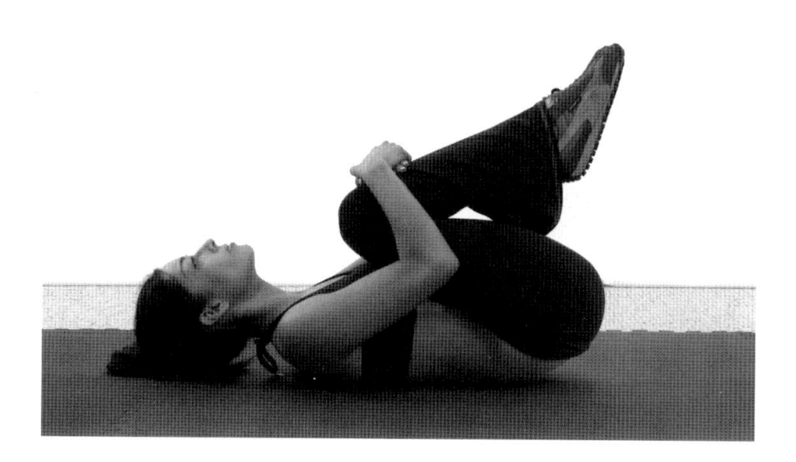

Lie on your back and bring both knees to your chest. From this position, grab your lower legs just below the knee, and gently hug your knees to your chest. Keep your neck lengthened. End the stretch by gently rocking back and forth 5 to 10 times.

## TRAINING TIPS

- Breathe into your lower back.
- Activate your inner core for the rocking.
- Initiate the movement from your center.

# KNEES-TO-SIDE

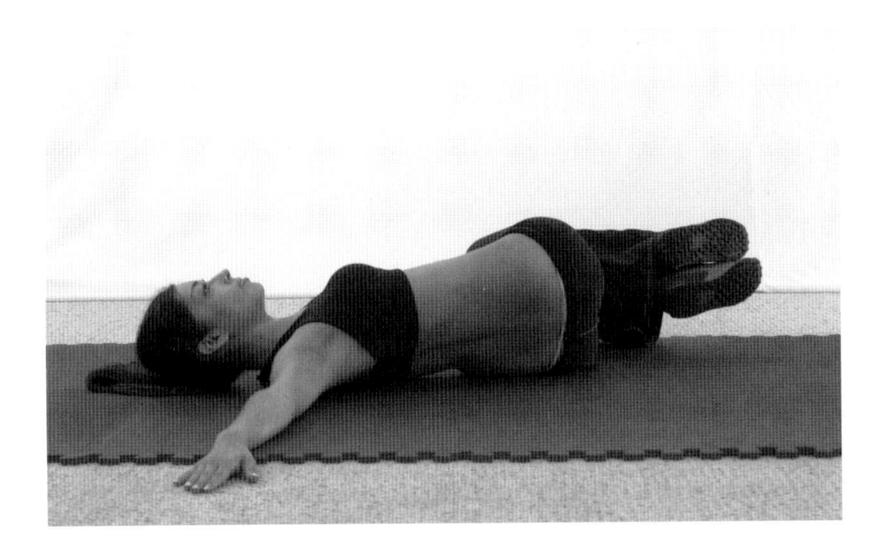

Lie on your back, knees bent, feet flat on the floor. Let both legs fall to one side. Then let the legs fall to the other side.

### TRAINING TIPS

- Let the rotation movement start from the center of your body.
- Work toward bringing your knees to a 90 degree angle with your upper body.
- Keep both shoulder blades on the ground.
- Initiate the movement from your center.

SEQUENCE FOUR

# HAMSTRING, HIP, AND GLUTE SERIES

Do the Hamstring Stretch, Swing Wide, and Across the Body stretches all with one leg, and then repeat the sequence with the other leg. After you're done with this series, complete the sequence with the glute stretch.

## HAMSTRING STRETCH

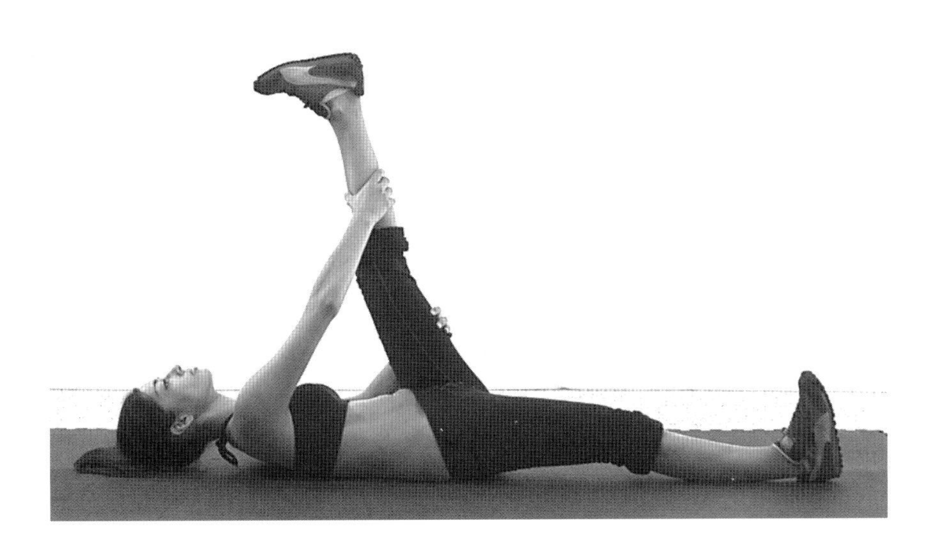

Lie on your back, legs extended. Raise your left leg and hold it just above and below your knee, pulling back as you straighten the leg. Gently pull it toward your head. If this is too difficult, bend your right leg. Hold stretch or move dynamically to the other leg.

### TRAINING TIPS

- Breathe into the stretch.
- Keep your leg straight and flex your toes.
- Focus on releasing your hamstring.

## SWING WIDE

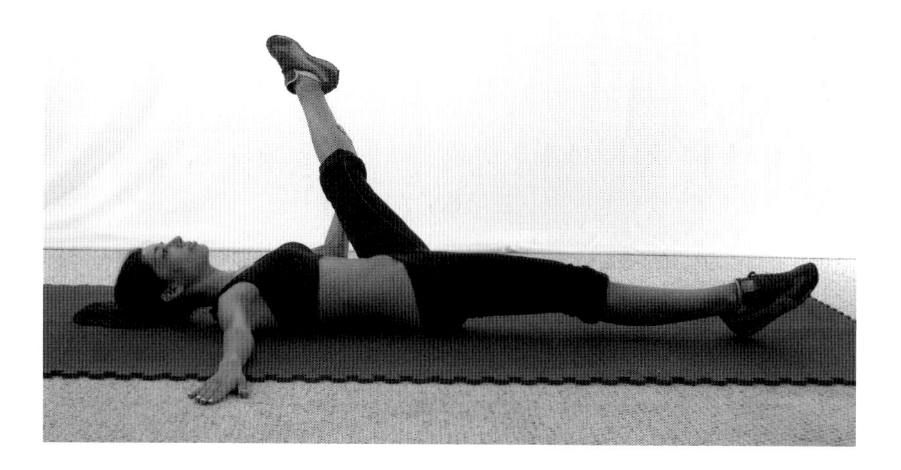

From the up position of the hamstring stretch, let your left leg swing out wide to the side, keeping both shoulder blades on the ground. Hold stretch or move dynamically into the next posture.

## ACROSS THE BODY

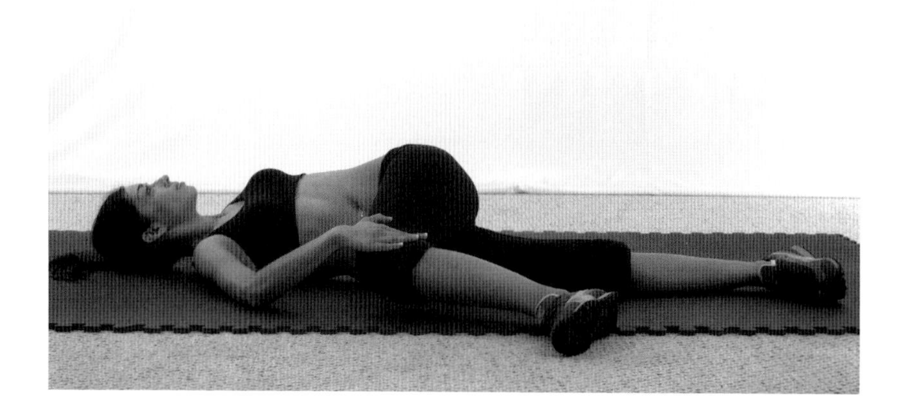

Bring your left leg across your body, letting your left arm rest extended straight out from your shoulder as your right hand assists lowering your left leg toward the floor. Bend your left leg at the knee once the leg is across your body. Hold stretch or move dynamically into the next posture. Repeat with the other leg.

# GLUTE STRETCH

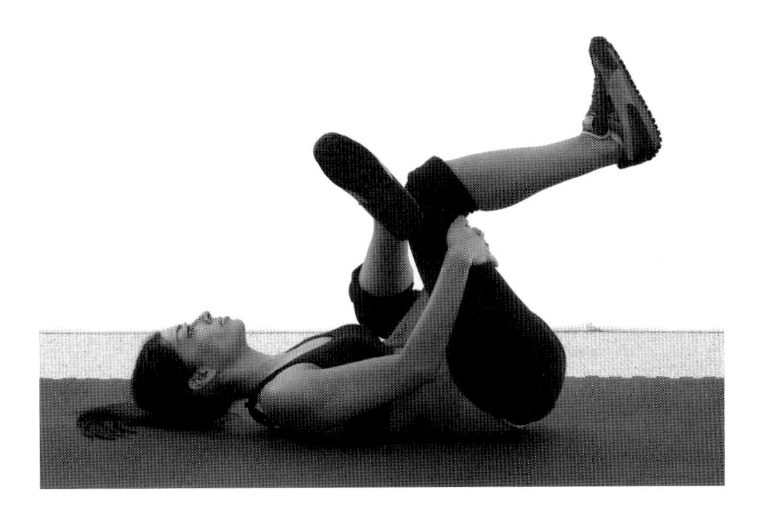

Lying on your back, bring both knees up so your thighs are perpendicular to your upper body. Then place your left ankle across just above your right knee, at the top of your thigh. Reach in between your legs and grab your right hamstring with both hands and pull the right leg toward your chest. Hold stretch or move dynamically into the next posture. Repeat on the other side.

# ON THE FLOOR: ON YOUR STOMACH

SEQUENCE FIVE

## BACK ARCH

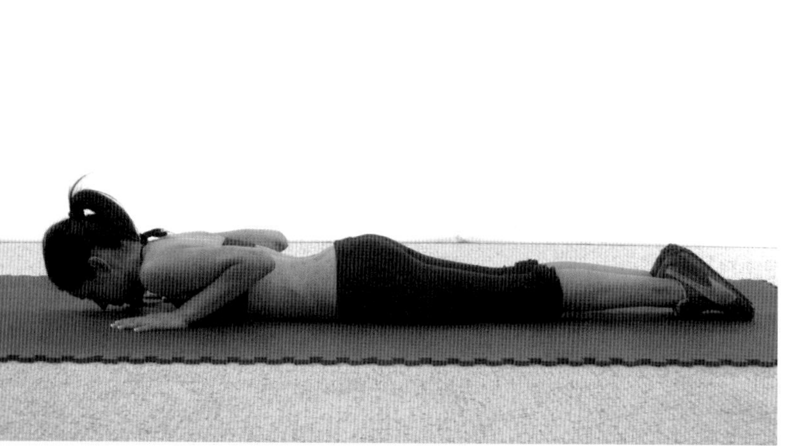

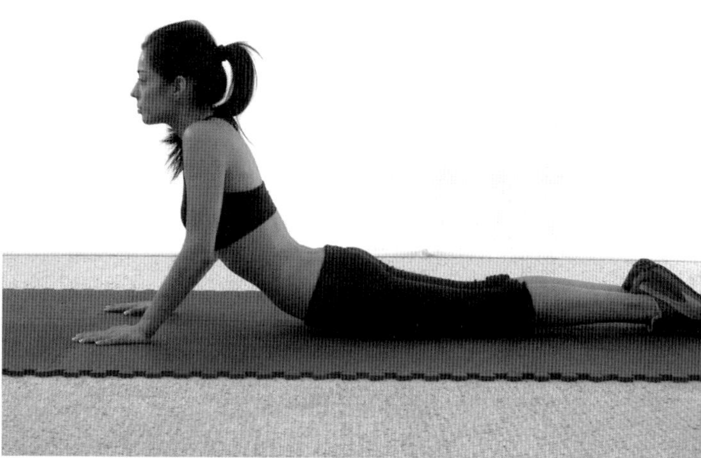

Lie on your stomach, hands under your shoulders (palms down). Slowly raise your torso off the floor, arching your back, using your arms to lightly assist the movement. Allow your back muscles to do most of the work, using the arms just to increase your range of motion. Hold stretch (or move dynamically), then slowly lower your torso back to the starting position.

TRAINING TIPS

- Let your neck and head follow the curve of your spine.
- Tighten your butt to protect your lower back.
- Initiate the movement from your center.

# PRONE QUADRICEPS STRETCH

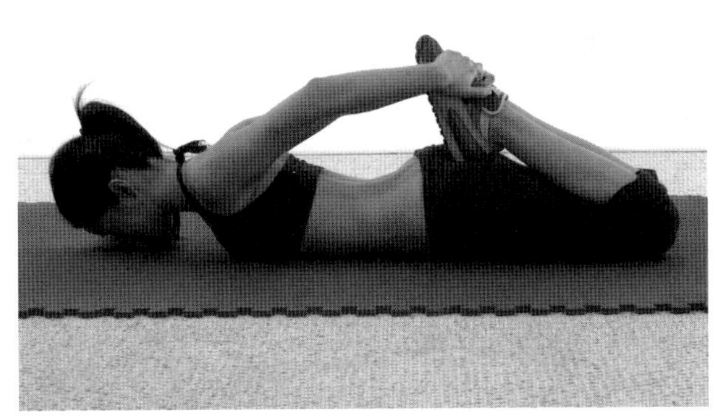

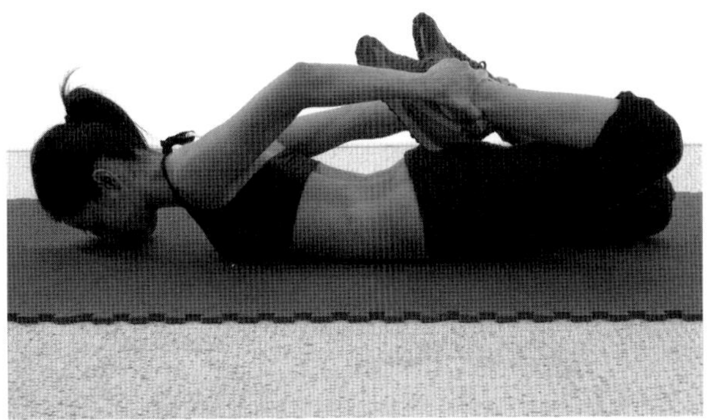

Reach back and grab both ankles, keeping your legs and feet together. Then gently pull your left knee off the floor. Hold stretch or move dynamically, repeating on the other leg.

### TRAINING TIPS

- Focus on your quadriceps.
- Breathe into the movement.
- Keep your upper body relaxed.

# ON ALL FOURS

SEQUENCE SIX

## CAT-COW

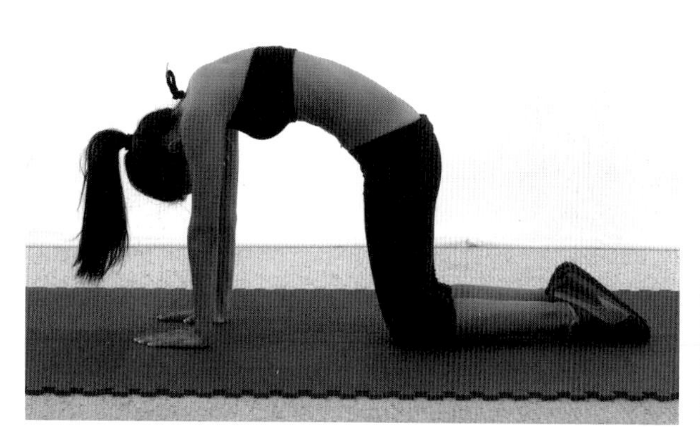

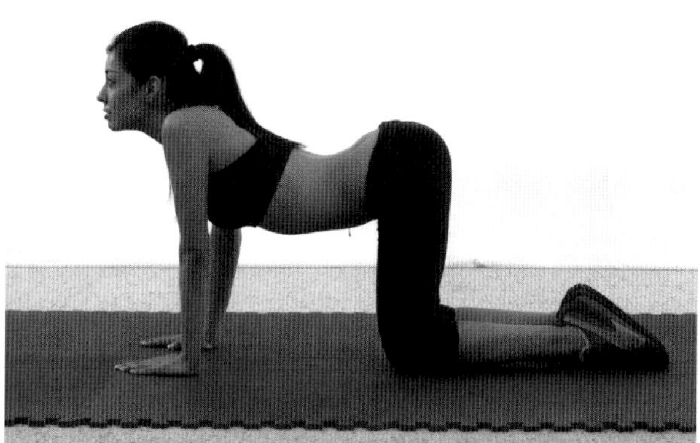

Begin on all fours with a flat back, your hands under your shoulders and your knees under your hips. Arch your back up like an angry cat, lowering your head to look between your legs.

Then arch your back in the opposite direction.

### TRAINING TIPS

- Initiate the movement from your center.
- Keep your arms aligned under your shoulders.
- Feel the movement in your spine.

# DEEP SQUAT TO STANDING

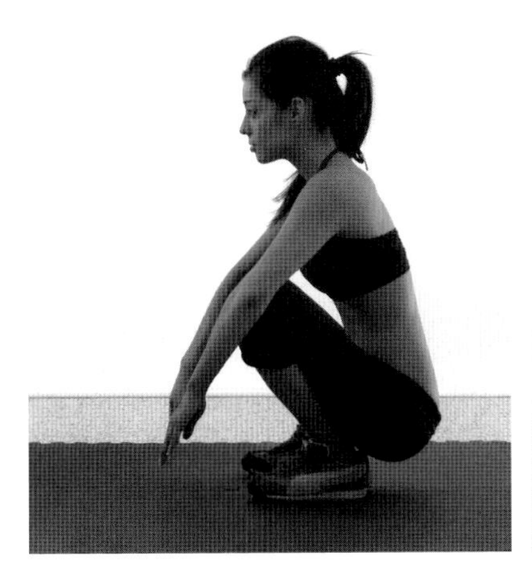
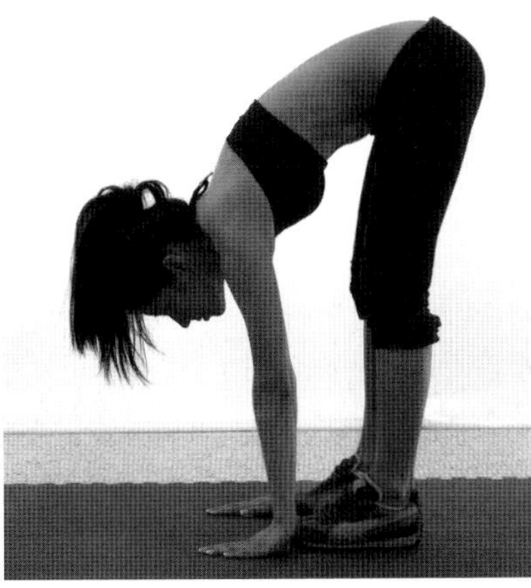
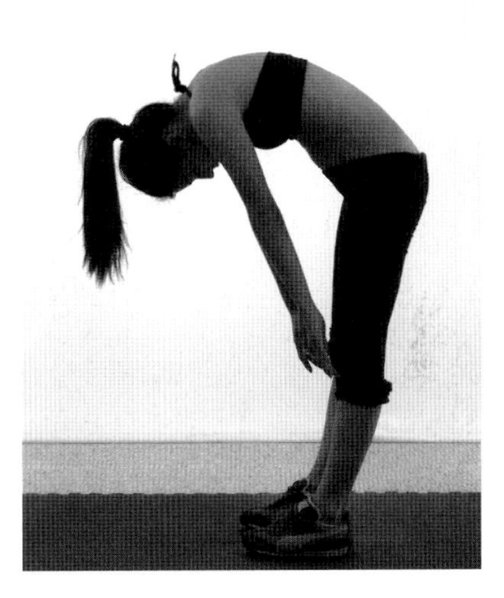

From all fours, push pack to a deep squat position. Pause for a stretch, then fully extend your legs, keeping your torso bent over. Lift your head up, then let it drop down relaxed. Pause for the stretch, then roll up vertebra on vertebra.

### TRAINING TIPS

- Initiate the movement from your center.
- Keep your weight on your heels during the squat stretch.
- Roll up slowly, feeling your vertebrae stack on top of each other like building blocks.

# 20

# CREATING YOUR OWN ROUTINE

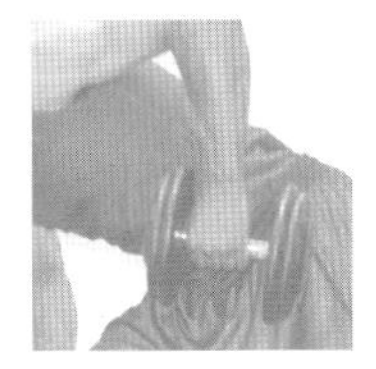

## THE DESIGN MODEL

This chapter will give you the tools you need to design your own core routine. When creating a core routine, you need a basic design model. A core routine has four design components you need to consider:

- Moving in all directions
- Isolation holds
- Inner core work
- Exercises for all the major muscles

The following template gives an easy fill-in-the-blank format.

**DESIGN ROUTINE TEMPLATE:** Your routine should contain at least one exercise for each of the five areas.

### UPPER BODY

1. Flexion move
2. Extension moves
3. Crossing and rotation moves

### LOWER BODY

4. Glute and hip move
5. Combo moves: moves that involve more than one area

### BUILDING A ROUTINE

To build a routine, you need to think about how you want to shape and strengthen your core area. This will depend on your individual needs and goals:

- **Weak areas**
- **The look you want to achieve**
- **Sports-specific goals, and so forth**

This can get tricky if you're training for a specific sport. You may need to emphasize certain moves for your sport. This does not mean, however, that you neglect training any area outlined in the design model. This would eventually lead to an imbalance.

The design template matches the way the exercises are categorized in the book, so you'll find it easy to plug in exercises and personalize your routine.

## BASIC CONCEPTS

The following principles will help you make smart design choices.

### BODY BALANCE

Your routine needs to work the important core muscles and train your body in all directions. If you have strong areas, keep training them but emphasize the weak areas, bringing them into balance. When one muscle or muscle group becomes considerably stronger than another, the potential for injury is greatly increased.

## EXERCISE ORDER

Train your weak areas first, when you are fresh. Also, shuffle the template order. For example, don't always work forward (flexion) and backward (extension) movements first.

## INTENSITY

The simplest way to think about intensity is, "How quickly do I reach failure in an exercise?" The faster you reach failure, the greater the intensity. Let's look at an example using the squat. On your first set, you do 20 reps with 40 pounds. On your second set, you do 5 reps with 100 pounds. This second set has greater intensity, using 100 pounds. You reach failure much quicker. There are three main ways to increase intensity:

- **Difficulty level of an exercise**
- **Amount of resistance or weights used in the exercise**
- **Increasing or decreasing the amount of rest time between exercises and sets**

## VOLUME

Volume is the combination of the total number of repetitions and sets. You don't want to increase volume and intensity at the same time. When you increase intensity, your volume needs to decrease, and vice versa. For example, you would not want to add a difficult exercise, like Supermans with Rotation, and increase your number of sets in your routines. Just add one challenging element at a time.

## VARIETY

Variety is the most neglected training principle. Training needs to be varied to:

- **Prevent overtraining through repetitive body use.**
- **Minimize training plateaus**
- **Alleviate the boredom and monotony**

When you first start working your core, it's easier to shock your muscles and cause positive adaptation. As you become more advanced, you will need to change your workouts more frequently.

The two basic ways to create variety and adaptation are intensity and volume. We discussed the three main factors for adjusting intensity. Now let's look for ways to increase volume. You add volume by:

- **Increasing the number of reps**
- **Increasing the number of sets**
- **Increasing the number of exercises**

Adjusting intensity and volume causes your body to adapt positively to the new stimuli.

### GUIDELINES FOR USING INTENSITY AND VOLUME

There are a number of ways to work with intensity and volume to add variety to your workouts. As a general rule of thumb, you want to employ these tools judiciously and you want your choices to fit your goals and training needs.

Here are some guidelines:

**ADD ONLY ONE VARIATION ELEMENT AT A TIME.** For example, don't *increase* weight on an exercise and *decrease* your rest time at the same time; this would be adding two intensity elements at once. By doing either one of these moves, you challenge your body to adapt and grow stronger. By adding both, you overstress your body and give away all your tricks at once. You want slow, steady progress, not burnout or injury.

**FIT YOUR CHOICES TO YOUR NEEDS.** If you are training for a sport that requires explosive movements with rest time between efforts, like golf, then you don't need to do a lot of high-volume work. This doesn't mean you don't do any high-volume work, but you emphasize explosive rotational movements.

**TRAIN FOR A VARIETY OF ENERGY SYSTEMS.** You need to train your full range of energy systems, from explosive to endurance. This means mixing your workouts between high-intensity days, medium-intensity days, and high-volume days. Variety should always be focused to serve your goals, not added simply for its own sake. With all of these energy systems you work to a breakdown in technique. The only difference is that on high-intensity days you reach this breakdown faster than on high-volume days. Here is a general repetition scheme for the different energy systems:

- **Explosive: 1 to 5 reps**
- **Medium: 5 to 10 reps**
- **Endurance: 10 to 30 reps (and beyond)**

## PERIODIZATION

Periodization is a systematic and progressive training method designed to aid planning and organization. This training philosophy helps you organize and customize your goals. It is used by the greatest athletes and by the world's top strength coaches. The following is a practical primer that you can apply when you are creating your routine and setting goals.

The basis for periodization was the General Adaptation Syndrome (GAS), developed during the 1930s. It was intended to describe a person's ability to adapt to stress. The three distinct phases of adaptation, according to GAS, are the following.

**ALARM STAGE:** This relates to the individual's initial response to training. This could result in a temporary drop in performance because of stiffness and soreness.

**ADAPTATION STAGE:** This is your target stage, when you positively adapt to the training stimulus by making gains in strength, endurance, and appearance.

**OVERTRAINING STAGE:** This occurs when you place too much stress on the body. It means you are overtraining. The following can happen:

- **Decreased performance level**
- **Chronic fatigue**
- **Loss of appetite**
- **Loss of body weight or lean body mass**
- **Increased illness potential**
- **Increased injury potential**
- **Decreased motivation and low self-esteem**

During this stage, the desired training adaptations will not occur. Outside stresses—for example, social life, nutrition, amount of sleep, work, and so forth—also need to be considered to avoid overtraining.

The goal is to remain in the resistance stage of training, where your body is positively adapting to the stress by making fitness gains. Helping you stay in this stage is the goal of periodization.

## THINKING IN CYCLES

After you have defined your goal, the next step is planning. The planning process can be divided into four training phases. Before going into these cycles, you will need a definition of the peaking period, which is the goal of all these cycles. These cycles are a precise, fitness-oriented look at goal setting.

## THE PEAKING PERIOD

This is the period in which all your training culminates, bringing out peak results. This will, of course, be different for everybody, depending on individual goals.

## MACROCYCLE

The macrocycle is the longest of the training phases. Its length depends on your goals. In general, the macrocycle lasts from the beginning of one peaking period through the transition period. The macrocycle defines long-term goals and a specific time frame in which you want to peak: six weeks, six months, or one year. The macrocycle contains four components: mesocycles, microcylces, peaking, and transition.

### MESOCYCLE

The next-largest phase is the mesocycle. Mesocycles make up a macrocycle. The number, length, and purpose of your mesocycles will depend on the goals of your macrocycle. Each mesocycle has specific goals. If you were on a four-month macrocycle, each mesocycle might last one month. The first month's mesocycle may be that of preparation, which might include high volume and fairly low-intensity training to build a base of strength. The second month's mesocycles might include an increase in intensity (more difficult exercises, shorter rest periods, and so forth) while maintaining volume requirements to build endurance. The third month's mesocycle might be geared toward high-intensity strength gains.

The fourth and final mesocycle, moving toward your peaking period, might require more intensive evaluation:

- **What areas are weak and need extra work**
- **What areas are strong**
- **What has worked best in the past**
- **Nutrition, and so forth**

### MICROCYCLE

Within each mesocycle are smaller units, called "microcycles." Microcycles further refine the objectives by manipulating training variables on a weekly and daily basis. One day you might train at high volume (lots of reps), while the next day you might train at a high intensity (fewer reps). This leads to the peaking phase, the goal of the macrocycle, which we defined earlier.

### TRANSITION

Unfortunately, maintaining peak anything for a long period of time is impossible. A transition phase needs to follow a peaking period. This allows for regeneration and recuperation, both mentally and physically. The transition phase allows you to move to a higher training level in the next macrocycle. Without a transition phase, the rigors of peaking will ultimately lead to overtraining. The body needs time off after a peaking phase. The transition phase allows you jump right back to a growth phase in your next macrocycle.

Recuperation doesn't mean you become a couch potato. You continue to train, but at lower volumes and intensities. This could be something as simple as taking four or five days off, then cutting back on your training days for a few weeks. This is also a good time to explore a new class or fitness interest, take a break from your normal routine, and have fun!

## USING THE DESIGN MODEL

Using the design model beginning on page 145 in this chapter, you can choose exercises from the book to create your own customized routine. Then, following the natural cycles of periodization, you can create a series of progressive routines to achieve your goals.

## A CASE EXAMPLE: SKI VACATION

Let's say your goal is to get into peak shape for a ski vacation in Aspen. You want a strong core for skiing and you want to look great in a swimsuit for the hot tub. You have three months to get in shape. This three-month time frame is your macrocycle.

You would break this down into one-month mesocycles with two-week microcycles for the first two months and one-week microcycles for the last month, as you prepare to peak.

Let's create a structure for your routine. The specifics would depend on your fitness level and your personal goals.

**FIRST MONTH:** This would be your preparation period. Build a safe foundation doing low-intensity exercises with high reps. During your two microcycles, gradually decrease your rest time.

**SECOND MONTH:** This mesocycle is broken down into two microcycles. During your first two-week microcycle a new exercise is added to each area. In the second microcyle, you would replace certain exercises with more difficult exercises.

**THIRD MONTH:** During this mesocycle, change your workouts more often, going to one-week microcycles. Your schedule might look like this:

- **Week One: High repetition with no rest time (up to 20 reps for each exercise)**
- **Week Two: Heavy resistance that allows you to do between 4 and 8 reps. This may vary with different exercises.**
- **Week Three: Mixing high- and low-intensity days**
- **Week Four: Increase your training volume and/or intensity daily. Add an extra training day to your schedule.**

Also, during this week all other facets of your training must peak (diet, cardio, and strength training).

These training principles and this design model will allow you to customize your routines. The applications of these principles will lead to ultimate success and longevity in training.

PART SIX

# THE ROUTINES

# 21
# INTRODUCTION TO THE ROUTINES

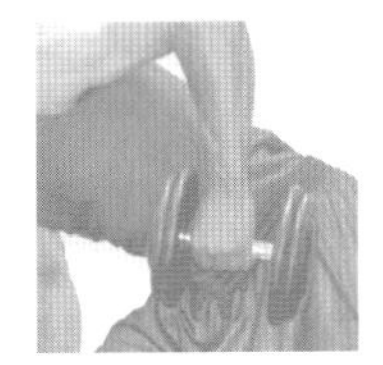

## THE ROUTINES

The routines in this book do all the workout planning for you. The following guidelines will help you get the best results.

One of the most important training principles is variety. You can't just stick with one routine forever, but you can always come back to a favorite routine after you've spent some time away. The important thing is to switch up your routines to keep your body and mind from getting bored. Chapter 20, "Creating Your Own Routine," gives you options and tools to customize a routine to fit your unique needs.

The routines in this section will give you a variety of choices. Here are some general training guidelines to help you negotiate these routines.

- **Don't stress out if you miss a workout during the week; you haven't destroyed the whole program. Just get back in pace with the program. Remember, the key is consistency over the long haul.**
- **Think maintenance when things get hectic. The goal of any maintenance program is to keep the gains you've worked to achieve. You could work out just twice a week, or go to an easier program that is less time consuming. The key is not to stop completely. Doing a little will go a long way toward maintaining your gains.**
- **Think variety when you get bored. Choose a new routine, or create your own routine.**
- **Add resistance to your routine: ankle weights, medicine balls, resistance bands, and so forth.**

# 22
# CORE ROUTINES

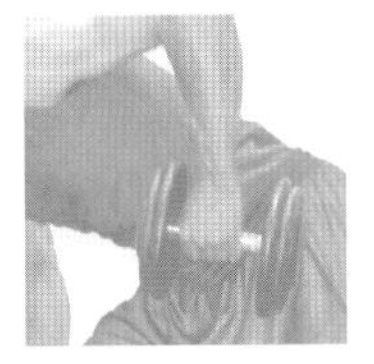

## DYNAMIC WARM-UP: A BEGINNER'S ROUTINE

The following dynamic warm-up will prepare your body to move in all directions. It will also improve your balance and agility. This is a beginner's routine and is a good introduction. Like any fitness workout, you can make it more complex and challenging.

During this workout you will be using the concept of the core clock. Imagine that you are standing in the center of an imaginary clock: Twelve o'clock is in front of you and 6 is behind you. Directly to your right is the 3 and to your left is 9.

1. Marching: 30 seconds. March in place. After the first 10 seconds, try to bring your knees up to waist level.
2. Heel to Butt: 30 seconds. Moving in place, bring your heels up, trying to touch your butt.
3. March with Cross: 30 seconds. Marching in place, add a twisting or crossing motion to your movement. As you raise your right knee, bring it across your body, simultaneously pumping your left arm across your body.
4. First Step Series: 45 seconds. From the ready position, imagine you are standing in the center of the core clock. Move with one quick step alternating your right, then left leg in the following directions on the clock (after each step move back to the starting position at the center of the clock): 12 o'clock, 6 o'clock, 3 o'clock, 9 o'clock, between 10 and 11 o'clock, between 1 and 2 o'clock, between 7 and 8 o'clock, and between 4 and 5 o'clock.
5. Twisties: 15 seconds. From the ready position, imagine you are standing in the center of the core clock. Then start to twist your lower body so your feet point toward the 3, then the 9. This movement is a combination of twisting and jumping with the emphasis on the twisting motion. Each time you twist both feet leave the ground.
6. Over Unders: 30 seconds. Moving along the line that connects 3 and 9 on the core clock, move to the left, crossing your right leg over (in front of) your left, and then move back to the starting position. Move your right leg behind the left leg and back to the starting position. Repeat the same motion, using your left leg. Keep alternating sides.
7. Lateral Drop Touches: 30 seconds. Moving along the line that connects 3 and 9 on the core clock, move to the left, crossing your right leg over (in front of) your left, as you lower your body toward the floor, reaching across your torso with your right hand, touching the ground outside and in front of your right foot.
8. Jumping Jacks: 30 seconds. Starting with your feet together and hands at your sides, simultaneously spread your legs and raise your arms above your head along the line that connects 3 and 9. Return to the starting position and repeat.
9. Jumping Jills: 30 seconds. Starting with your feet together and hands at your sides, simultaneously move your legs and arms forward and backward along the line that connects 6 and 12 on the core clock. Alternate legs and arms with each repetition. This exercise is just like a jumping jack, except the movement is forward and backward instead of side to side.
10. Windmills: 30 seconds. Stand with your legs spread wide and your arms extended straight out to your sides at shoulder level. With your right hand, reach across your body

and down toward your left foot, touch your toes if you can. Return to the starting position and repeat to the other side.

## PRE-CORE ROUTINE

This routine is designed for the first-time exerciser. Its purpose is to ease you into Level One of the Complete Core Workout. When you can achieve the prescribed repetition goals three times in a row, advance to Level One of the Complete Core Workout.

## THE ROUTINE

1. Standing Bicycles: 10 reps each side, p. 334
2. Knee Touch—Crossing: 10 reps each side, p. 226
3. Heel Touch: 10 reps each side, p. 257–59
4. Leg Over: Bent-Knee Single Leg: 10 reps each side, p. 260
5. Side Leg Raise: All Fours: 10 reps each side, p. 278
6. Opposite Arm/Opposite Leg: All Fours: 10 reps each side, p. 247
7. Tummy Tucks: 10 reps, p. 302
8. Plank: All Positions: Hold each position for five seconds, p. 314

    **Down Plank**

    **Side Planks**

    **Up Plank**

# ON THE BALL CORE: BEGINNER

**INTRODUCTION:** This is the first level of a three-part program designed to introduce you to ball work. This routine will give you a foundation of strength in your inner core, help you gain confidence on the ball, and improve you balance on the ball.

## TRAINING TIPS FOR BALL WORK

- **Exercise balls should be purchased according to your body height. The manufacturer will give you guidelines.**
- **Inflate to the point where it becomes firm, but not hard.**
- **When sitting on the ball, your hips and knees should be bent at approximately 90 degrees.**
- **If you have any medical condition or if you are pregnant, please consult your doctor before doing exercises.**
- **Start slowly. Ball work requires more strength, balance, and coordination than you realize.**
- **Never combine bouncing with bending and twisting of the spine.**
- **Wear gym shoes to prevent your feet from slipping.**
- **Have a clear, safe space surrounding the ball and your workout area.**

## THE EXERCISES

1. OTB: Knee Raise, p. 336
2. OTB: Side-to-Side Tilt, p. 337
3. OTB: Forward and Backward Tilt, p. 311
4. OTB: Reverse Hyperextension, p. 284
5. OTB: Back Extension, p. 254
6. OTB: Russian Twists, p. 267

**PRESCRIPTION:** Work up to 20 repetitions on each exercise. For exercises where you alternate sides, do 10 reps on each side.

# ON THE BALL CORE: INTERMEDIATE

**INTRODUCTION:** This is the second level of a three-part program. This routine introduces you to a more advanced series of moves to challenge your core area.

## THE EXERCISES

1. OTB: 45 degree Leg Extension, p. 308
2. OTB: Glute Bridge, p. 283
3. OTB: Reverse Glute Bridge, p. 289
4. OTB: Roll Out, p. 241
5. OTB: Roll In, p. 240
6. OTB: Back Extension (feet against wall), p. 254
7. OTB: Glute Bridge with Hip Rotation, p. 274
8. OTB: Torso Corkscrew, p. 309

**PRESCRIPTION:** Work up to 20 repetitions on each exercise. For exercises where you alternate sides, do 10 reps on each side.

# ON THE BALL CORE: ADVANCED

**INTRODUCTION:** This is the third level of a three-part program. This routine introduces you to advanced variations of moves you learned in level two, plus a couple of new moves.

### THE EXERCISES

1. OTB: 45 degree Leg Extension, p. 308
2. OTB: Glute Bridge, Single Leg, p. 294
3. OTB: Reverse Glute Bridge, p. 289
4. OTB: Roll Out with a Cross, p. 321
5. OTB: Roll In with a Cross, p. 320
6. OTB: Back Extension with Rotation (feet against wall), p. 335
7. OTB Glute Bridge with Hip Rotation with ankle weights, p. 274
8. OTB: Plank Twist, p. 268
9. OTB: Straight Leg Bridging, p. 285
10. OTB: Plank—Hands on Ball, p. 317

**PRESCRIPTION:** Work up to 20 repetitions on each exercise. For exercises where you alternate sides, do 10 reps on each side.

## GOING DEEPER: THE INNER CORE ROUTINE

# INTRODUCTION

Getting in touch with your inner core is not easy—it's a deep muscle that you normally don't isolate. You're used to working and isolating the bigger external muscles, like the six-pack muscle or the biceps. This routine will take you through this process one step at a time, until inner core activation is second nature.

This sounds complicated and in a way it is. On the other hand, it's not. Your body is made to function this way. Your transverse abdominis muscle is a postural muscle, which means that it's made up of endurance fibers designed to hold contractions to keep you upright and supported throughout the day. Your body wants to work this way. The inner core is designed to fire a millisecond before you move to give you that support. Core work trains these often neglected muscles, making them stronger, increasing their endurance, and improving their functionality.

Often, clients overtrain their big external muscles. This is especially true of the six-pack muscle. Everyone wants great abs, so they overwork them. Overtraining one area creates an imbalance in the body. The stronger muscles can become dominant, taking over. When this happens, other muscles begin to suffer from disuse. These smaller muscles begin to atrophy. This causes a functional imbalance. A body that is out of balance, that lacks good teamwork, cannot function with peak efficiency and is vulnerable to injury. Also, if you've ever suffered from lower back pain, your body may not be firing in an efficient and optimal pattern. This work will retrain your muscles for balance and the correct firing order. The goal of core training and all this work on the inner core is to create a balanced body that is working as it is designed to work.

## ACTIVATING YOUR INNER CORE

The following tips are important for all the exercises in this routine:

- **When you are lying on your back, use a pillow, towel, or foam roller to support your head so you can observe your belly.**
- **Place a towel or light medicine ball between your knees. Squeezing your knees together will activate your adductor muscles, which will help activate the pelvic floor, hence the transverse abdominis. You can also place something between your knees when you are on all fours.**
- **Remember, contract your inner core at level 3 intensity.**

- Ultimately, you want to break your dependence on squeezing an object between your legs as in the above guideline. So gradually phase out this prop.
- In any position, you can place your hand on your belly to get some direct sensory feedback. But don't get dependent on this touchy-feely method—it can become a crutch. Your hands need to be free to play.
- The goal of this progression of exercises is to integrate inner core activation independent of breath and movement, so it naturally supports your movements.

## INNER CORE ACTIVATION: PHASE ONE

The first step in this process is to isolate your transverse abdominis so you can strengthen and improve the muscle's endurance. Practice this activation in five different positions.

# INNER CORE ACTIVATION: LYING ON YOUR BACK

**STARTING POSITION:** Lie on your back, knees bent, feet flat on the floor, and hands at your sides. Place a small weight plate (2½ pounds), a teacup and saucer, or any small light object on top of your belly button. Relax your rectus abdominis (your six-pack muscle).

**THE MOVEMENT:** Use your transverse abdominis muscle to lower your belly button toward your spine, so the object sinks downward. Hold the contraction for the prescribed amount of time, then release. Repeat.

### TRAINING TIPS

- Do this while maintaining a neutral spine. In other words, don't let your powerful six-pack muscle tilt your pelvis backward, moving your lower back toward the floor.
- Focus your mind on a point one to two inches below your belly button.
- Breathe naturally and don't hold your breath during the inner core contraction.
- Your stomach may slightly expand on the inhale and hollow out more on the exhale.

### REPETITION GUIDELINES

REPS: **5 REPETITIONS**

**HOLD:** Hold each repetition for 3 breaths.

## INNER CORE ACTIVATION: ALL FOURS

**STARTING POSITION:** Get in an all-fours position, hands under your shoulders, your knees under your hips, and your back flat.

**THE MOVEMENT:** Let your abdomen drop toward the floor, then use your transverse abdominis to pull your belly button toward your spine.

### TRAINING TIPS

- Don't arch or round your back; keep it level as you draw your belly button toward your spine.
- Focus your mind on a point one to two inches below your belly button.
- Your stomach may slightly expand on the inhale and hollow out more on the exhale.
- Breathe naturally and don't hold your breath during the inner core contraction.

### REPETITION GUIDELINES

REPS: **5 REPETITIONS**

**HOLD:** Hold each repetition for 3 breaths.

## INNER CORE ACTIVATION: LYING ON BELLY

**STARTING POSITION:** Lying facedown, place a tennis ball or rolled towel under your belly button.

**THE MOVEMENT:** Use your transverse abdominis to lift your belly button off the ball or towel and up toward your spine.

### TRAINING TIPS

- Try to breathe into the back of your ribs.
- Focus your mind on a point one to two inches below your belly button.
- Breathe naturally and don't hold your breath during the inner core contraction.

### REPETITION GUIDELINES

REPS: **5 REPETITIONS**

**HOLD:** Hold each repetition for 3 breaths.

## INNER CORE ACTIVATION: STANDING WITH HANDS ABOVE HEAD

**STARTING POSITION:** Stand in your ready position, raise your arms above your head.

**THE MOVEMENT:** Use your transverse abdominis to bring your belly button toward your spine. Hold the contraction for the prescribed time, then release. Repeat the action.

### TRAINING TIPS

- Focus your mind on a point one to two inches below your belly button.
- Breathe naturally and don't hold your breath during the inner core contraction.

### REPETITION GUIDELINES

REPS: **5 REPETITIONS**

**HOLD:** Hold each repetition for 3 breaths.

## INNER CORE ACTIVATION: STANDING

**STARTING POSITION:** Stand in the ready position.

**THE MOVEMENT:** Use your transverse abdominis to bring your belly button toward your spine. Hold the contraction for the prescribed time, then release. Repeat the action.

### TRAINING TIPS

- Focus your mind on a point one to two inches below your belly button.
- Breathe naturally and don't hold your breath during the inner core contraction.

### REPETITION GUIDELINES

REPS: **5 REPETITIONS**

**HOLD:** Hold each repetition for 3 breaths.

## INNER CORE ACTIVATION: PHASE TWO: ADDING MOVEMENT

Now you're ready to add movement to inner core activation. This is like juggling—you're adding another ball. The first phase had two main goals:

- **To integrate inner core activation with movement.**
- **To strengthen and increase the endurance of the transverse abdominis**

Now add movement. In the following exercises, simple movements are added to the process. The goal is to integrate inner core activation, movement, and breath. Inner core activation needs to happen independent of your breathing. It is a constant, like wearing a weight belt. If you were getting ready to squat, you would activate your inner core and maintain the contraction as you do your entire set of squats. Your breathing would follow a pattern that would support your squatting motion, inhaling as you bend your knees and exhaling as you extend your legs back to standing. You breathe to support the movement; breathing fuels the movement. Breath and inner core support are there throughout to support the movement. An activated inner core brings stability and deep support to movement.

# INNER CORE ACTIVATION: LYING ON BACK WITH ARM MOVEMENT

**STARTING POSITION:** Lie on your back, knees bent, feet flat on the floor, and hands at your sides. Relax your rectus abdominis (your six-pack muscle).

**THE MOVEMENT:** Use your transverse abdominis muscle to lower your belly button toward your spine, then raise and lower your arms from your waist to above your head for the prescribed number of repetitions.

### TRAINING TIPS

- Do this while maintaining a neutral spine. In other words, don't let your powerful six-pack muscle tilt your pelvis backward, moving your lower back toward the floor.
- Focus your mind on a point one to two inches below your belly button.
- Breathe naturally and don't hold your breath during the inner core contraction.

### REPETITION GUIDELINES

REPS: **WORK UP TO 12 REPS.**

# INNER CORE ACTIVATION: LYING ON BACK WITH LEG MOVEMENT

**STARTING POSITION:** Lie on your back, knees bent, feet flat on the floor, and hands at your sides. Relax your rectus abdominis (your six-pack muscle).

**THE MOVEMENT:** Use your transverse abdominis muscle to lower your belly button toward your spine, then raise your right leg, bringing your thigh perpendicular to your upper body. Then lower it back to the floor and raise your left leg. Alternate for the prescribed number of repetitions. Next Step: Raise both legs to perpendicular and then lower. Repeat for the prescribed number of repetitions.

### TRAINING TIPS

- Do this while maintaining a neutral spine. In other words, don't let your powerful six-pack muscle tilt your pelvis backward, moving your lower back toward the floor.
- Focus your mind on a point one to two inches below your belly button.
- Breathe naturally and don't hold your breath during the inner core contraction.

### REPETITION GUIDELINES

REPS: **WORK UP TO 12 REPS WITH EACH LEG. THEN 12 REPS WITH BOTH LEGS.**

# INNER CORE ACTIVATION: LYING ON BACK WITH ARM AND LEG MOVEMENT

**STARTING POSITION:** Lie on your back, knees bent, feet flat on the floor, and hands above your head. Relax your rectus abdominis (your six-pack muscle).

**THE MOVEMENT:** Use your transverse abdominis muscle to lower your belly button toward your spine, then raise your right leg, bringing your thigh perpendicular to your upper body, while simultaneously raising your left arm even with your chin. Then, at the same time, lower your arm and leg back to the starting position. Alternate sides for the prescribed number of repetitions.

### TRAINING TIPS

- Do this while maintaining a neutral spine. In other words, don't let your powerful six-pack muscle tilt your pelvis backward, moving your lower back toward the floor.
- Focus your mind on a point one to two inches below your belly button.
- Breathe naturally and don't hold your breath during the inner core contraction.

### REPETITION GUIDELINES

REPS: **WORK UP TO 10 REPS ON EACH SIDE.**

# INNER CORE ACTIVATION: ALL FOURS WITH ARM MOVEMENT

**STARTING POSITION:** Get in an all-fours position, hands under your shoulders, knees under your hips, and back flat (level, not rounded or arched), head in neutral.

**THE MOVEMENT:** Use your transverse abdominis to pull your belly button toward your spine, then extend your right arm out. Hold for the prescribed count, then return to the starting position. Repeat the movement with the other arm.

### TRAINING TIPS

- Don't arch your back; keep it level as you draw your belly button toward your spine.
- Focus your mind on a point one to two inches below your belly button.
- Maintain inner core activation as you integrate movement and breathing.
- Breathe naturally and don't hold your breath during the inner core contraction.

### REPETITION GUIDELINES

REPS: **10 WITH EACH ARM**

**HOLD:** Pause for 2 seconds when arm is extended.

# INNER CORE ACTIVATION: ALL FOURS WITH ARM AND LEG MOVEMENT

**STARTING POSITION:** Get in an all-fours position, hands under your shoulders, knees under your hips, and back flat (level, not rounded or arched).

**THE MOVEMENT:** Use your transverse abdominis to pull your belly button toward your spine, then simultaneously extend your right arm out and your left leg up and out. Hold for the prescribed count, then return to the original position. Repeat the movement with the other arm and leg.

### TRAINING TIPS

- Don't arch your back; keep it level as you draw your belly button toward your spine.
- Focus your mind on a point one to two inches below your belly button.
- Maintain inner core activation as you integrate movement and breathing.
- Breathe naturally and don't hold your breath during the inner core contraction.

### REPETITION GUIDELINES

REPS: **10 WITH EACH ARM**

**HOLD:** Pause for 2 seconds when arm and leg are extended.

## INNER CORE ACTIVATION: STANDING WITH ARM MOVEMENT

**STARTING POSITION:** Stand in the ready position.

**THE MOVEMENT:** Use your transverse abdominis to bring your belly button toward your spine. Hold the contraction as you raise and lower your arms from your waist to above your head for the prescribed number of repetitions.

### TRAINING TIPS

- Focus your mind on a point one to two inches below your belly button.
- Breathe naturally, inhaling and exhaling as you move your arms. Try different breathing patterns: inhale as you raise up and exhale as you lower, then the opposite, exhale as you raise and inhale as you lower.
- Maintain inner core activation as you integrate movement and breathing.
- Breathe naturally and don't hold your breath during the inner core contraction.

### REPETITION GUIDELINES

REPS: **10 REPETITIONS**

# INNER CORE ACTIVATION: BALANCE BEND

**STARTING POSITION:** Stand in the ready position

**THE MOVEMENT:** Bring your belly button toward your spine, then bend your torso to the side directly over your right hip, as you simultaneously, in a controlled motion, swing your left leg laterally out to the side. Your leg should swing out approximately one foot.

### TRAINING TIPS

- Focus your mind on a point one to two inches below your belly button.
- Breathe naturally, inhaling as you bend and exhaling as you straighten back to the starting position.
- Maintain inner core activation as you integrate movement and breathing.
- Breathe naturally and don't hold your breath during the inner core contraction.

### REPETITION GUIDELINES

REPS: **5 REPS ON EACH SIDE**

**HOLD:** Hold the finish position for 2 seconds.

# INNER CORE ACTIVATION: STANDING KNEE RAISE

**STARTING POSITION:** Stand in the ready position.

**THE MOVEMENT:** Use your transverse abdominis to bring your belly button toward your spine, activating your inner core; then bend and raise your right knee so your thigh makes a 90 degree angle with your upper body. Lower the leg back to the floor and repeat. Hold the inner core activation as you raise and lower your leg for the prescribed number of repetitions, then switch legs.

**VARIATION:** Alternate legs, as if you were walking in place.

## TRAINING TIPS

- Focus your mind on a point one to two inches below your belly button.
- Breathe naturally, inhaling and exhaling as you move your arms. Try different breathing patterns: inhale as you raise up and exhale as you lower, then the opposite, exhale as you raise and inhale as you lower.
- Maintain inner core activation as you integrate movement and breathing.
- Breathe naturally and don't hold your breath during the inner core contraction.

## REPETITION GUIDELINES

REPS: **5 REPS ON EACH SIDE**

**HOLD:** Hold the finish position for 2 seconds.

# INNER CORE ACTIVATION: STANDING: OPPOSITE ARM AND LEG

**STARTING POSITION:** Stand in the ready position.

**THE MOVEMENT:** Use your transverse abdominis to bring your belly button toward your spine, activating your inner core, as you bend and raise your right knee so your thigh makes a 90 degree angle with your upper body. Simultaneously, raise your left arm so your elbow is even with your ear. Then, at the same time lower your arm and leg. Repeat on the opposite side.

**EXTRA CREDIT:** Raise and lower the arm and leg on the right side of your body, then the arm and leg on the left side of your body.

### TRAINING TIPS

- Focus your mind on a point one to two inches below your belly button.
- Breathe naturally, inhaling and exhaling as you move your arms. Try different breathing patterns: inhale as you raise up and exhale as you lower, then the opposite, exhale as you raise and inhale as you lower.
- Maintain inner core activation as you integrate movement and breathing.
- Breathe naturally and don't hold your breath during the inner core contraction.

### REPETITION GUIDELINES

REPS: **5 REPS ON EACH SIDE**

**HOLD:** Hold the finish position for 2 seconds.

# INNER CORE ACTIVATION: STANDING ARM AND LEG MOVEMENT WITH ROTATION

**STARTING POSITION:** Stand in the ready position.

**THE MOVEMENT:** Use your transverse abdominis to bring your belly button toward your spine, activating your inner core, as you simultaneously bend and raise your right leg so your thigh makes a 90 degree angle with your upper body and raise both arms above your head while you rotate your torso and head to the right (looking over your shoulder). Then, at the same time, turn back to the left, lowering your arms and leg. Repeat to the other side.

### TRAINING TIPS

- Focus your mind on a point one to two inches below your belly button.
- Breathe naturally, inhaling and exhaling as you move your arms. Try different breathing patterns: inhale as you raise up and exhale as you lower, then the opposite, exhale as you raise and inhale as you lower.
- Maintain inner core activation as you integrate movement and breathing.
- Breathe naturally and don't hold your breath during the inner core contraction.

### REPETITION GUIDELINES:

REPS: **5 REPS ON EACH SIDE**

**HOLD:** Hold the finish position for 2 seconds.

## REVIEW

The goal is to make inner core activation a habit, so you don't have to think about it. By isolating and strengthening your inner core, you will have greater support as breath and movement work together to create power and grace.

# THE JOSEPH PILATES TEASER

**INTRODUCTION:** This routine offers a way to build up to one of the famous and difficult Pilates moves, the teaser. This can also be potentially dangerous for the beginner. This routine will give you a method for gradually and safely working up to a full teaser.

**BASIC HOLD PRESCRIPTION:** Work up to holding the balance position for 30 seconds without using your hands for support.

## THE MOVES

### BALANCE HOLD

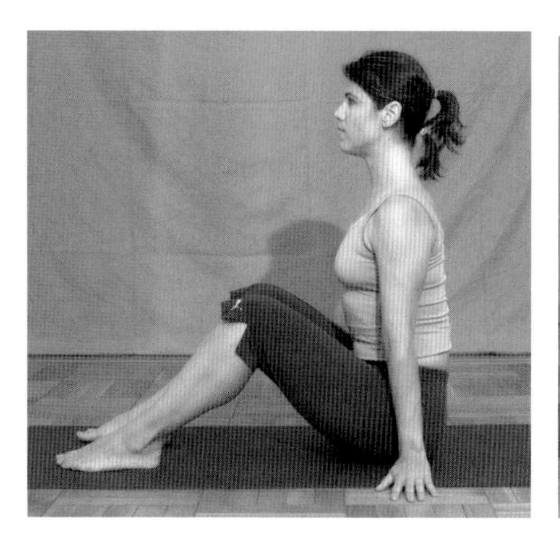

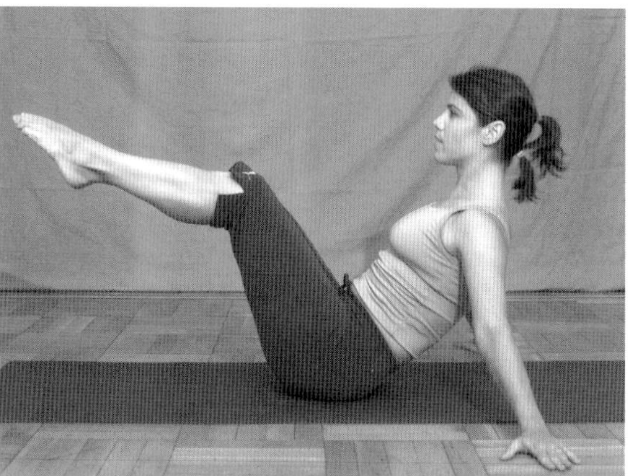

**STARTING POSITION:** Sit with a neutral pelvis, spine and neck lengthened, and your hands at your sides.

**THE MOVE:** Lean back in balanced position, hands extended back and out to the sides.

### WALK UP AND DOWN

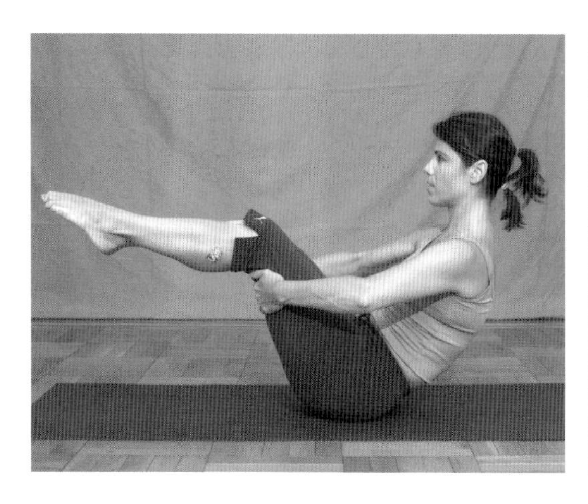

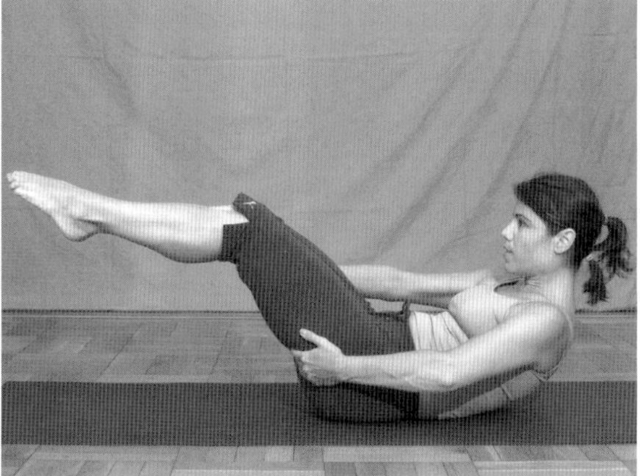

**STARTING POSITION:** Balance on your sit bones, grabbing your legs behind your knees.

**THE MOVE:** Lower your body down by walking your hands down your legs. Then repeat the motion walking back up to the starting position.

**PRESCRIPTION:** Work up to 10 reps for each phase of the sequence. If you are not strong enough to do the walk up phase, just do the walk down phase.

**TRAINING TIPS**

- **Engage the muscles of the center of your body, your "powerhouse" muscles.**
- **"Scoop in your belly," drawing your belly button toward your spine.**
- **Keep your neck long and lengthened during the entire movement**
- **Keep your spine in neutral (neither unnaturally arched or rounded) throughout the entire movement.**

## THE "KI" ROUTINE

**INTRODUCTION:** This routine will get you in touch with power of "ki" energy and the center of your body. The movement drills will help you initiate movements from the center of your body. These moves can be done with a partner or alone. If you're doing them alone, use a wall to create a spatial contact point, as if the wall was your partner.

## THE MOVES

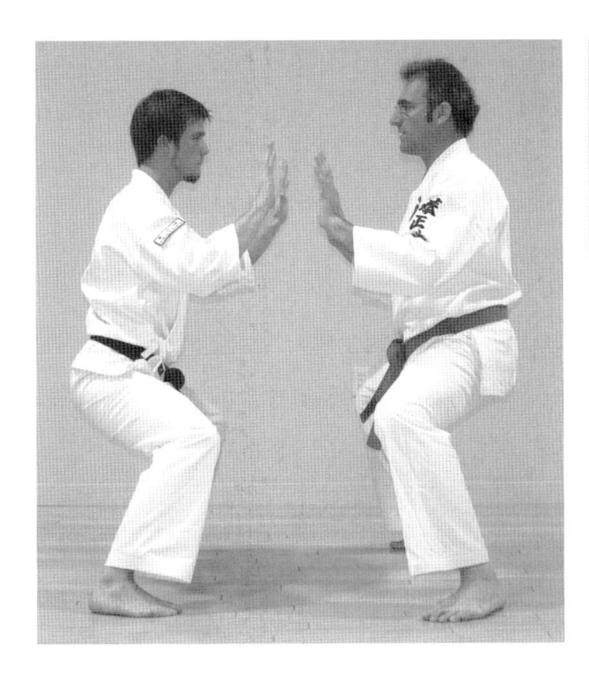

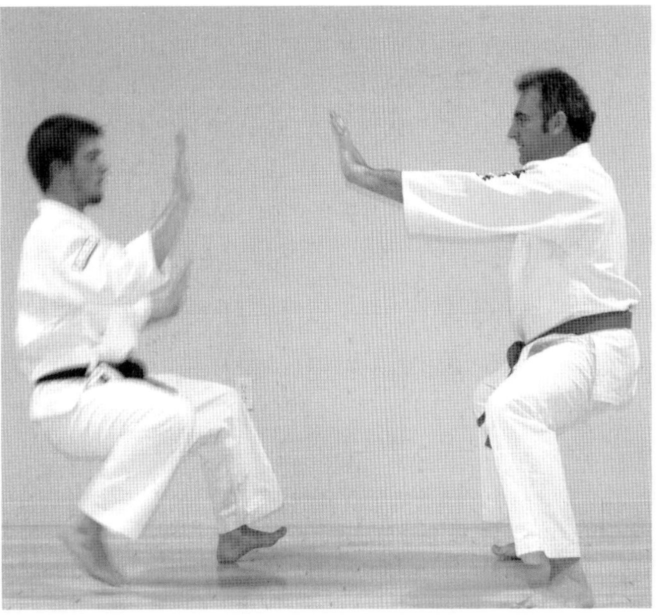

**CENTERED HAND PUSH: Both partners face each other in a ready stance, hands at chest level. They try to knock each other off balance through hand contact.**

- **Use single pushing strikes.**
- **Use sustained pushing pressure where your hands stay in contact.**

#### TRAINING TIPS

- Keep your center activated.
- Let the force from your partner move through your center and down into your feet.
- If you are using a wall it is best not to strike the wall; instead play with sustained pressure, getting a feel for the force being transferred into your center and into your feet.

**WORKOUT:** Work up to 10 push battles, not resting between battles.

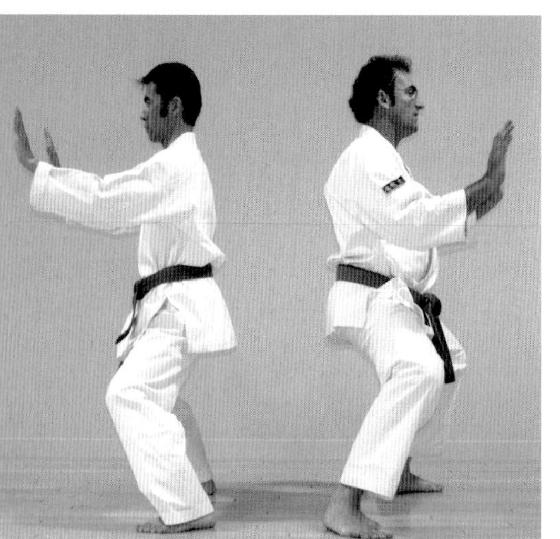

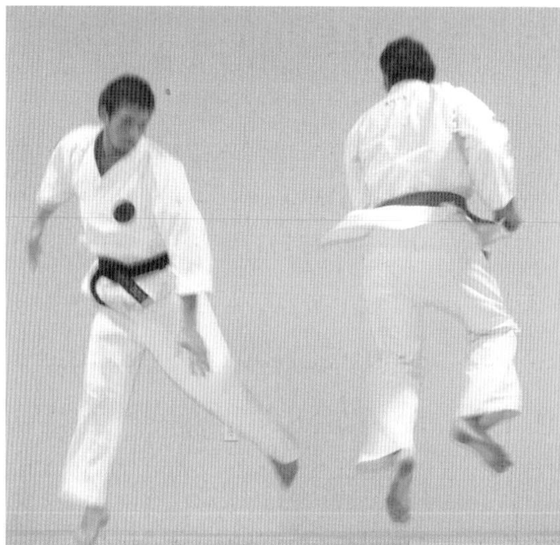

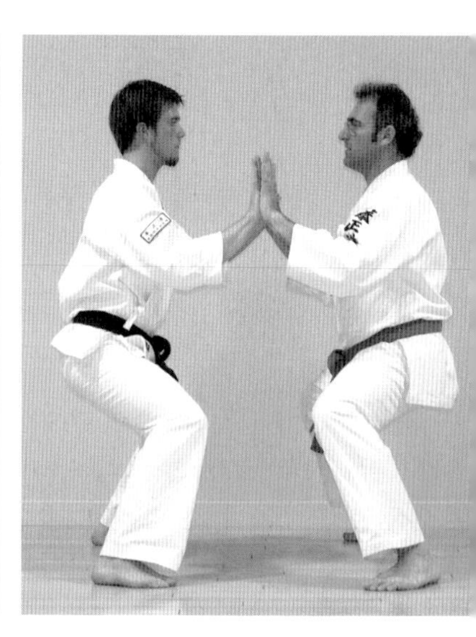

**RISE AND SPIN:** Stand in a ready position with your partner, so you are positioned back-to-back. In one powerful motion jump straight up and rotate 180 degrees, facing your partner. When you land, engage in hand pushing, immediately trying to knock your partner off balance. Alternate rotation motion with each repetition.

- Control the movement from your center.
- Make the motion powerful and efficient, trying to land your feet in the exact position you started in.

**WORKOUT:** Do 10 reps, 5 spins in each direction

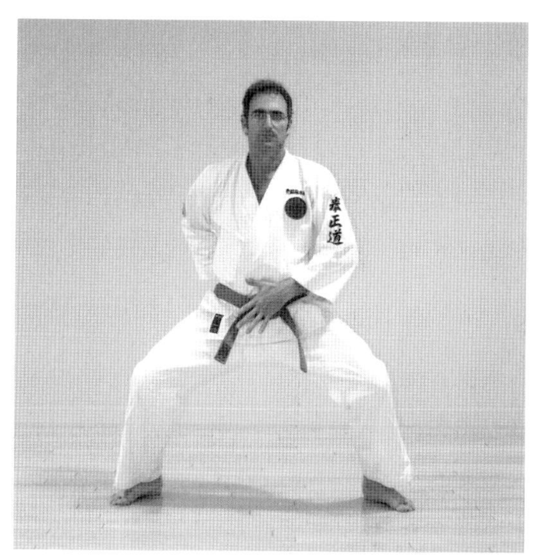

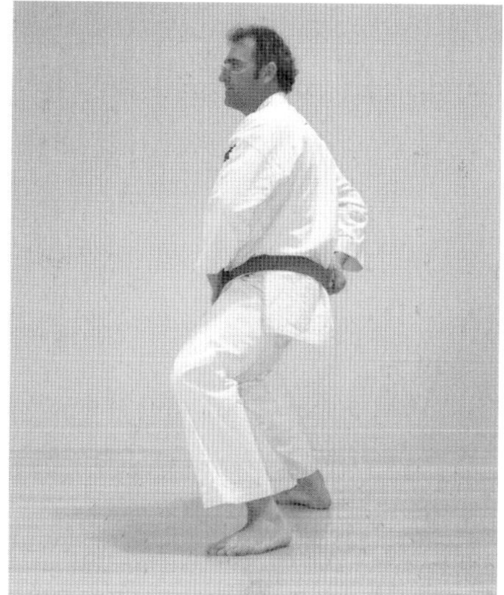

**SQUARE TO BLADE:** Begin in the ready position, in a square stance, with one hand in front of your body and one hand behind your body (both hands centered in the middle of your body). If you were standing on a clock face, your feet would be on the 3 and the 9, spread wide.

Then in a smooth circular motion, move your right leg back to the 6 o'clock position, directly behind your right foot. The goal of this exercise is to learn to move from the center of your body.

### TRAINING TIPS

- Initiate the movement from your center, not your foot and leg.
- Maintain the ready position throughout the movement.

**WORKOUT:**

- Do 10 reps with each leg, then switch legs.
- Once you've become efficient with the move, alternate legs each time.

## PRIME TIME CIRCUIT, BY BRYAN HOLMES

**INTRODUCTION:** This routine is designed for senior citizens. It will strengthen your core area: your abs, lower back, butt, and hips. Having a strong core will help you enjoy all of your favorite physical activities and enhance your balance.

### THE EXERCISES

Standing Knee Flexion with hold, p. 243

Glute Bridge, p. 277

Knee Touch—Crossing, p. 226

Lying Hip Rotation, p. 292

Back Extension, p. 252

### PRESCRIPTION

**LEVEL ONE:** Work up to 20 reps. For exercises where you alternate sides, do 10 on each side.

**LEVEL TWO:** Rest one minute and repeat the routine.

**FREQUENCY:** 3 to 6 times a week.

## YOGA CORE ROUTINE, BY STEVE FALK

### YOGA EXPERIENCE

All too often, new Yoga students expect their Yoga practice to be some extensive form of stretching. Depending upon the style of Yoga you practice, this expectation could be very accurate or one could be in for quite a rude awakening. In Bikram Yoga, we often characterize the physical aspects of our practice as the balance between strength and flexibility.

Historically, I believe Yoga has attracted a majority of students with a predisposition toward flexibility. Naturally, we tend to gravitate toward activities in which we excel and quickly develop confidence. As Yoga has grown in popularity in the past decade, we teachers are now seeing larger amounts of students who don't have this great natural flexibility, but on the other hand are often quite strong. The majority of this stronger and tighter group of students are men and ex-athletes (both male and female), who are realizing the tremendous healing power of Yoga and its balanced approach to fitness.

### MY STORY

I came to Yoga to alleviate the back and knee pain that I had developed from years of basketball, along with lots of heavy weight training and almost no stretching. As I was quite inflexible, I knew that I needed a structured flexibility program to complement my lifting. Like most of my contemporaries in the gym, I would not dedicate sufficient time to stretching if left to my own devices. I had been doing light stretching after workouts for years but had made zero progress. I finally realized that to truly improve my flexibility and hopefully relieve my pain, I needed to allot an equal amount of time (or more) to my flexibility. Five minutes a day of stretching was no balance for five hours a week of weight training. So I turned to Yoga.

What I found after my first Yoga class was that not only was I inflexible, but quite weak as well. Like many large athletes, I had a very hard time merely manipulating my body weight. And balance? It was not a pretty sight. As I continued my practice, Yoga did wonders for my back and knees, burned off body fat, and even improved my sleep quality.

## OBSERVATIONS AS A TEACHER

I realize the low back pain that brought me and so many others to Yoga cannot merely be attributed to a lack of flexibility. In fact, researchers are now noting that low back pain is often the result of too much low back flexibility and not enough core stability. While everyone's individual case is different, I continue to see the following physical deficiencies (the same ones that I had) with our students:

1. Tight hip flexors
2. Tight shoulder girdle—especially pecs and front delts
3. Tight hamstrings
4. Weak core—low back, hip flexors, hip extensors, abdominals
5. Hypermobile low back—usually noted by excessive spinal rounding in forward bends and the inability to sit up straight in a seated straddle stretch.

## THE CHALLENGE

The low back often becomes hypermobile to compensate for tight hip flexors and hamstrings. Even if we add flexibility to these areas, it will often only be temporary because this tightness is the body's protection response for the spine. If the body feels weak and unstable, especially around the spine, then it will contract the supporting muscles in order to add a degree of tension and stability. This, then, begs the question, how do we fix this? We approach these deficiencies with a progressive, balanced program that stresses gaining flexibility in tight muscles and strength in weak muscles, and yes, these are often the same muscles.

**THE WORKOUT:** This program can be done as a stand-alone workout, or ideally at the end of another workout when you are warm. As with any form of exercise, finding quality, hands-on instruction and coaching is always the best approach.

# THE VACUUM

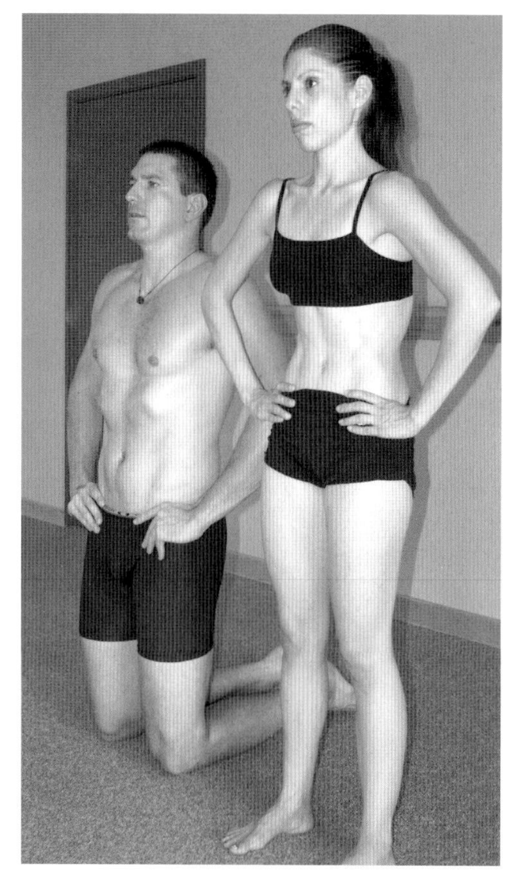

**AREA:** Activate your transverse abdominus.

**THE MOVE:** From a standing or kneeling position draw your belly button inward and upward.

# DOWNWARD DOG

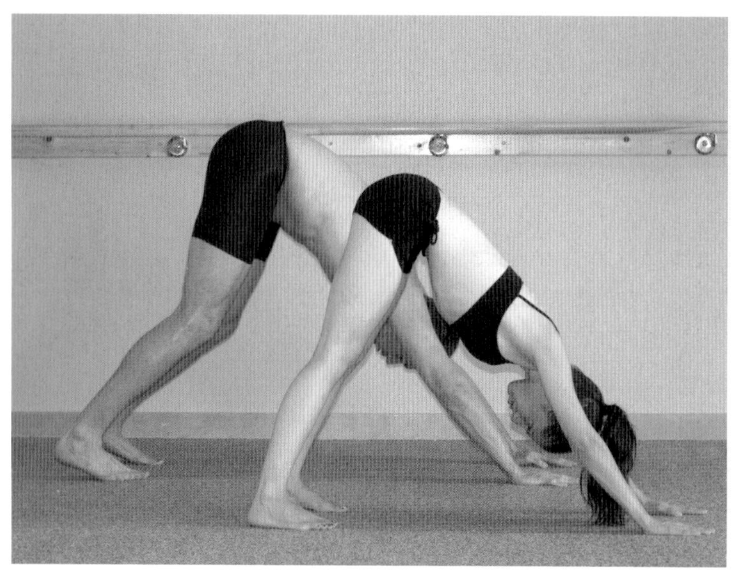

**THE MOVE:** Create an angled pike position, distributing your body weight on your hands and feet. Keep your back from rounding by bending your knees in order to keep a straight spine. As you gain flexibility over time, your legs will straighten and your heels will drop to the floor.

# KNEELING HIP FLEXOR AND STRETCH TO BACKWARD BEND

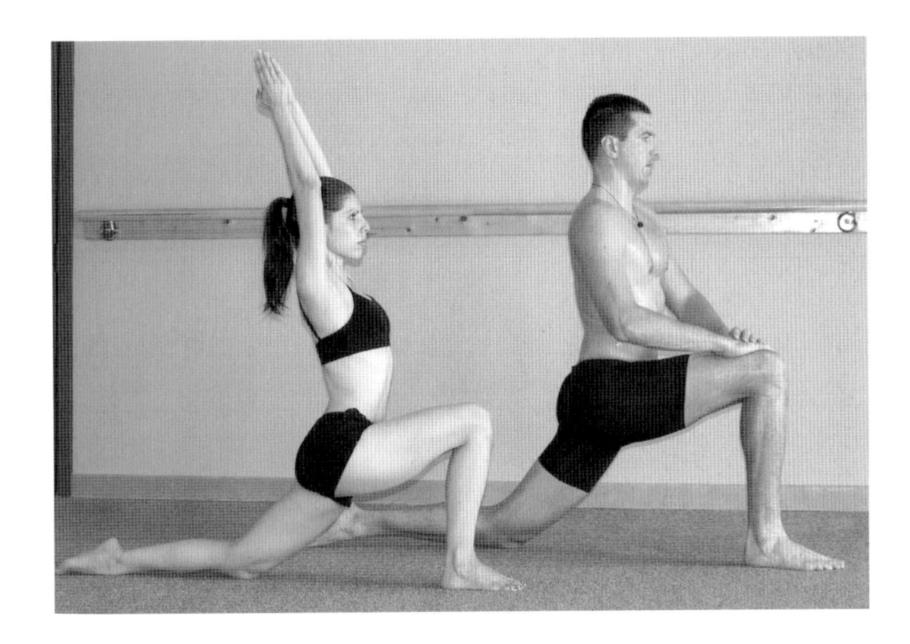

**THE MOVE:** Lunge forward on your right leg, resting your hands on your thigh or extending them above your head. Try to drop your hips to the ground and don't sink to one side. Tight hip flexors will tilt your pelvis and are a big cause of tight hamstrings and bad backs.

# COBRA

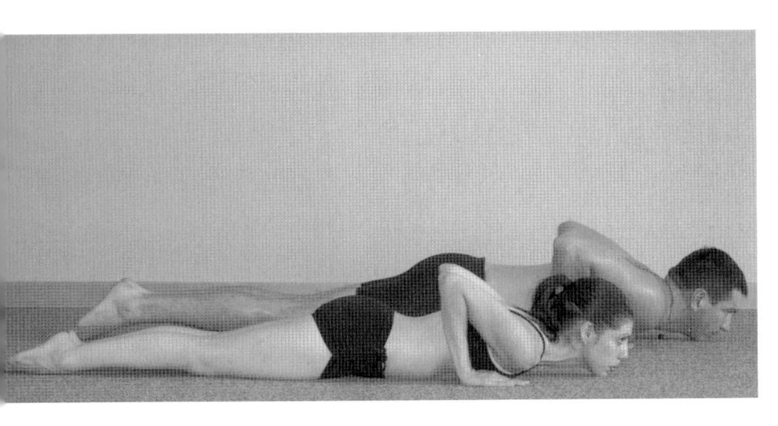

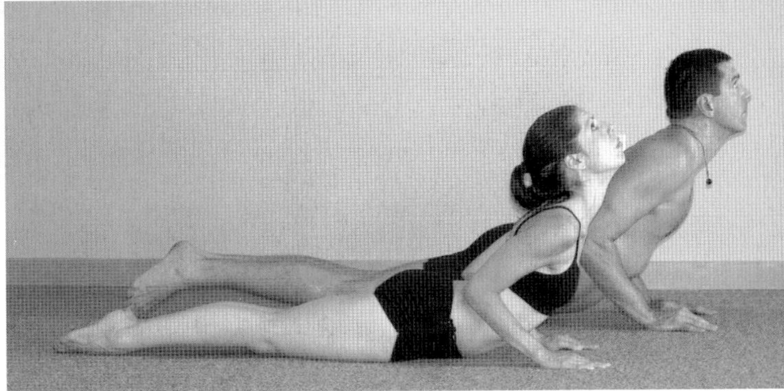

**THE MOVE:** Place your hands under your shoulder blades and gently arch your body up. Minimize your arm contribution by squeezing your glutes and lifting with your low back. Resist the urge to shrug or crunch your neck. Think of wrapping your spine backward around a beach ball.

# BOAT

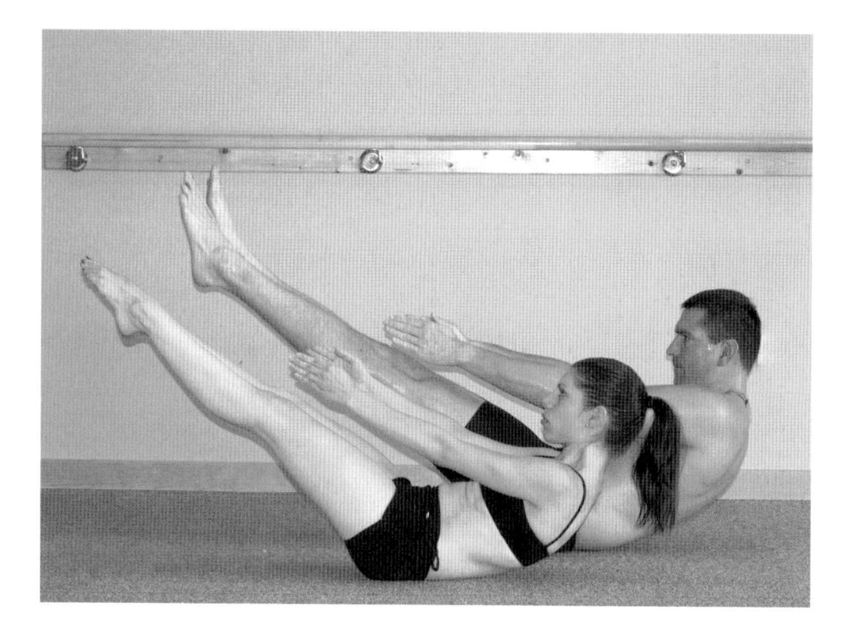

**THE MOVE:** Using your core muscles to balance in a modified V shape, raise your arms and legs, balancing on your sit bones.

# THE V SIT-UP

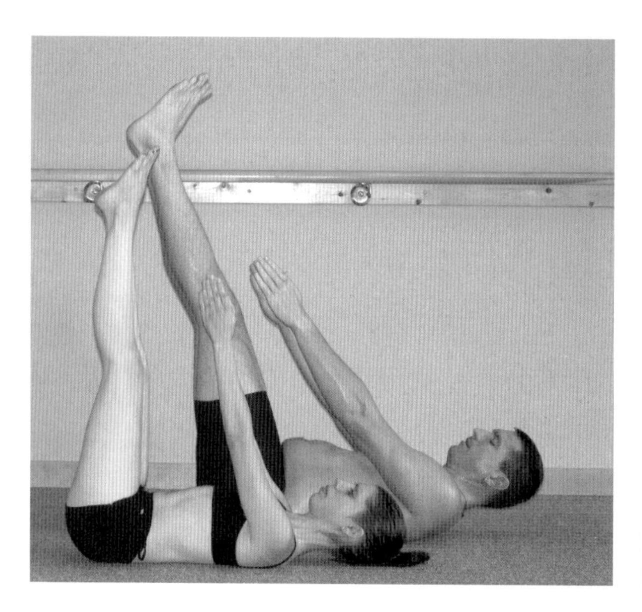

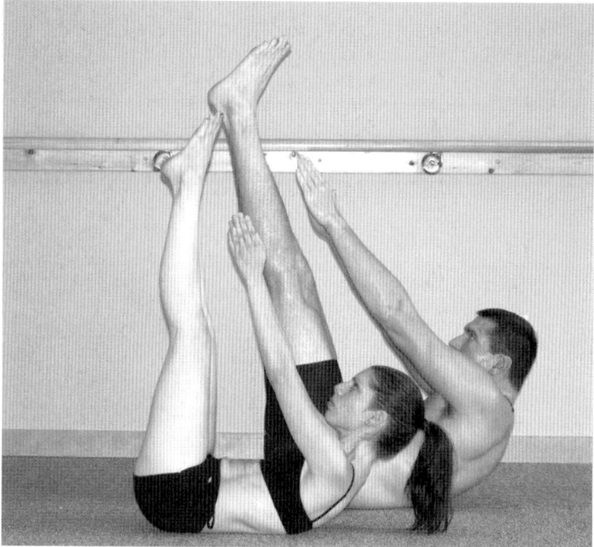

**THE MOVE:** Lying on your back with legs perpendicular to your upper body, arms extended straight, raise your torso and hands toward your feet. The classic v-sit crunch.

# CAMEL

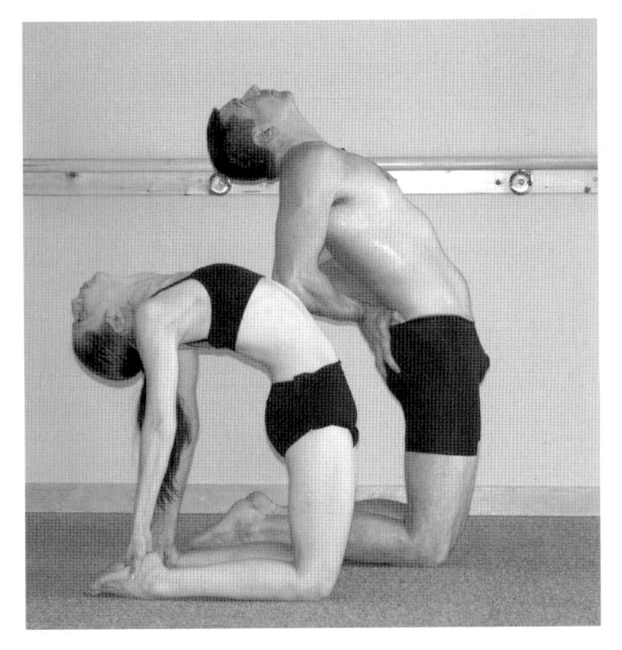

**THE MOVE:** Stand up on your knees with your lower legs approximately hip width apart. Place your hands on your glutes/lower back. Squeeze your glutes and push your hips forward and then slowly bend backward as you lift your chest up to the sky. In the more advanced version, reach back and hold on to your feet.

# SPINE TWIST

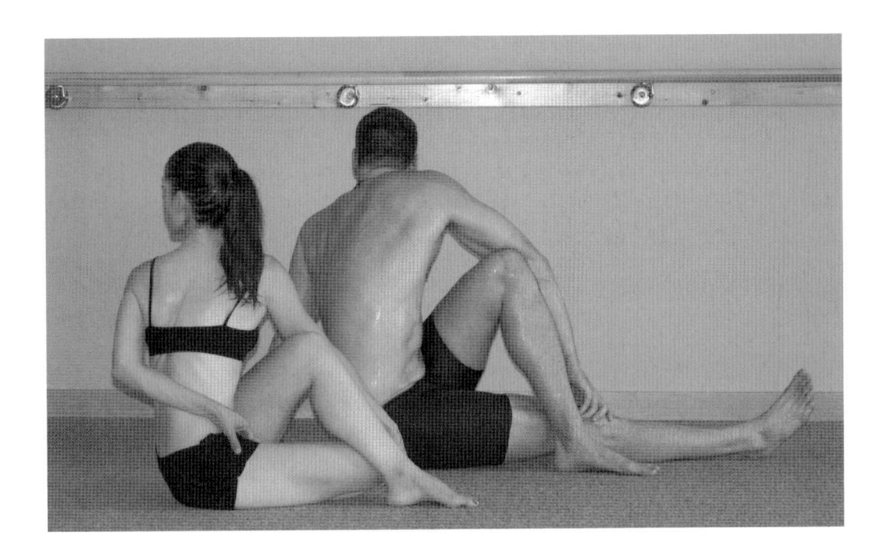

**THE MOVE:** In a seated position extend your right leg out in front of you, bring the sole of your left foot over your right thigh, and place the sole of your left foot flat on the floor. Place your left hand on the floor behind you or wrap it around your waist. Bring your right arm up and around your left knee and twist; looking over your left shoulder. Focus on lengthening your spine and growing taller as you twist. Repeat on the other side.

# COBBLER'S POSE

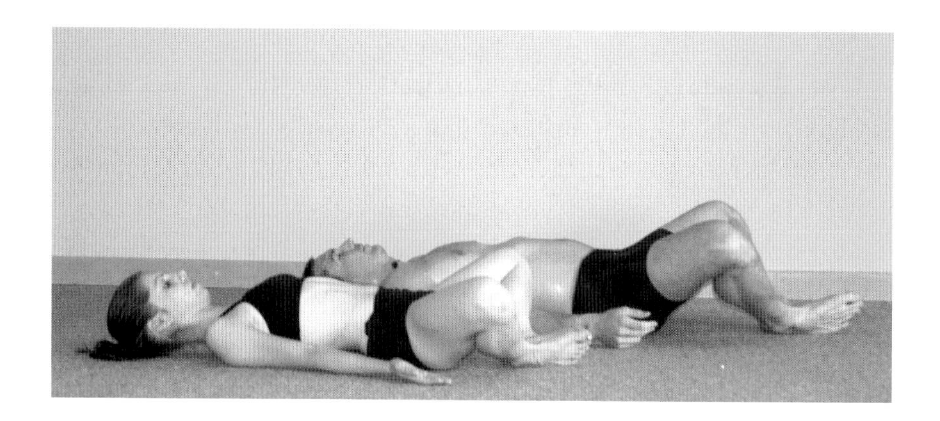

**THE MOVE:** **A relaxing finishing pose that lets gravity gently open your hips and groin. Lie down on your back and bring the soles of your feet together like a classic butterfly stretch. Relax and let gravity do the work.**

**PROGRAM PROGRESSION AND PRESCRIPTION**

**FREQUENCY:** 3 times a week

**WEEK 1:** hold each pose for 15 seconds, Week 2–20 seconds, Week 3–30 seconds, Week 4–45 seconds, Week 5–60 seconds. After week 5, one can advance by adding more sets and/or a greater frequency per week. Always listen to your body and progress at a conservative pace.

# CORE BALL ROUTINE, BY MIKE BRUNGARDT

## INTRODUCTION

This program has two elements. Stage one strengthens the core area and stage two adds a cardio conditioning component. To do stage one of this program you will need a solid wall and floor to bounce the ball against. For stage two, you'll need approximately half the length of a basketball court for the cardio conditioning drills. When you get fatigued technique suffers. It is best to master the exercises in stage one before adding the conditioning element to the workout. If you are dealing with conditioned athletes you can combine the two elements from the start. To increase the intensity, use a heavier medicine ball. I use this routine with the Spurs, but it would work to build a foundation of core strength for almost any sport.

Most sports take place on your feet, standing. This routine is designed to increase core strength, power, and endurance while standing, instead of doing exercises on the floor or on all fours.

# STAGE ONE: BALL THROWS

**GETTING SET-UP:** You want to stand 3 to 10 feet away from the wall depending on your core strength.

# OVER THE SHOULDER THROW

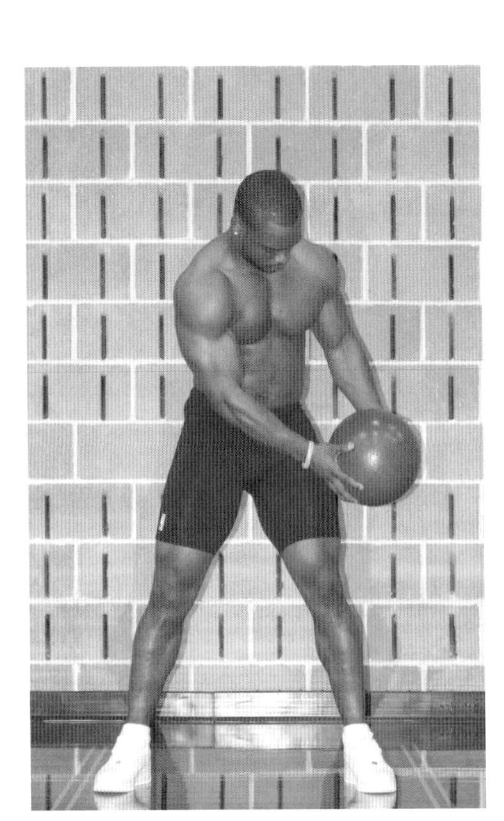

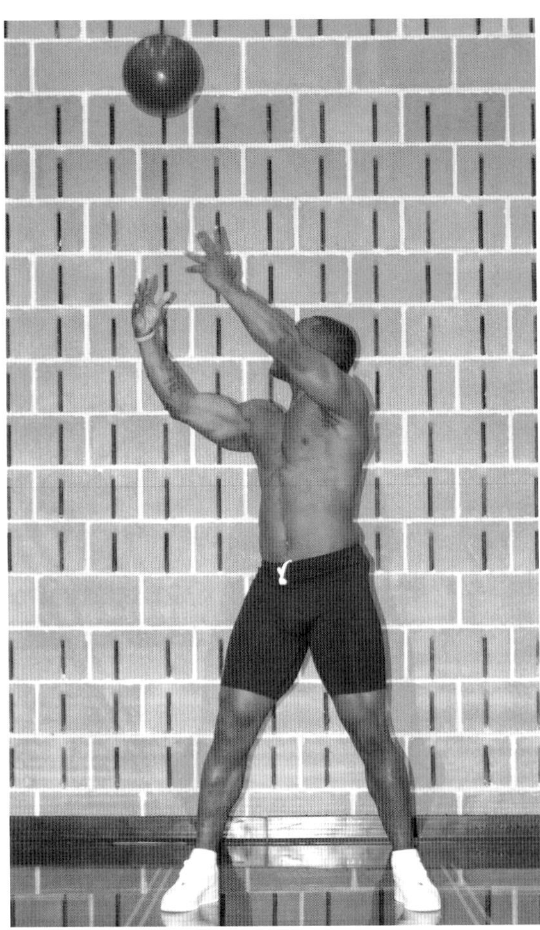

**STARTING POSITION:** Start in the ready position with your back to the wall. Lower the ball to your left hip.

**THE THROW:** Rotate your torso and throw the ball over your right shoulder. Catch the ball in the air off the bounce. Return to the starting position and repeat.

# SIDE HIP THROW

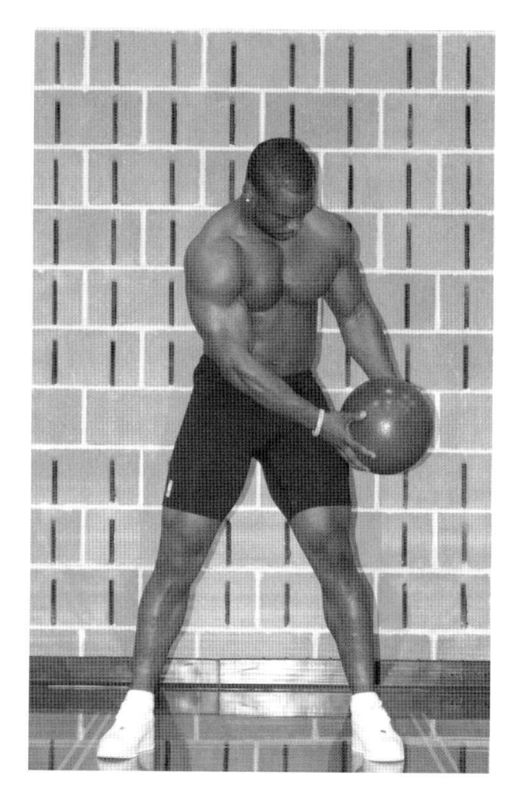

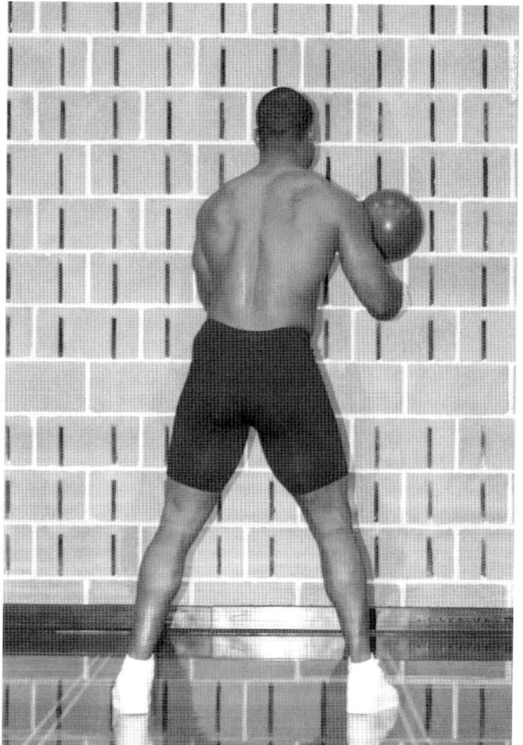

**STARTING POSITION:** Start in the ready position with your back to the wall. Lower the ball to your left hip.

**THE THROW:** Rotate your torso and throw the ball at hip level off the wall. Turn and catch the ball in the air off the bounce. Return to the starting position and repeat.

# OVERHEAD THROW

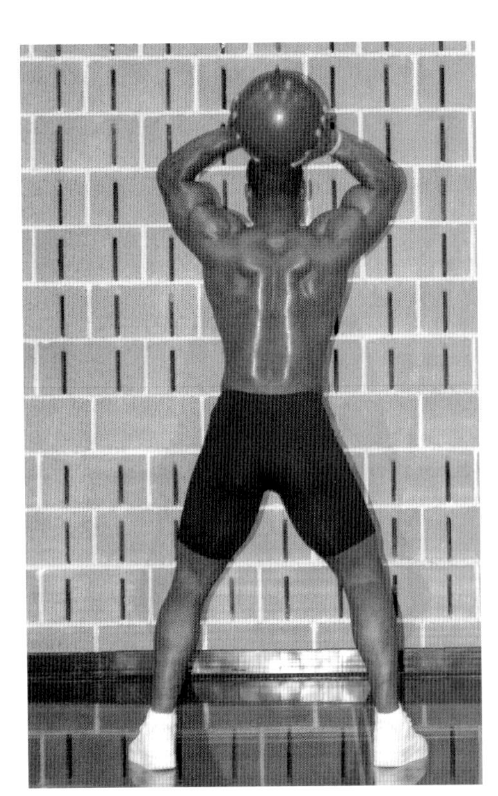

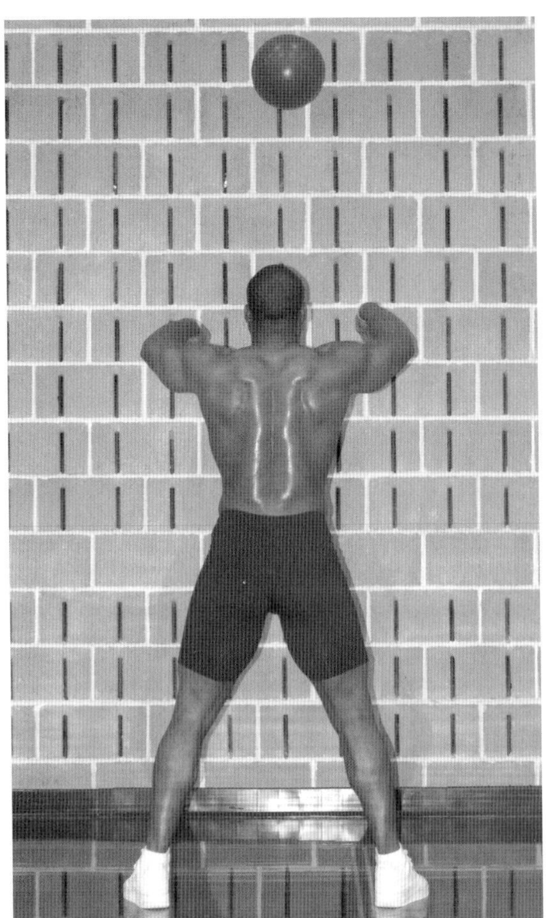

**STARTING POSITION:** Start in the ready position facing the wall. Raise the ball over your head.

**THE THROW:** From the overhead position throw the ball off the wall and catch it in the air. Repeat.

# CHEST PASS

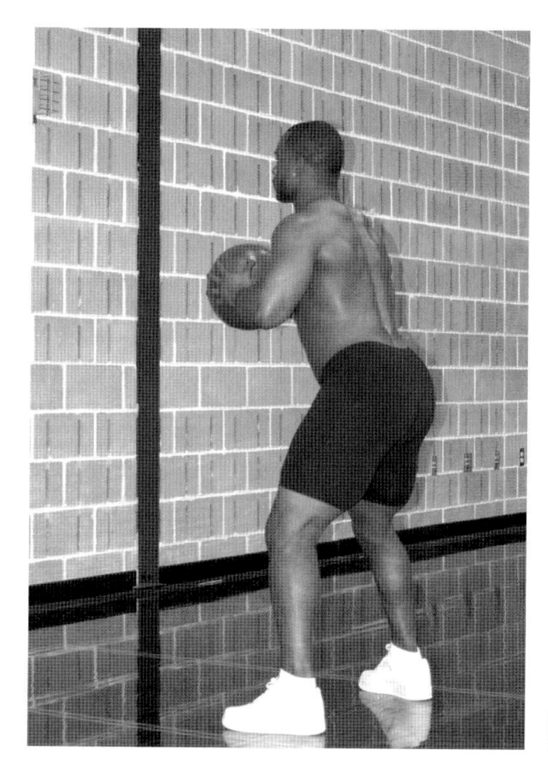

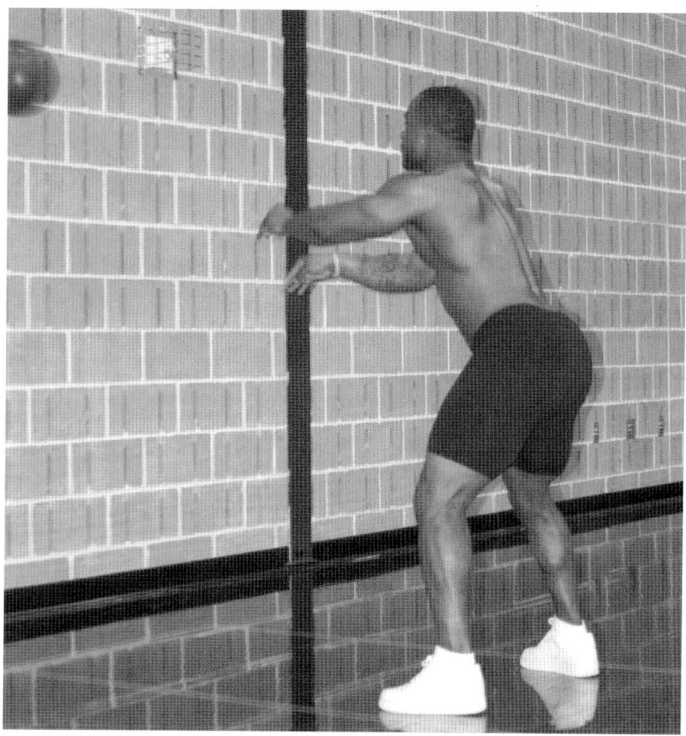

**STARTING POSITION:** Start in the ready position facing the wall. Bring the ball to your chest.

**THE THROW:** From the chest position throw the ball off the wall and catch it in the air. Repeat.

# SQUAT THROWS

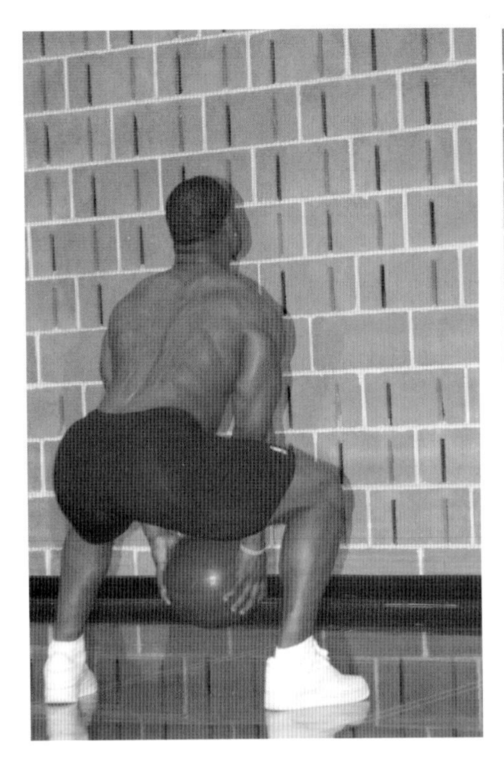
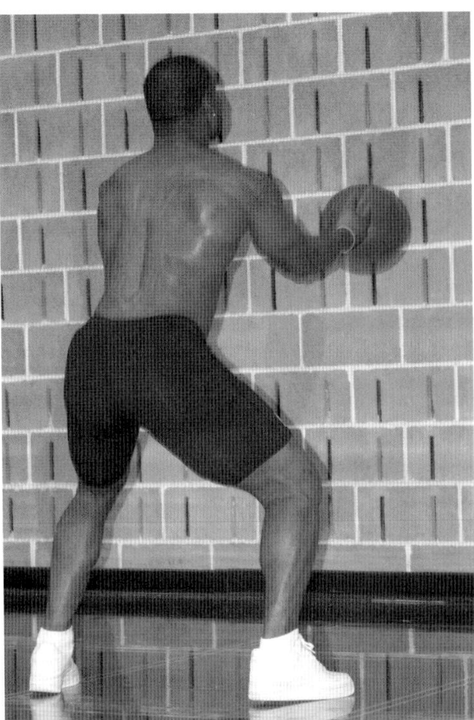

**STARTING POSITION:** Start in the ready position facing the wall. Lower into a quarter squat bringing the ball between your legs.

**THE THROW:** Explode out of the squat position popping your hips forward as you throw the ball off the wall. Catch it in the air and repeat.

# ONE ARM THROW AND CATCH

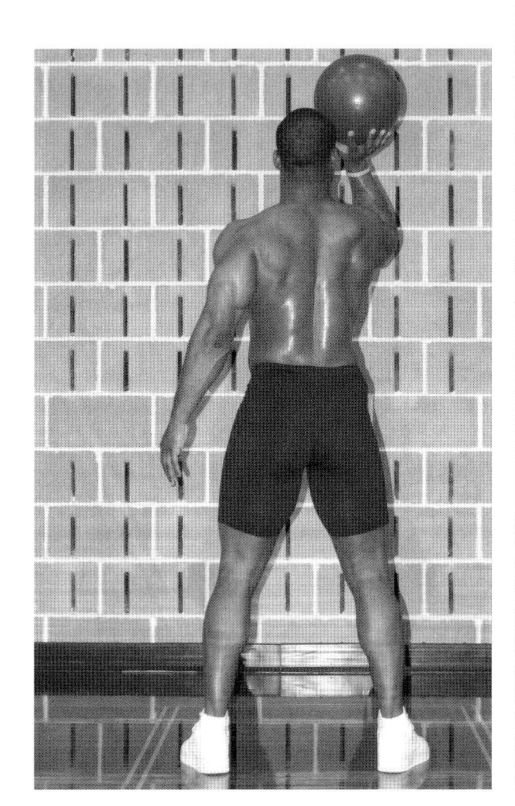

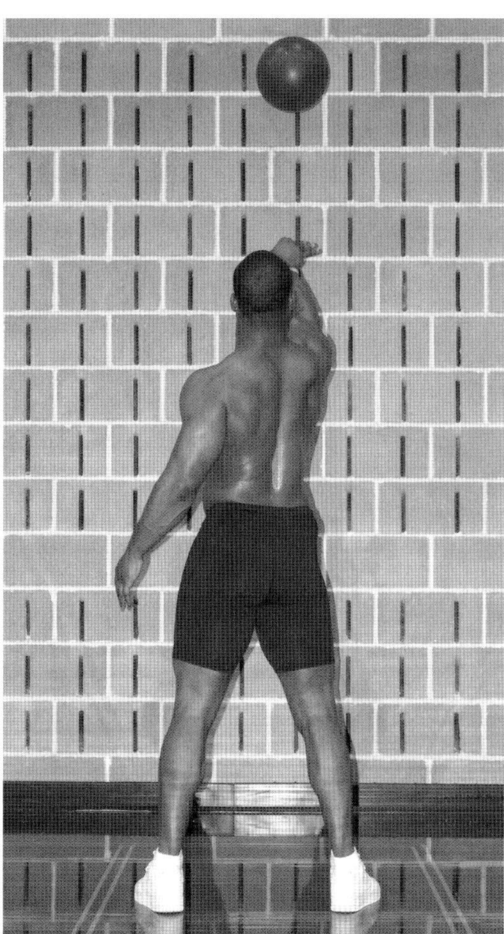

**STARTING POSITION:** Start in the ready position facing the wall. Hold the ball at shoulder level with one arm.

**THE THROW:** From the one arm position throw the ball off the wall and catch it in the air. Repeat, then switch to the other arm.

# COCK AND THROW

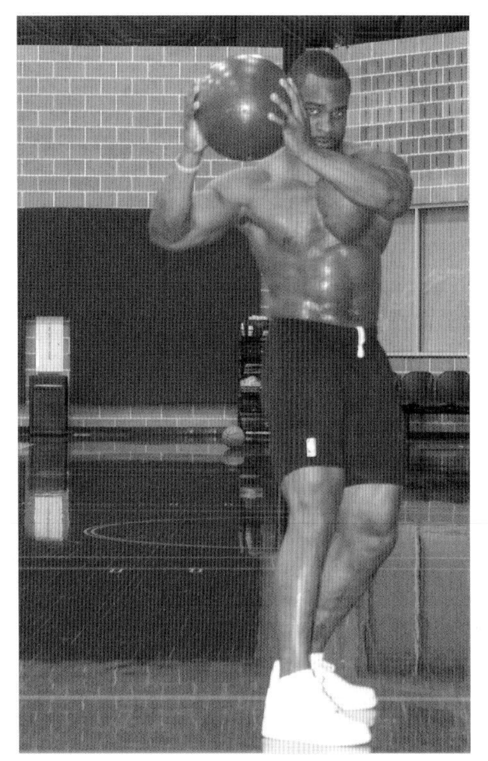

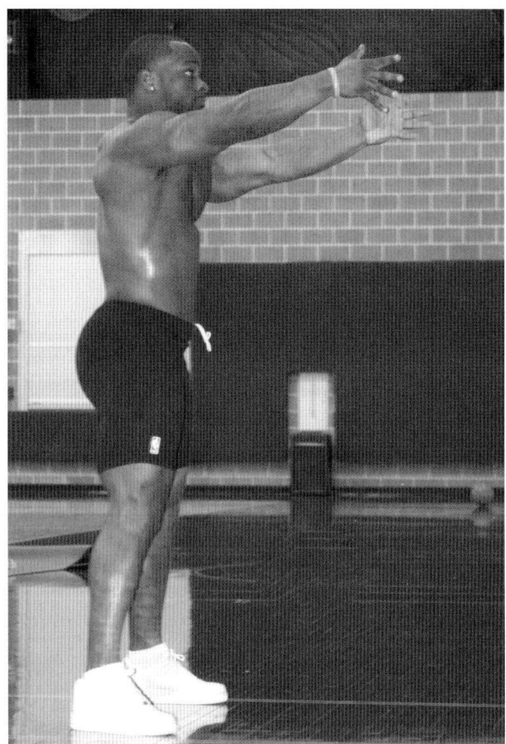

**STARTING POSITION:** Start in the ready position facing the wall. Raise the ball to the right side of your head, level with your ear.

**THE THROW:** From this position turn and look to the right, then back to center, as you throw the ball off the wall and catch it in the air. Repeat.

# FORWARD HIP THROW

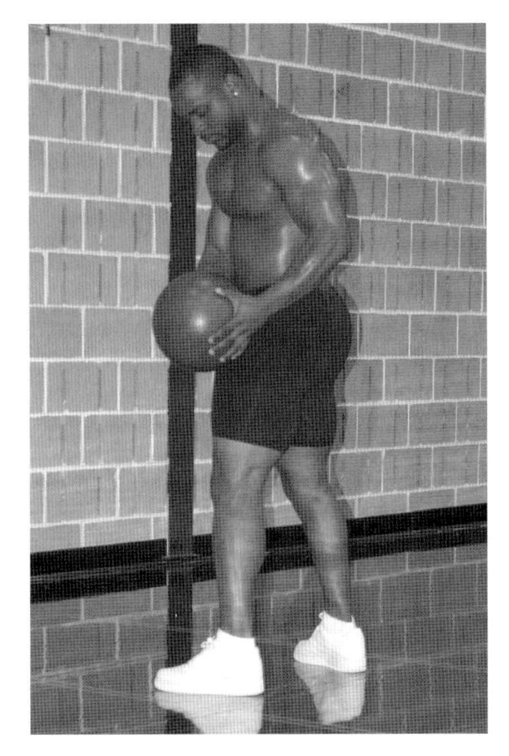

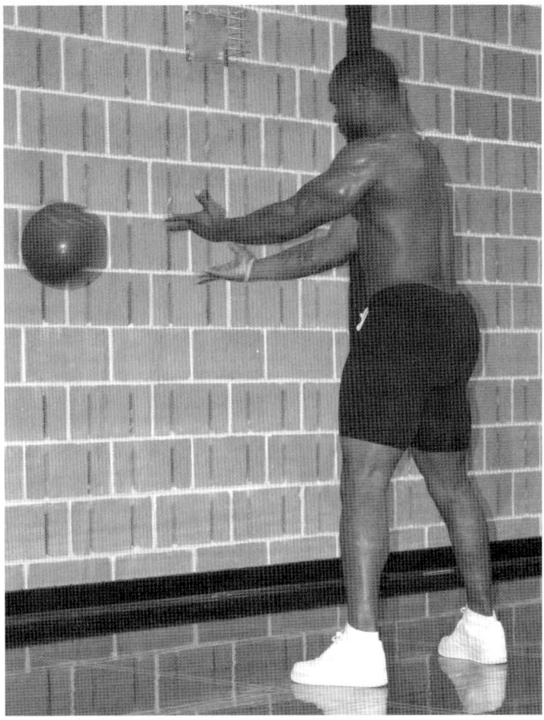

**STARTING POSITION:** Start in the ready position facing the wall. Lower the ball to the left side of your hip.

**THE THROW:** From this position turn your hip to the left, then pop it back to center as you throw the ball off the wall and catch it in the air. Repeat.

# OVERHEAD WOODCHOPPER

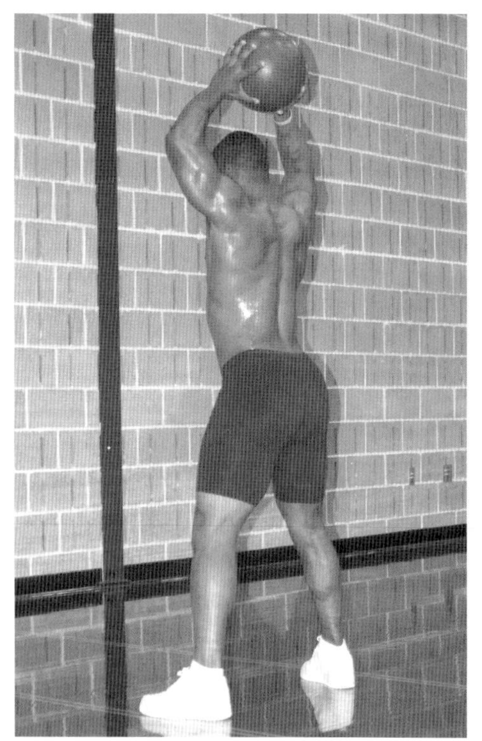

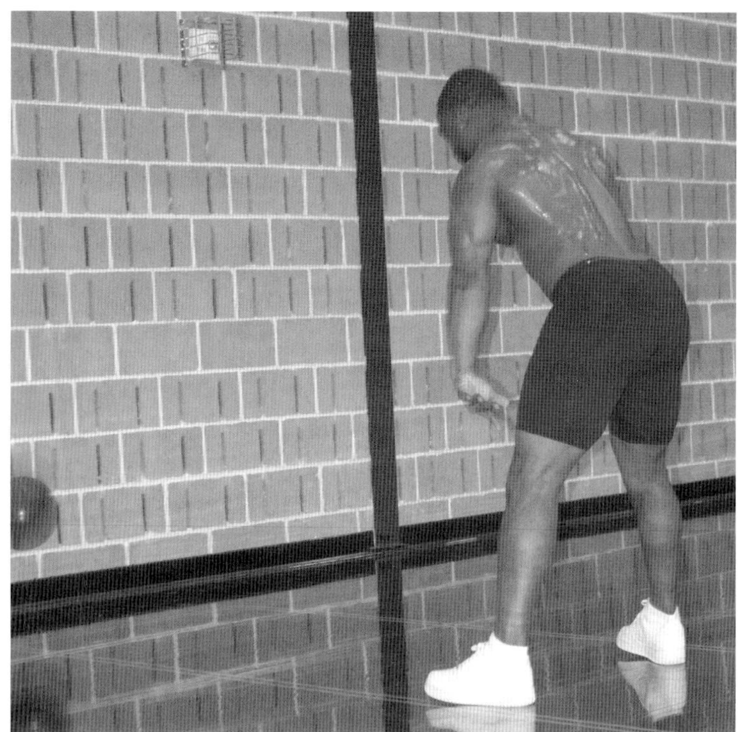

**STARTING POSITION:** Start in the ready position facing the wall. Raise the ball over your head.

**THE THROW:** From the overhead position throw the ball straight down and bounce it off the floor. Catch and repeat.

# OVERHEAD WOODCHOPPER WITH ROTATION

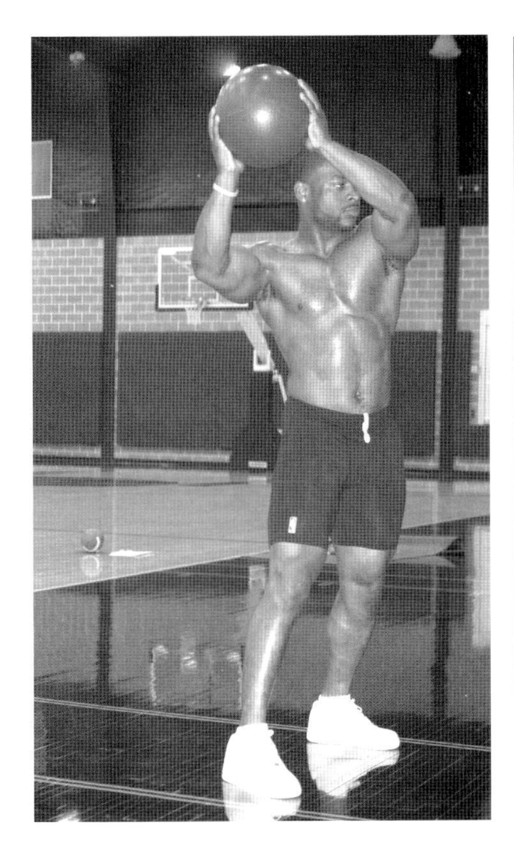

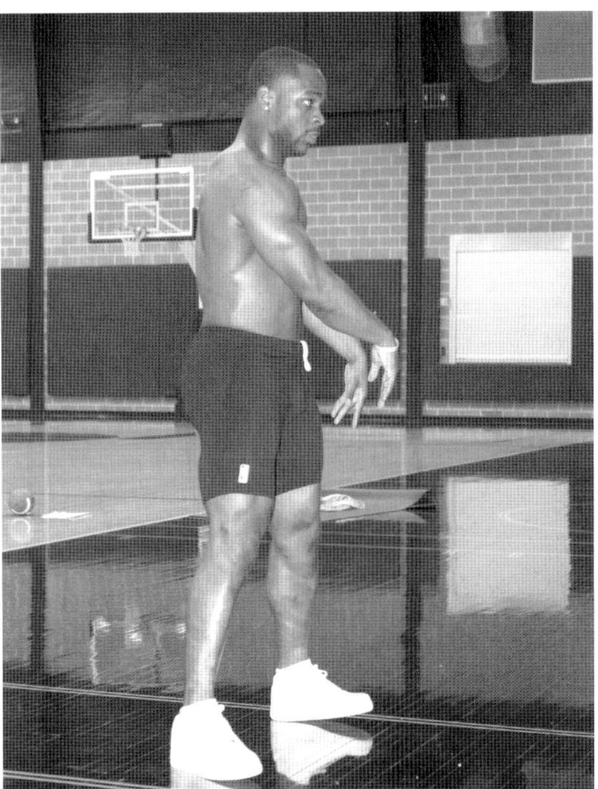

**STARTING POSITION:** Start in the ready position facing the wall. Raise the ball above your head and out at an angle over your shoulder. Rotate that shoulder away from the wall.

**THE THROW:** From this position rotate and throw the ball straight down and bounce it off the floor. Catch and repeat.

## STAGE TWO: CONDITIONING DRILLS

**INTRODUCTION:** The conditioning stage is designed to work in conjunction with the throws. After each throwing drill you move on to the next conditioning drill. The drills get progressively more intense. They are designed to go half the distance of a basketball court, so the up and back distance equals the length of a court.

### CONDITIONING DRILLS

1. Jog
2. Butt Kicks (bring your heel to your butt as you run).
3. Skip
4. Lateral Shuffle: (move sideways in a shuffle motion, not letting your feet cross).
5. Over Unders: (move sideways in a shuffle motion, crossing one leg in front then in back of the other leg. Make sure you switch the over under leg).
6. Backward Jog
7. 80% Sprint
8. 80% Skip Sprint
9. 80% Lateral Sprint
10. 80% Backward Sprint

## THE ROUTINE

**LEVEL ONE:** Do 10 reps for each throw. If you're alternating sides do 5 on each side.

**LEVEL TWO:** Add conditioning drills.

**LEVEL THREE:** Increase your sets for both ball throws and conditioning drills. Depending on your fitness level and goals you can progress up to a maximum of five sets with no rest between sets.

## MEDICINE BALL PARTNER ROUTINE, BY BRETT BRUNGARDT

**INTRODUCTION:** This is a challenging routine you can do with a partner. It will dynamically train your core, building a foundation of strength for your favorite sport.

# STANDING: ROTATE AND SIDE HANDOFF

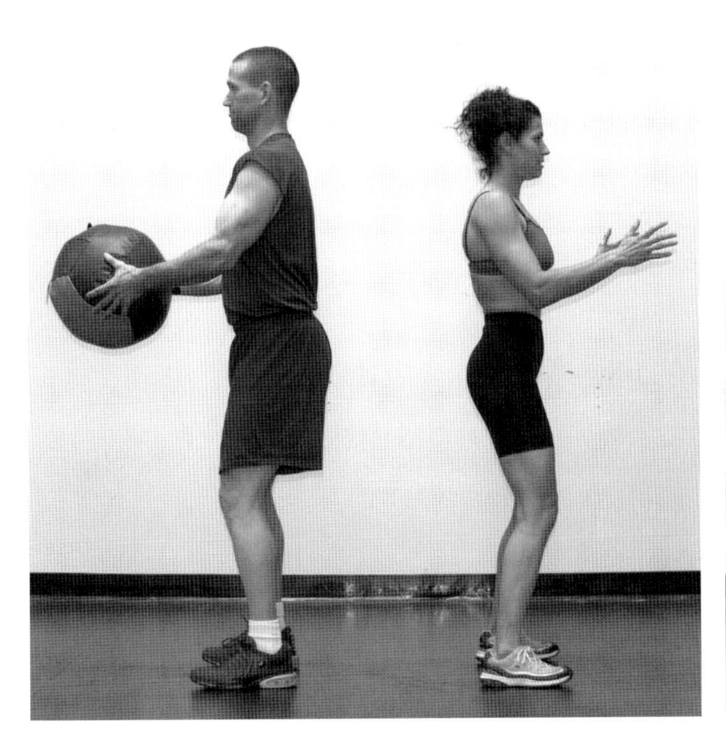

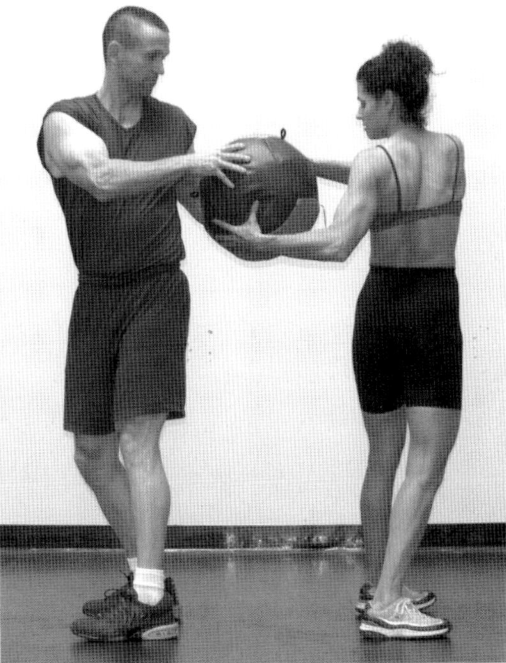

**STARTING POSITION:** Stand in the ready position with your back to your partner, approximately arm's length away from your partner. One person holds the medicine ball at chest level.

**THE MOVE:** Rotate toward each other, handing the ball to your partner. Then rotate in the opposite direction, turning toward each other and handing the ball back to your partner. Repeat until you have completed the prescribed number of reps for that direction, then switch directions.

## TRAINING TIPS

- Keep your inner core activated throughout the movement.
- Initiate the movement from your center, not your arms.
- Maintain a balanced ready stance throughout the exercise.

# HI-LO HANDOFF

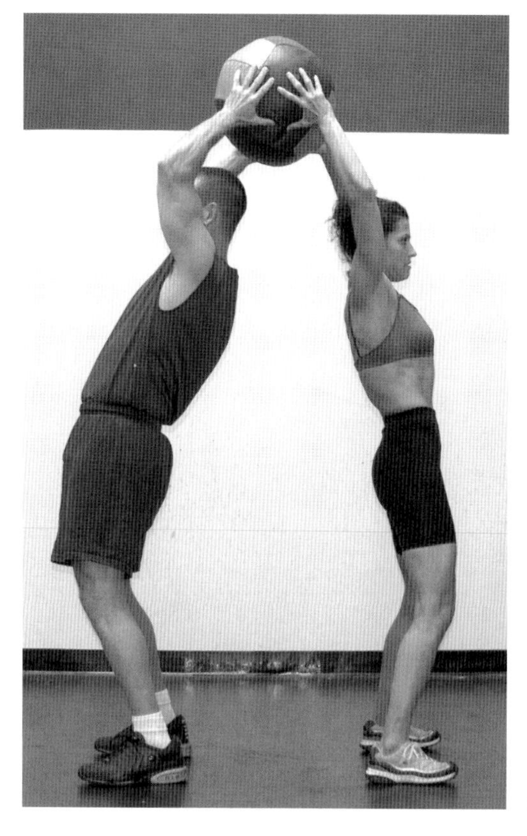

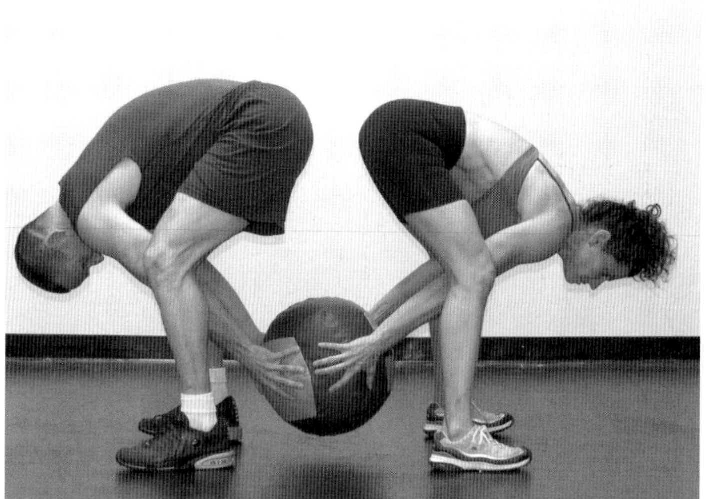

**STARTING POSITION:** Stand in the ready position with your back to your partner, approximately a foot away from each other. One person holds the medicine ball at chest level.

**THE MOVE:** The person with the ball raises it above his head and back toward his partner, handing the ball off. The partner then takes the ball down and hands it off between his legs to his partner. Repeat the movement for the prescribed number of repetitions, then switch the movement pattern.

### TRAINING TIPS

- Keep your inner core activated throughout the movement.
- Initiate the movement from your center, not your arms.
- Maintain a balanced ready stance throughout the exercise.

# HI-LO HANDOFF WITH ROTATION

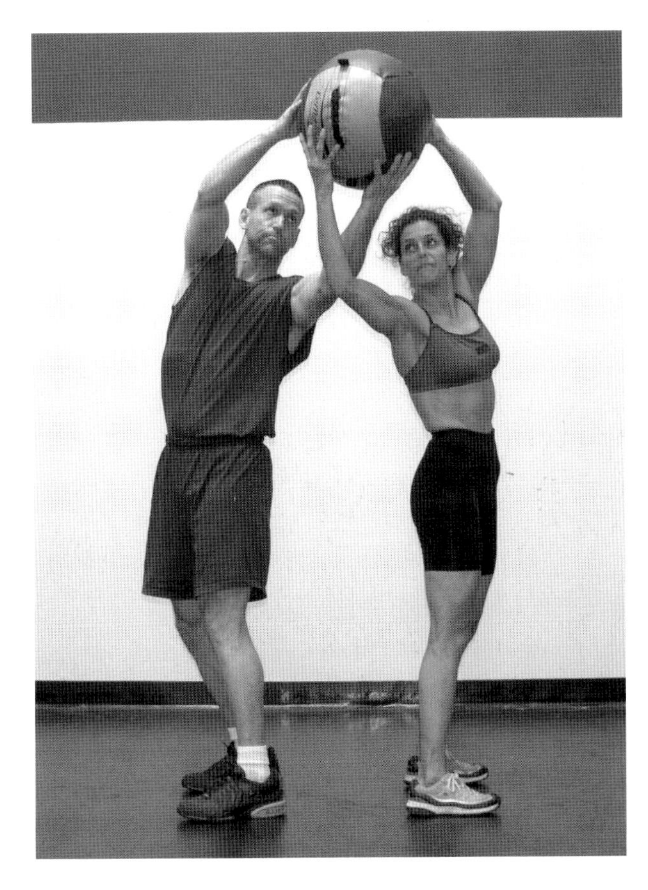

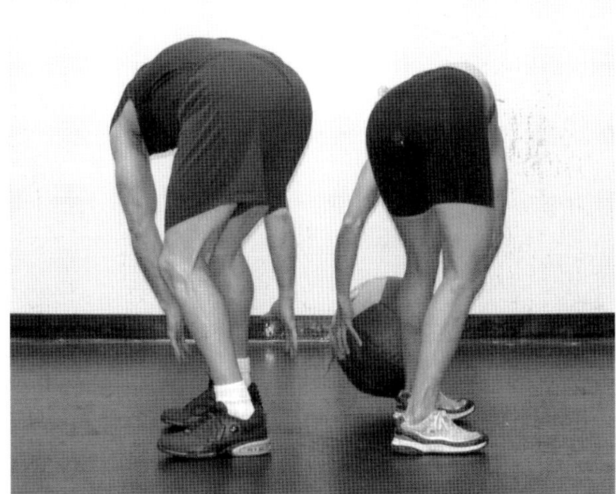

**STARTING POSITION:** Stand in the ready position with your back to your partner, approximately a foot away from your partner. One person holds the medicine ball at chest level.

**THE MOVE:** The person with the ball lowers it to the outside of his ankle, as he and his partner move simultaneously, mirroring the downward rotational movement. Then both exercisers rotate and move upward and diagonally to the opposite side of their bodies, handing the ball off. The other person repeats the motion with the ball. Perform the movement for the prescribed number of repetitions, then switch and train the other side.

**TRAINING TIPS**

- Keep your inner core activated throughout the movement.
- Initiate the movement from your center, not your arms.
- Maintain a balanced ready stance throughout the exercise.

## SEATED

# BALANCE TOSS

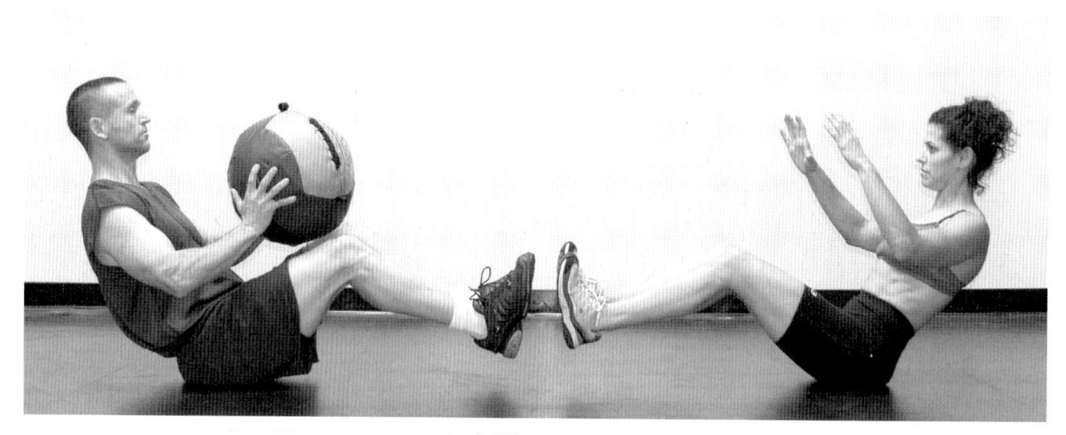

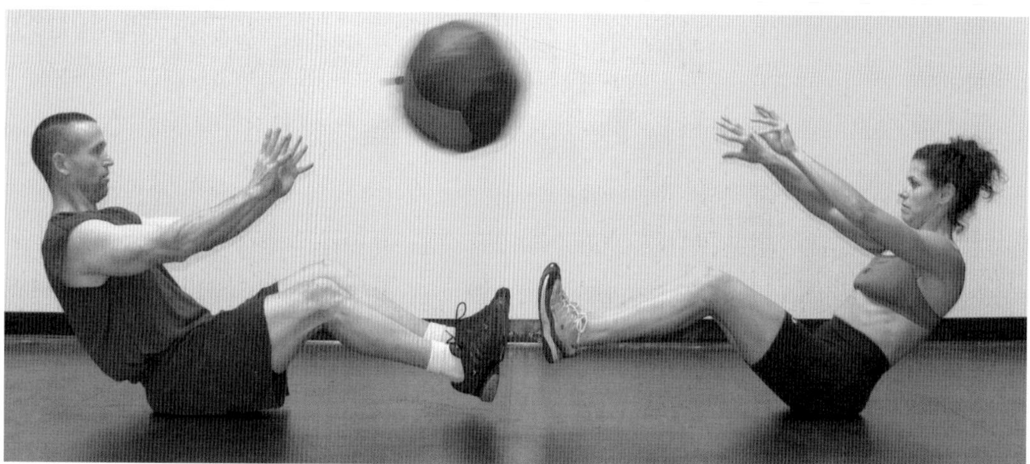

**STARTING POSITION:** Face each other in a seated position, balanced on your butt with your feet off the ground.

**THE MOVE:** Pass the ball to your partner. He catches it and passes it back.

### TRAINING TIPS

- Keep your inner core activated throughout the movement.
- Initiate the movement from your center, not your arms.
- Maintain a balanced ready position throughout the exercise.

# FULL SIT-UP WITH HANDOFF

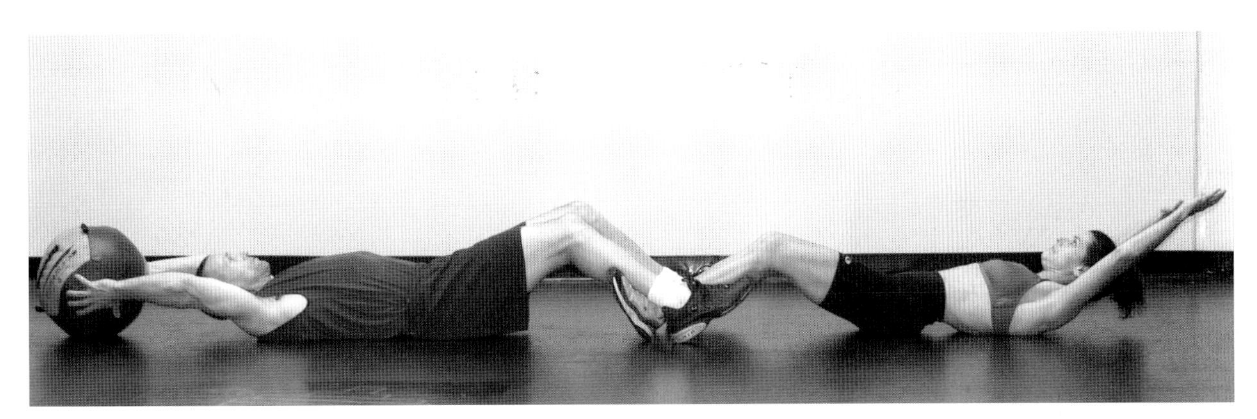

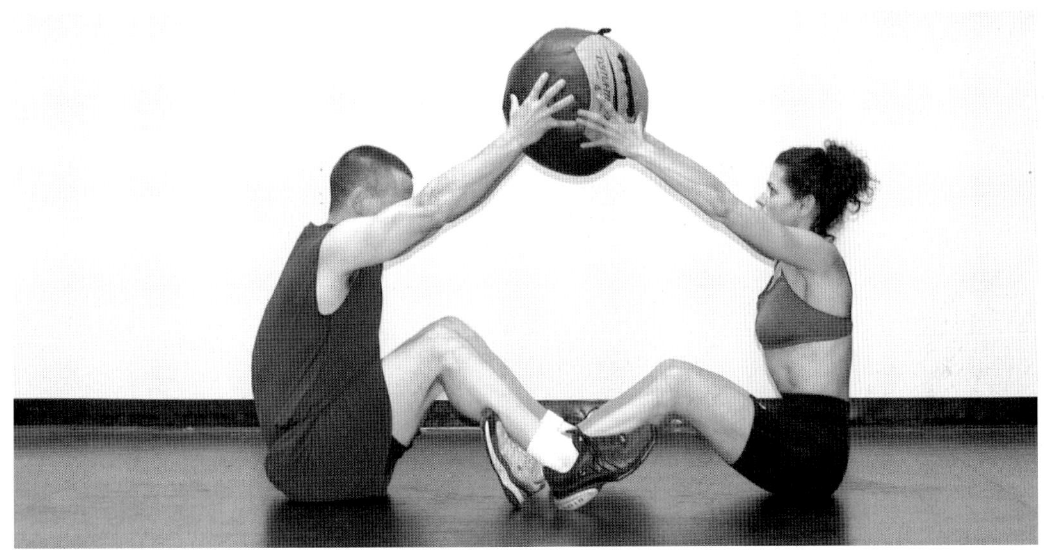

**STARTING POSITION:** Face each other in a seated position with your ankles interlocked, then lower your torso to the floor.

**THE MOVE:** Both exercisers simultaneously roll up to a seated position. The person with the ball completes the handoff and both exercisers return to the starting position. Repeat with the other person performing the roll-up with the ball and completing the handoff.

## TRAINING TIPS

- Keep your inner core activated throughout the movement.
- Initiate the movement from your center, not your arms.
- Maintain a balanced ready position throughout the exercise.

# BALANCE POSITION: SIDE PASS

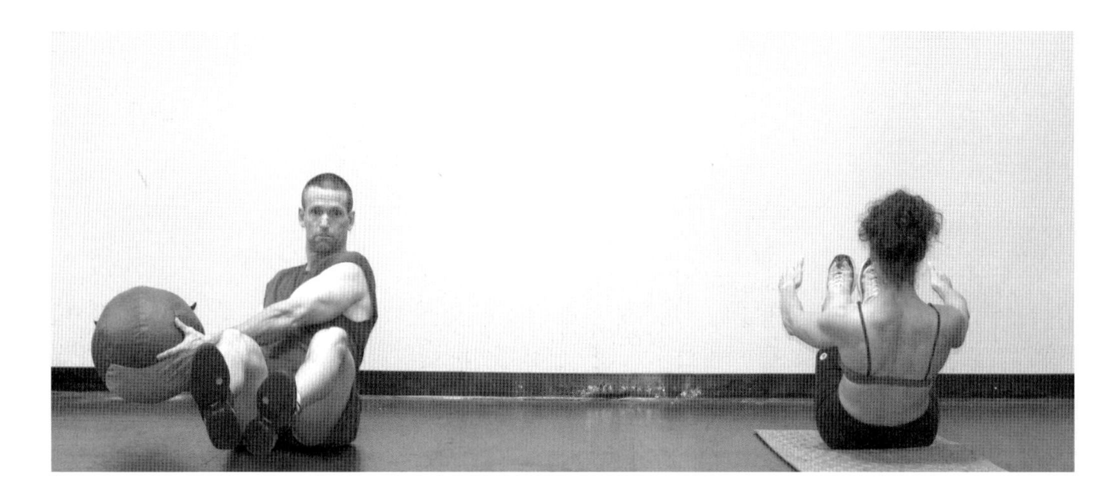

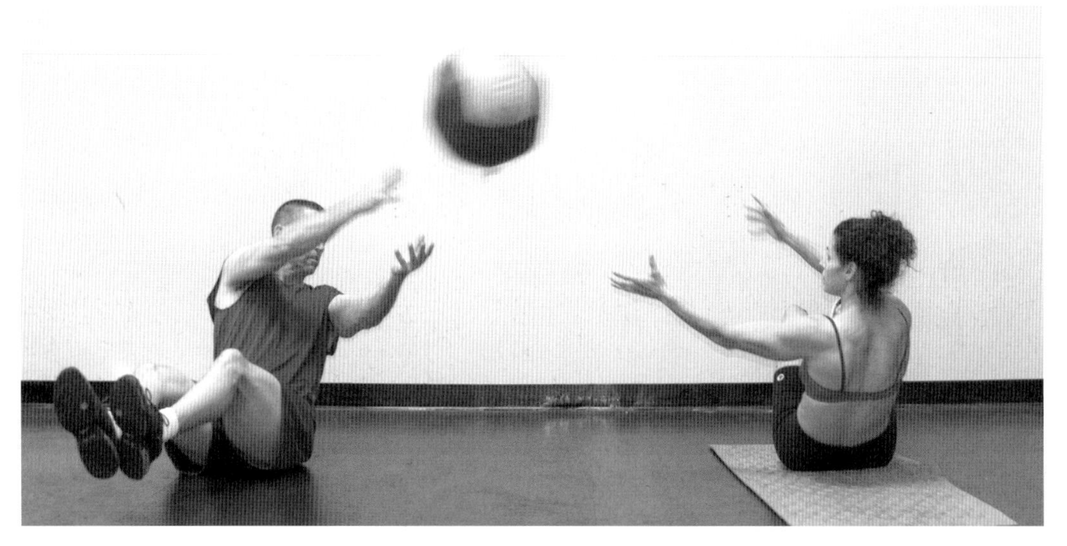

**STARTING POSITION:** Sit in a balance position side to side with your partner, approximately five feet away from your partner. One person holds the medicine ball at chest level.

**THE MOVE:** Move the ball out to the side away from your partner, then in a high arcing motion, toss the ball to your partner. Your partner will repeat the motion and toss back to you.

### TRAINING TIPS

- Keep your inner core activated throughout the movement.
- Initiate the movement from your center, not your arms.
- Maintain a balanced ready position throughout the exercise.

# BALANCE POSITION: SIDE HANDOFF

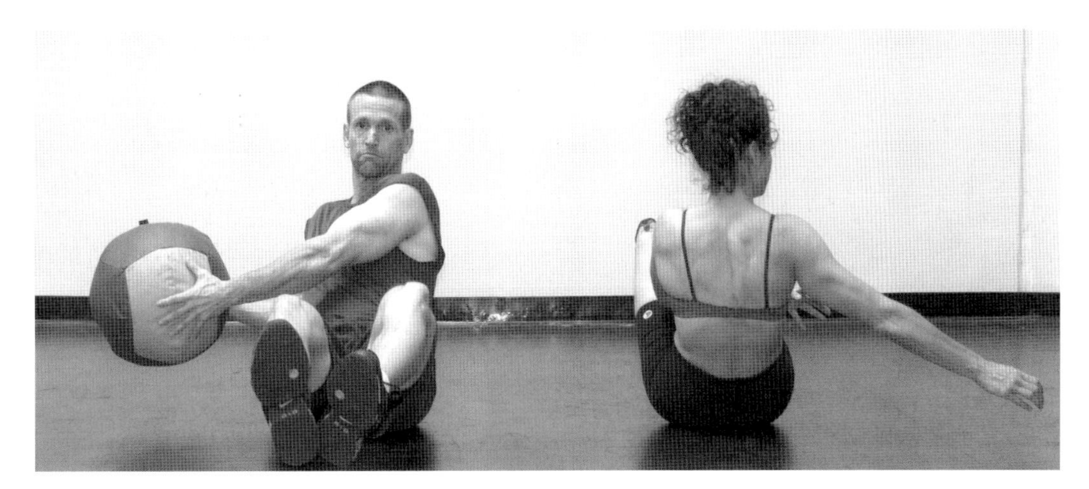

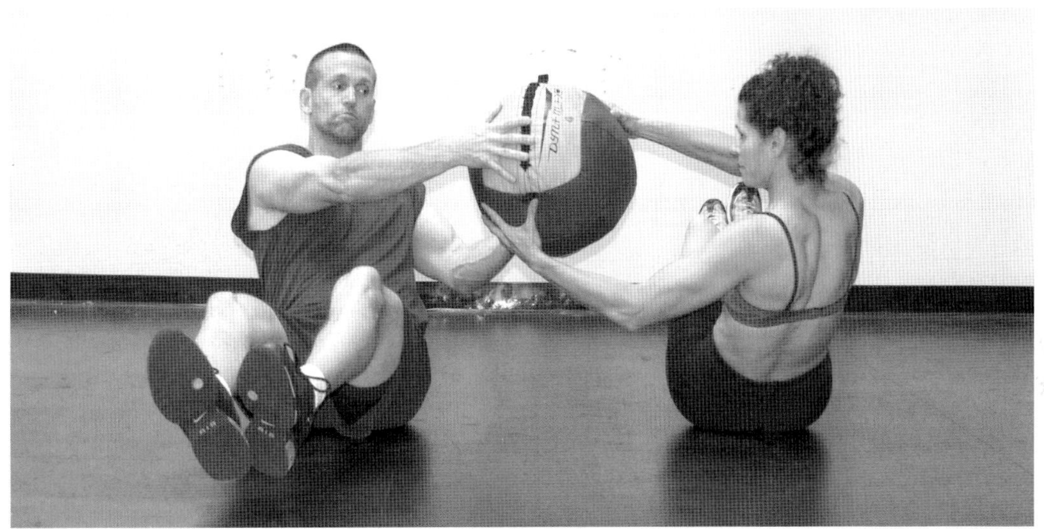

**STARTING POSITION:** Sit in a balance position side to side with your partner, approximately a foot apart. One person holds the medicine ball out to his side away from the partner.

**THE MOVE:** Rotate toward each other, handing the ball to your partner. Then rotate back to center and repeat.

### TRAINING TIPS

- Keep your inner core activated throughout the movement.
- Initiate the movement from your center, not your arms.
- Maintain a balanced ready position throughout the exercise.

## LYING

# FULL SIT-UP WITH TOSS

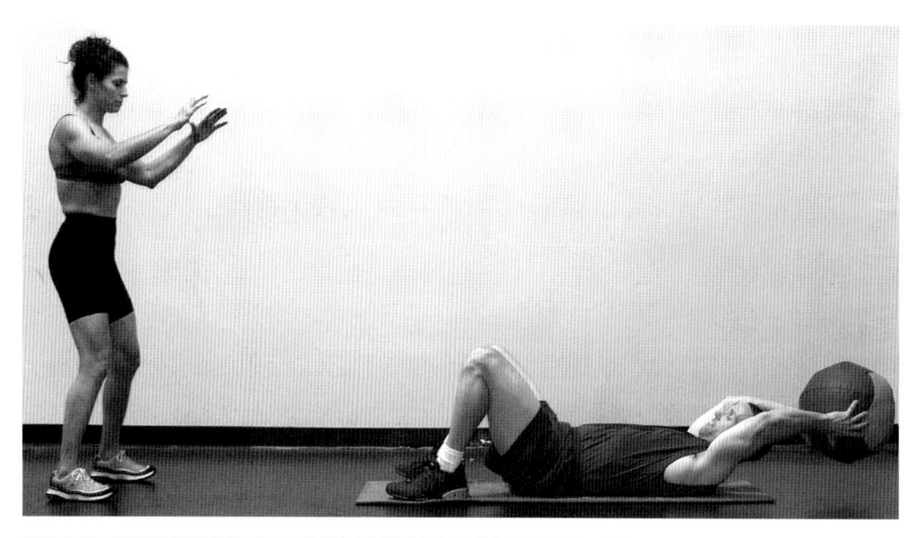

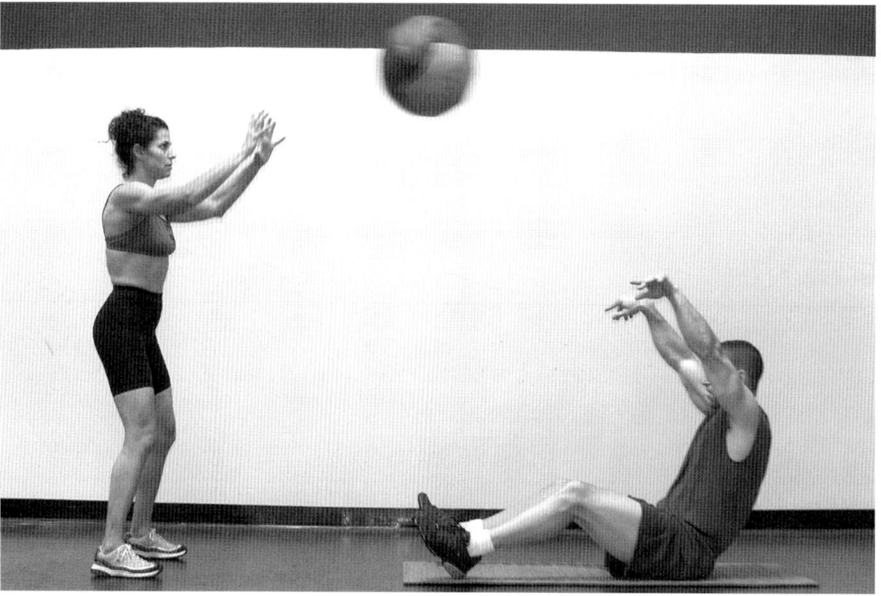

**STARTING POSITION:** Face each other, one person holding the ball and lying on his back with his knees bent and feet flat on the floor. The other person stands in the ready position three to five feet away.

**THE MOVE:** The person on the floor rises in a sit-up motion as he passes the ball to his partner. His partner catches it and passes it back. The person on the floor lowers his body back to the starting position and repeats.

### TRAINING TIPS

- **Keep your inner core activated throughout the movement.**
- **Initiate the movement from your center, not your arms.**
- **Maintain a balanced ready position throughout the exercise.**

### PRESCRIPTION

- **Level One: Work up to ten reps for each exercise. If you're alternating sides, then do 5 reps on each side.**
- **Build up slowly; start out by working on proper technique and form, resting when needed between repetitions and sets.**
- **Level Two: Rest three minutes and repeat entire routine.**

## CORE ROTATION, BY STEVEN WILDE

### INTRODUCTION

This routine trains your core to be strong in all directions with exercises that emphasize rotation and side-to-side movements.

### THE EXERCISES

Plank—Swinging Gate, p. 316

OTB: Lateral Back Extensions, p. 254

On the Ball—Shoulder Roll, p. 269

Woodchop—Low Cable (do all the repetitions on one side then switch to the other side), p. 332

### THE ROUTINE

- **Work up to 15 reps on each side for each exercise.**
- **Work up to 3 sets, resting one minute between sets.**

## SOCCER ROUTINE, BY BRETT BRUNGARDT

### INTRODUCTION

This routine is designed to improve performance and endurance, emphasizing the muscles used in soccer.

### EXERCISES

V-ups with a Cross, p. 304

Superman with Rotation, p. 306

Side Superman, p. 238

Woodchop: Low Cable, p. 332

Woodchop: High Cable, p. 333

Balance T-Bend, p. 327

Glute Bridge: 45 Degree with Hip Rotation, p. 274

Leg Overs: Double Leg, p. 262

### PRESCRIPTION

- **Work up to 30 reps for each exercise. If you are alternating sides in a move then do 15 reps on each side.**
- **Work up to 2 sets in the off season, resting 1 minute between sets. In season do one set for maintainence.**

## POSTPARTUM CORE ROUTINE, BY DEBBIE HOLMES

This routine will help you get your core strength back after giving birth. Do not start this routine until you have been cleared by a doctor. Understand that every birth experience is unique and will require more or less healing. Be patient with your body after giving birth.

I'd encourage you to begin walking before you start these exercises. Concentrate on keeping your abdominal muscles tight while you walk by pulling your belly button toward your spine. This is a great way to begin your core training. Once your body feels good in your walking routine, you can begin your core routine.

Lastly, it is normal for your abdominal muscles to be extra sore for the next several months; they've been stretched and challenged the last several months. It will take a few months of muscle, tendon, and ligament repair before you will be pain-free again. Don't begin your core routine if you are experiencing abdominal or pelvic pain, bleeding or spotting, cramping, or dizziness. If you do experience any of the above symptoms, stop immediately, and discuss your exercise routine with your doctor.

## THE ROUTINES

### LEVEL ONE

Standing Knee Flexion, p. 243

Pelvic Rock, p. 275, with Kegels, p. 53

Knee Touch, Crossing, p. 226

Opposite Arm and Leg—All Fours, p. 247

Lying Side Leg Raise, p. 290

Lying Inside Leg Raise, p. 291

### LEVEL TWO

Standing Knee Flexion, p. 243

Glute Bridge with Kegels, p. 277

Knee Touch—Crossing, p. 226

Back Extensions, p. 254

Lying Side Leg Raise, p. 290

Lying Inside Leg Raise, p. 291

Tummy Tucks, p. 302

Down Plank, p. 314

Side Plank, p. 314

## PRESCRIPTION

- **Work up to 20 repetitions for each exercise. If you're alternating sides on an exercise do 10 reps on each exercise.**
- **Once you've achieved that goal, add a second set.**
- **When you can do 2 sets at Level One with confidence and ease, move on to Level Two.**
- **When you've achieved the repetition goals for Level Two, add a second set.**

# KID CORE, BY DAVE JOHNSON

### INTRODUCTION

This routine is designed for kids. It will train the core muscles, building a strong foundation for health, sports, and fun activities.

### EXERCISES

Knee Touch, crossing, p. 226

Heel Touches, p. 257–59

Ankle Reaches, p. 250

Glute Bridge, p. 277

### PRESCRIPTION

- **Work up to 10 reps for each exercise. If you are alternating sides, do 5 on each side.**
- **For an added challenge, rest one minute and then repeat the entire routine.**

# CORE FOOTBALL, BY BAY McCLINTON

**INTRODUCTION:** This routine will train your core muscles to perform better in game situations. These simple drills will increase the strength in your stabalization muscles and improve your balance.

# THE EXERCISES

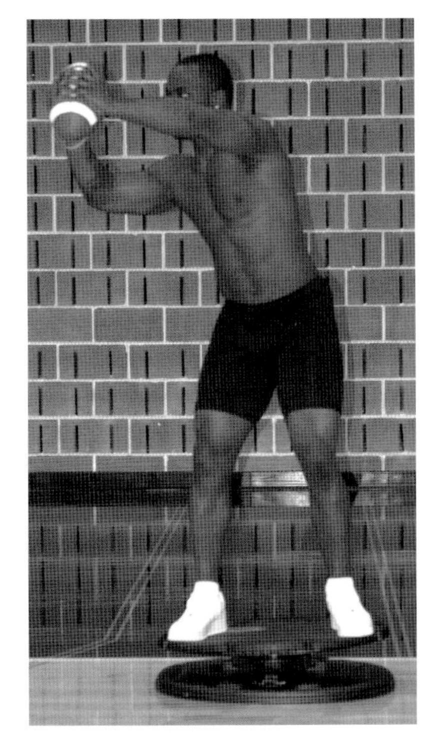
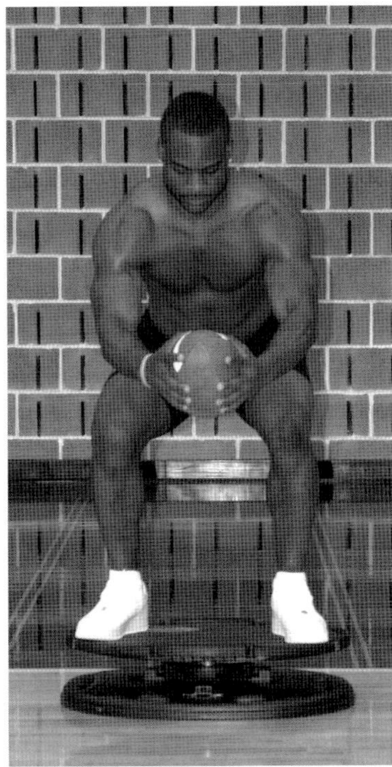
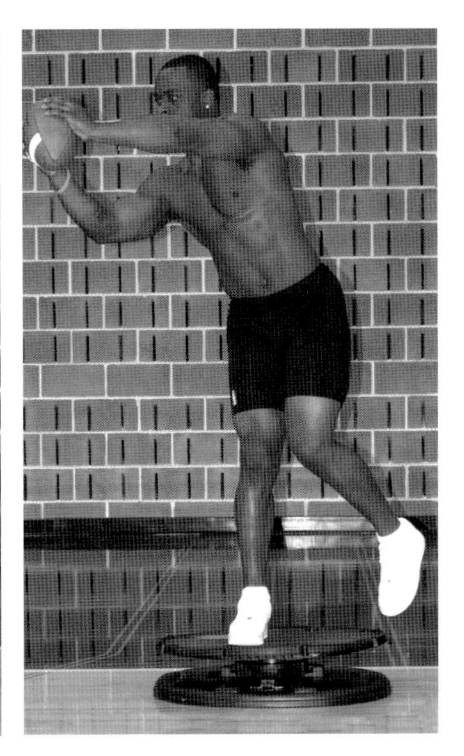

In all of these exercises someone throws the ball to the athlete on the core board.

**CATCH-1:** **Catch the ball high and to your right with both feet planted on the core board. Alternate sides each time.**

**CATCH-2:** **Catch a low pass in the center of your body with both feet planted on the core board.**

**CATCH-3:** **Catch the ball high and to your right, balancing on one leg. Alternate catch sides, then switch legs and alternate catch sides.**

### THE WORKOUT

- **Do 10 repetitions for each catch (this means 10 on each side).**

# DYNAMIC MEDICINE BALL ROUTINE, BY MARTIN KAMMLER

## INTRODUCTION

This routine changes your center of gravity, challenging your core and improving your mind-muscle connection. The shifting positions of balance will improve your functional strength in life and in sports.

## THE EXERCISES

# STATIC LUNGE WITH ROTATION

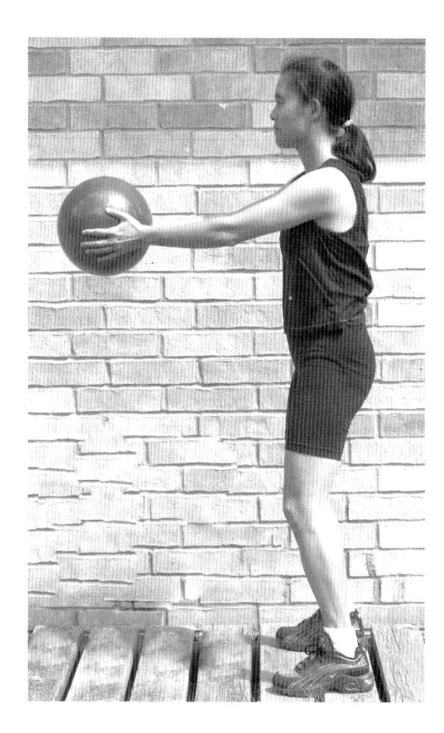

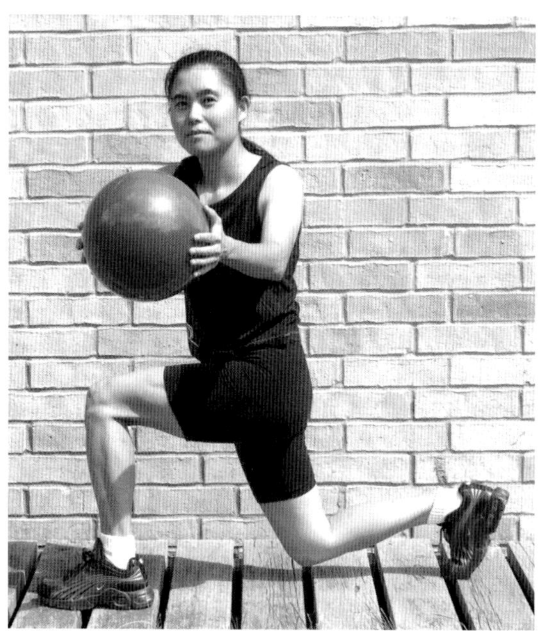

**STARTING POSITION:** In the ready position, hold a medicine ball in front of your chest, arms extended.

**THE MOVEMENT:** Lunge, leading with your left leg, bending your right knee toward the floor, but keep your knee about 2 to 3 inches off the floor. Stay in this position and rotate the ball from left to right, back and forth across your body for the prescribed number of repetitions. Repeat on other side, switching lead legs.

## DYNAMIC LUNGE WITH ROTATION

This exercise is the same as the Lunge with Rotation, except you walk forward with each lunge, as you rotate the ball out to the side.

## LUNGE WITH OVERHEAD RAISE

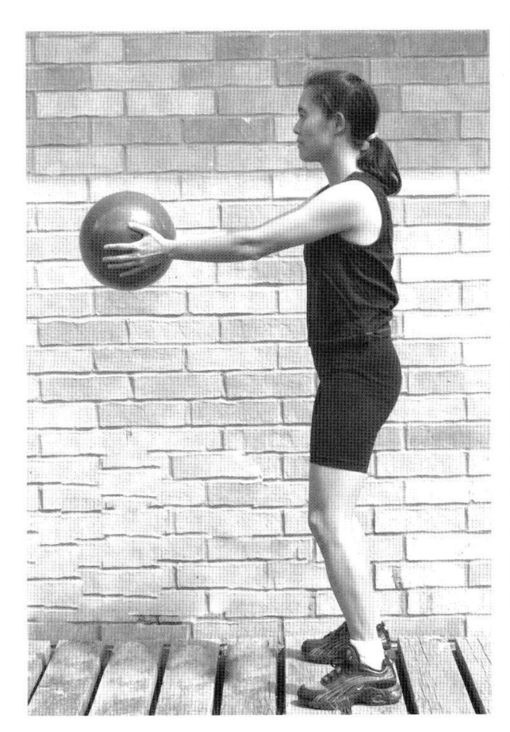

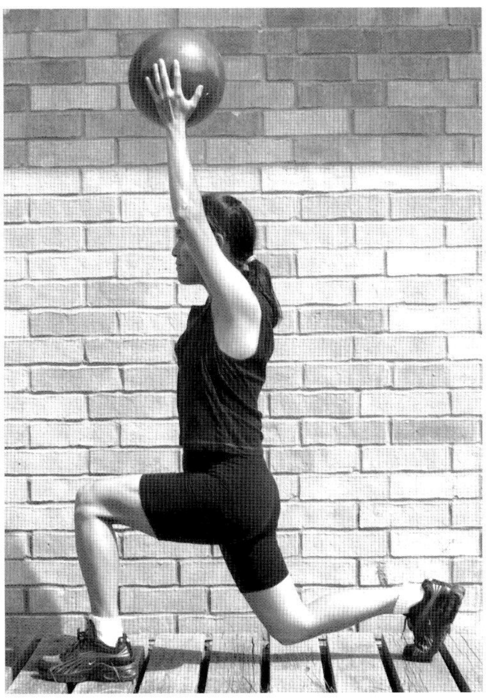

**STARTING POSITION:** In the ready position, hold a medicine ball in front of your chest.

**THE MOVEMENT:** Lunge, leading with your left leg, bending your right knee toward the floor as you raise the ball over your head, then lowering it as you return to the starting position. Complete your set, then switch lead legs.

# WALKING LUNGE WITH OVERHEAD RAISE

This exercise is the same as the Lunge with Overhead Raise, except you walk forward with each lunge, as you raise the ball over your head.

### THE ROUTINE

- **For each exercise work up to 15 reps for each leg.**
- **You can also add sets, working up to three sets for each exercise.**
- **After you have mastered the static moves, progress to the dynamic variations. Stay with the same repetition scheme. If you are working in an area with limited space you may have to turn around a couple of times to get 15 reps on each leg.**

# GOLF ROUTINE, BY BRETT BRUNGARDT

### INTRODUCTION

This routine exercises the key core muscles that are essential for achieving your full potential on the course.

### EXERCISES

Woodchop: High Cable, p. 333

Standing Woodchop: Low Cable, p. 332

Leg Over: Single Leg, p. 261

Superman with Rotation, p. 306

On the Ball: Glute Bridge, Single Leg, p. 294

Plank—Swinging Gate, p. 316

### PRESCRIPTION

- **Work up to 20 reps for each exercise. If you alternate sides on move, do 10 reps on each side.**
- **To increase the intensity, rest one minute and repeat the circuit.**

PART SEVEN

# THE EXERCISES

# 23
# INTRODUCTION TO THE EXERCISES

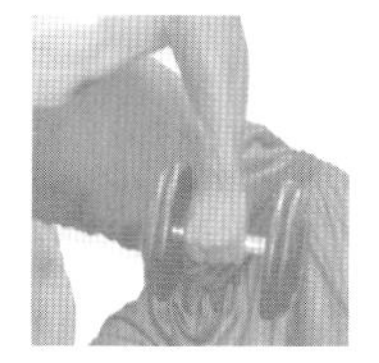

## THE EXERCISES

We know that all these exercises and variations can be maddening. The goal of this book is to give you a range of choices, so you can always have variety in your workouts. At the same time, we want the exercise section to be ordered and easy to use.

These chapters are broken down by movement direction and muscle area. There are five categories: Flexion Movements (forward bending moves and side-to-side bending moves), Extension Movements (backward bending moves and raising up moves), Rotation and Crossing Movements, Combination Moves (movements that combine more than one of the above categories), and Hip and Butt Moves.

## EXERCISE INFORMATION

The following is an explanation of the guidelines for each exercise.

**DIFFICULTY LEVEL.** This gives you guidance on how difficult the exercise is—1 being the easiest and 3 being the hardest. If you've been training consistently for a year and have a strong and healthy lower back, you should be able to do most of the exercises in this book. Some exercises will present more of a challenge. Safety must always come first. If you are unsure, consult a qualified professional.

**LOWER BACK.** This gives you guidance on the risk of injury to the lower back—low, moderate, or high. If you have a history of lower back problems, you need to proceed with extra care and consult a specialist for advice on your specific condition.

The Difficulty Level and Lower Back guidelines cannot be objective standards for everyone. Certain movements are going to be easy or difficult, low or high risk, depending on your personal history and strengths and weaknesses. But the guidelines can be a helpful starting place.

**STARTING POSITION.** This heading explains the proper starting position.

**THE MOVE.** This section outlines correct movement for the exercise.

**TRAINING TIPS:** This section acts as a personal trainer, giving you exercise tips. Some of the tips will be specific to the exercise; others will be constant reminders, tips that are true for every exercise. Like having a personal trainer at your side, hearing these tips over and over may get annoying, but hearing them repeated will make them second nature. The following tips are essential for core work:

1. Activate your inner core.
2. Keep the motion controlled for both the positive and negative phases of the movement—no bouncing or jerking.
3. Don't rest at the beginning of each new repetition before you begin the next one.
4. Focus your mind on feeling your core muscles do the work, putting your mind in the muscle. Don't just go through the motions.
5. Maintain proper posture and Ready Position.
6. Initiate the movements from your center.
7. Breathe!

**VARIETY:** Many of these exercises can be done in a variety of ways: on an exercise ball, using weights, a resistance band, machines, a medicine ball, a core board, and so forth. As you build a foundation of strength, you can experiment with these variations and create your own unique variations.

# 24
# FLEXION MOVES

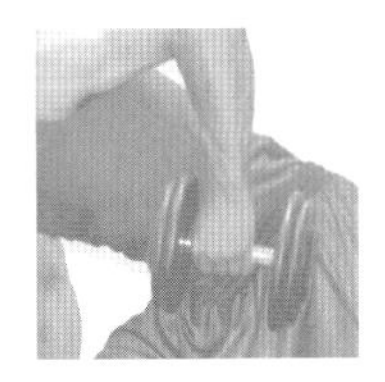

# EXERCISE: MODIFIED V-UP

DIFFICULTY: **2** LOWER BACK: **MODERATE RISK**

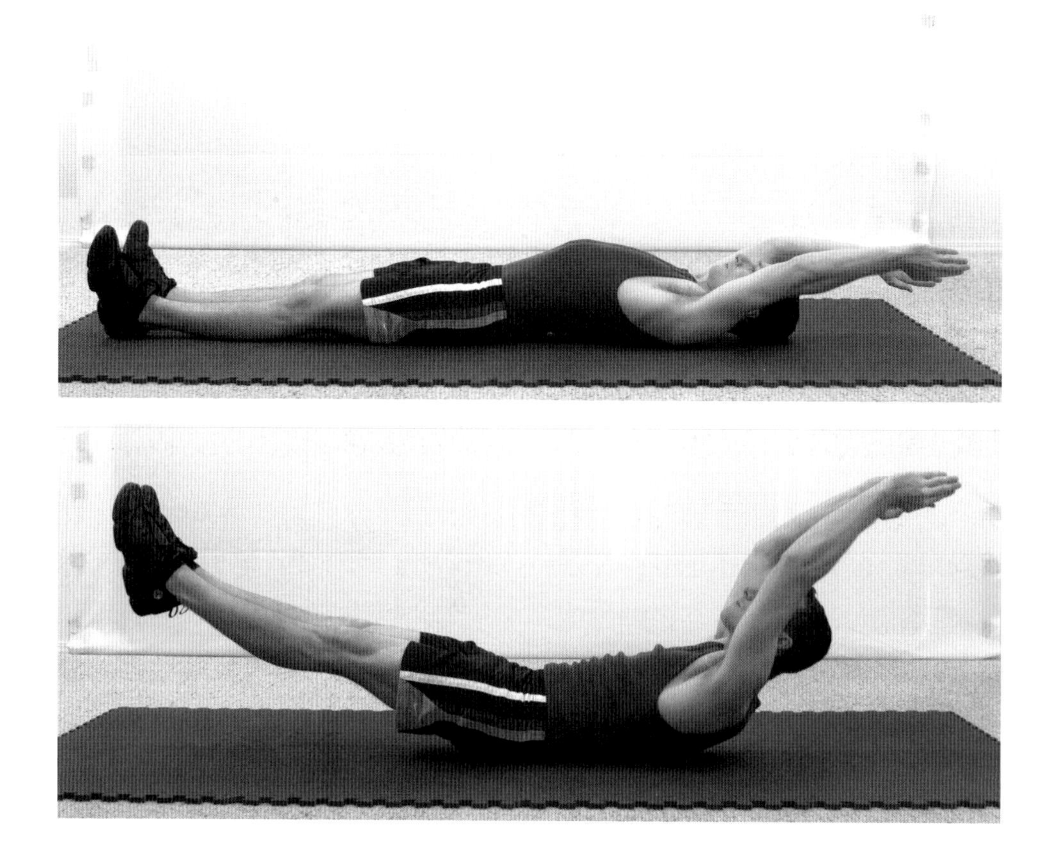

**STARTING POSITION:** Lie on your back with your legs fully extended on the floor and your arms extended over your head.

**THE MOVE:** Simultaneously raise your arms, torso, and legs off the floor. Hold the contraction at the top of the movement. Lower the arms and legs, lightly touching the floor.

### TRAINING TIPS

- Before you raise the arm, extend the spine by lengthening your arms and legs, as if someone was pulling on them.
- Feel the movement initiating from the center of your body.
- Control both the up and down phases of the movement.

# EXERCISE: V-UPS

DIFFICULTY: **3** LOWER BACK: **HIGH RISK**

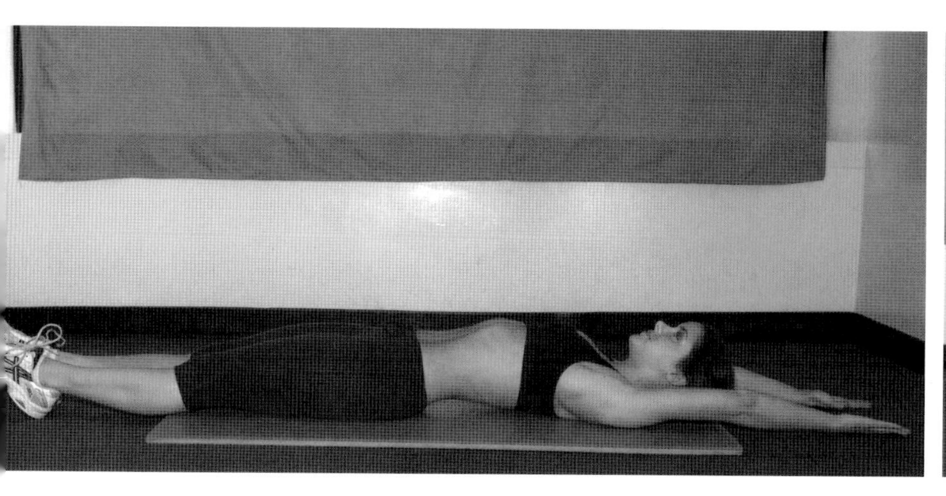

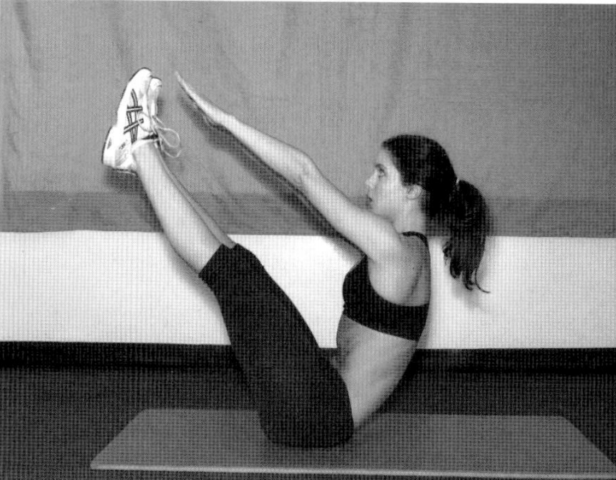

**STARTING POSITION:** Lie flat on your back, legs extended straight (knees unlocked), heels resting on floor, arms extended over your head.

**THE MOVE:** Use your core to simultaneously raise your torso and legs together like the closing of a hinge. Your hands touch your feet at the top of the movement. Then, in a controlled motion, lower your legs and torso back to the starting position. Repeat.

### TRAINING TIPS

- Focus on feeling your inner core pull your torso and legs together.
- Keep the movement controlled—don't jerk yourself up.
- Don't rest your arms and legs at the bottom of the movement.
- Focus your mind on feeling your core muscles do the work.

# EXERCISE: KNEE TOUCH—CROSSING

DIFFICULTY: **1** LOWER BACK: **LOW RISK**

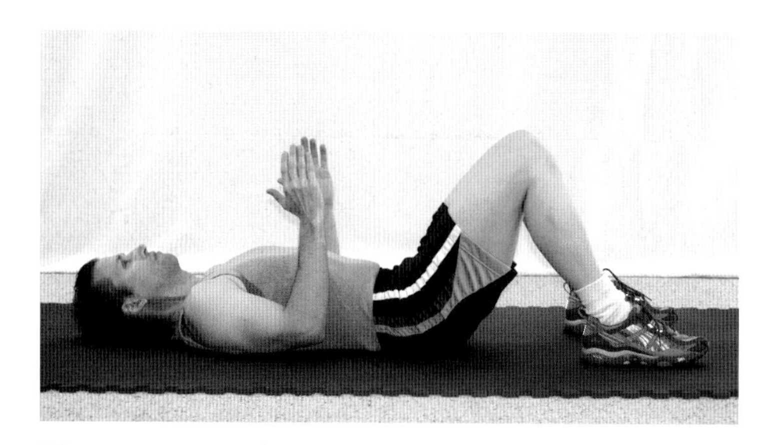

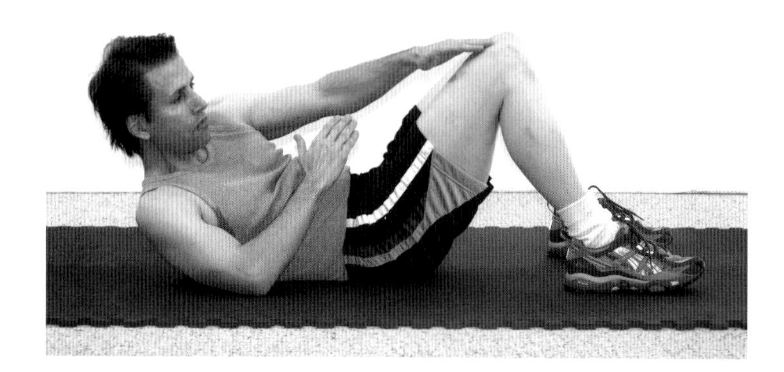

**STARTING POSITION:** Lie flat on your back, knees bent, feet flat on the floor, and hands pointing up.

**THE MOVE:** Raise your shoulder blades off the floor, crossing your left hand to touch the top of your right knee. Repeat to the other side.

**TRAINING TIPS**

- Keep your inner core activated.
- Keep a neutral spine.
- Initiate the movement from the center of your body, not your arms and legs.
- Don't rest at the bottom of the movement.

# EXERCISE: CRUNCHES—RAISED HIPS

DIFFICULTY: **2** LOWER BACK: **MODERATE RISK**

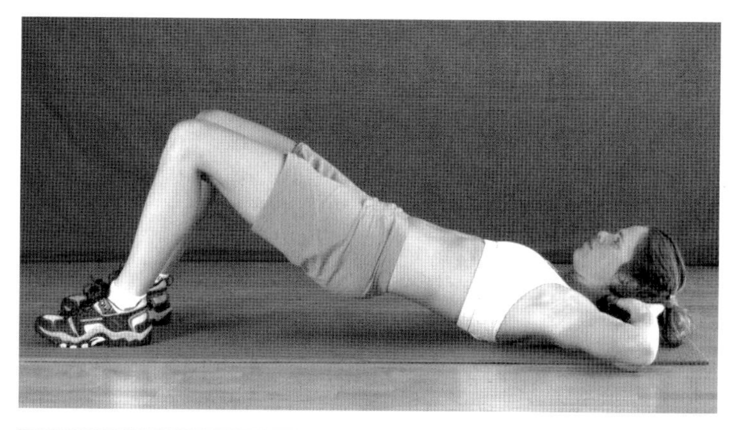

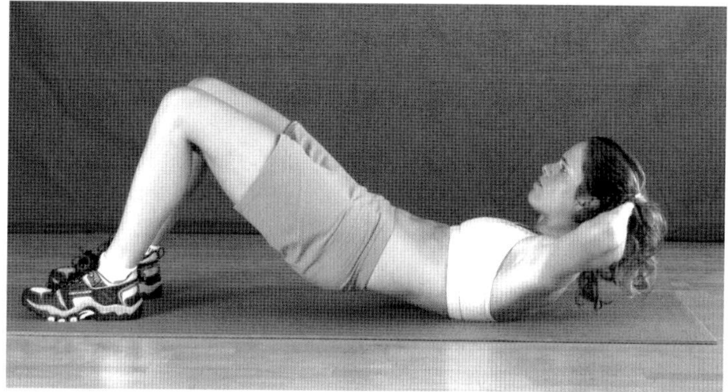

**STARTING POSITION:** Lie on your back, knees bent, feet flat on the floor. Raise your hips off the floor into a glute bridge position. Hold this position throughout the exercise.

**THE MOVE:** Use your core to raise your shoulder blades off the floor. Lower and repeat. Your range of motion will be only a few inches.

### TRAINING TIPS

- Keep your inner core activated.
- Make sure your shoulder blades come off the floor.
- Don't rest at the bottom of the movement.
- Don't let your hips drop.

# EXERCISE: TOE TOUCH 1

DIFFICULTY: **1** LOWER BACK: **LOW RISK**

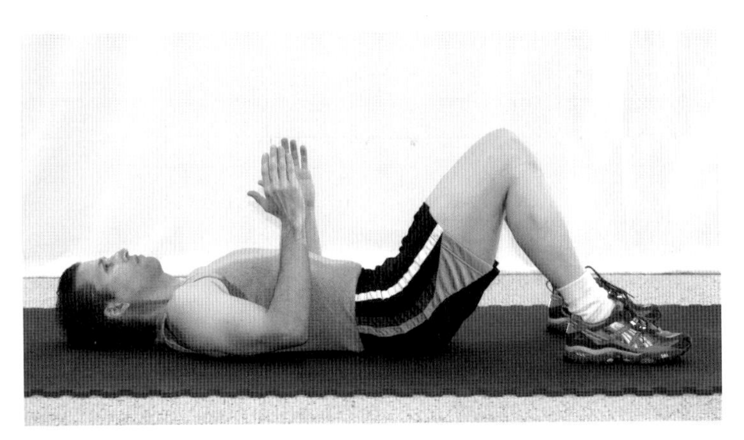

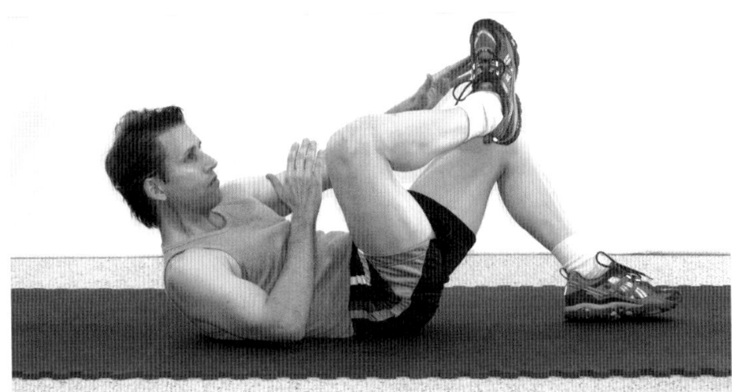

**STARTING POSITION:** Lie flat on your back, knees bent, feet flat on the floor, and hands pointing up.

**THE MOVE:** Simultaneously raise your torso and your right leg off the floor, reaching your left hand to your right toe. Return to the starting position and repeat to the other side.

### TRAINING TIPS

- Keep your inner core activated.
- Keep a neutral spine.
- Initiate the movement from the center of your body, not your arms and legs.
- Don't rest at the bottom of the movement.

# EXERCISE: TOE TOUCH 2

DIFFICULTY: **2** LOWER BACK: **LOW RISK**

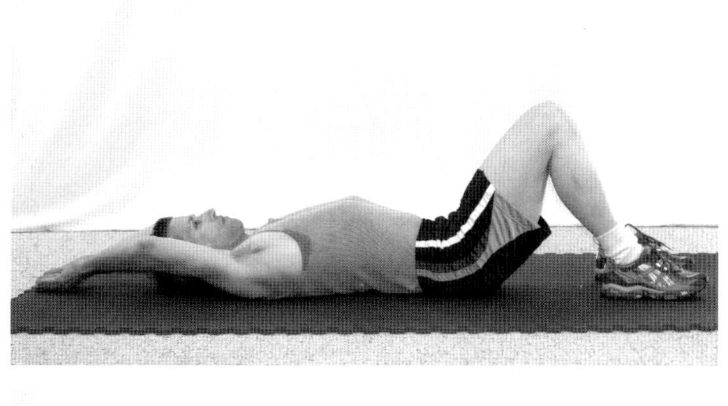

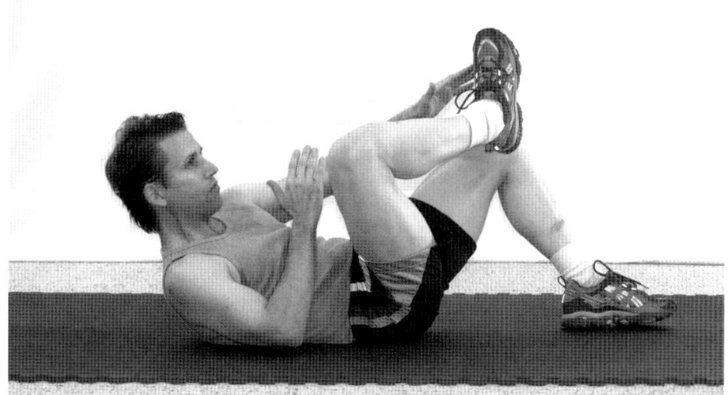

**STARTING POSITION:** Lie flat on your back, knees bent, feet flat on the floor, and hands extended over your head.

**THE MOVE:** Simultaneously raise your torso and and your right leg off the floor, reaching your left hand to your right toe. Return to the starting position and repeat to the other side.

### TRAINING TIPS

- Keep your inner core activated.
- Keep a neutral spine.
- Initiate the movement from the center of your body, not your arms and legs.
- Don't rest at the bottom of the movement.

# EXERCISE: TOE TOUCH 3

DIFFICULTY: **3** LOWER BACK: **MODERATE RISK**

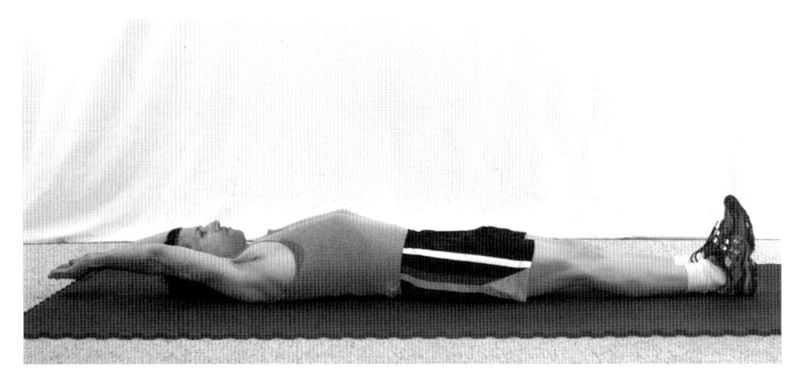

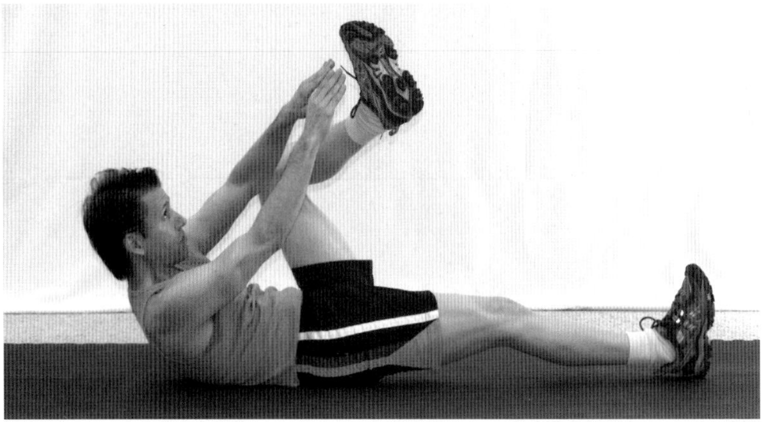

**STARTING POSITION:** Lie flat on your back, legs fully extended and hands extended over your head.

**THE MOVE:** Simultaneously raise your torso and and your right leg off the floor, reaching both hands to your right toe. Return to the starting position and repeat to the other side.

### TRAINING TIPS

- Keep your inner core activated.
- Keep a neutral spine.
- Initiate the movement from the center of your body, not your arms and legs.
- Don't rest at the bottom of the movement.

# EXERCISE: ROLL-UP

DIFFICULTY: **3** LOWER BACK: **MODERATE RISK**

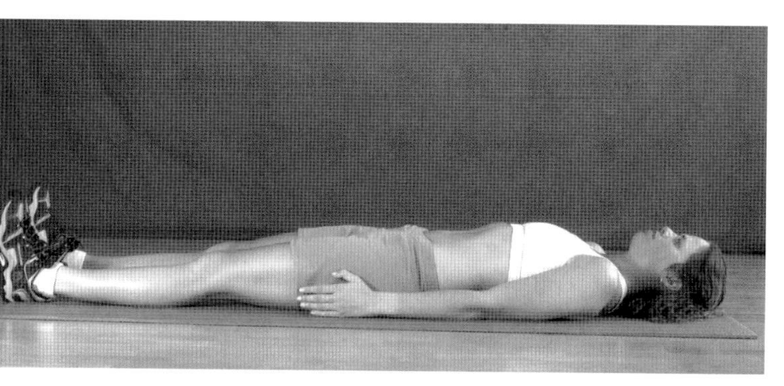

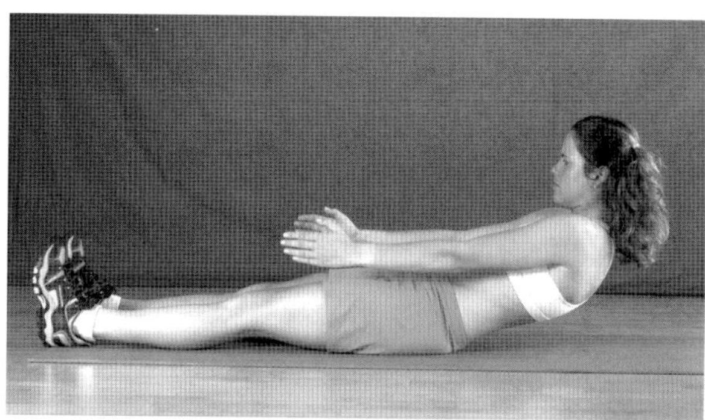

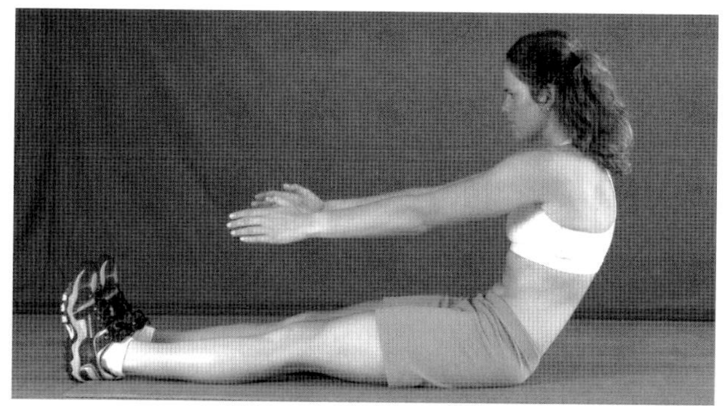

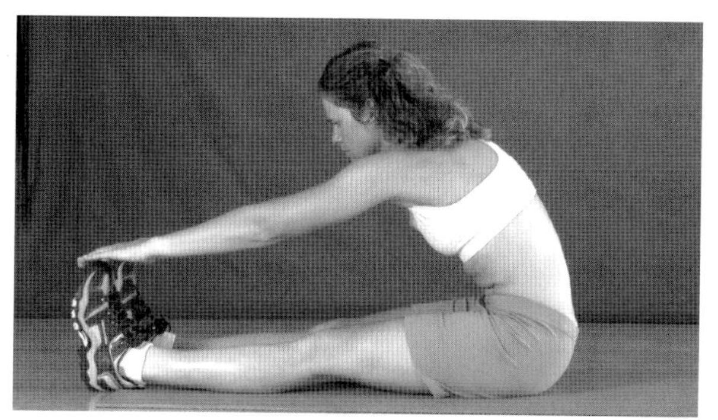

**STARTING POSITION:** Lie on your back, hands at your sides, legs extended straight out.

**THE MOVE:** Use your core to raise your torso vertebra by vertebra off the floor as your hands reach to your feet.

### TRAINING TIPS

- Keep reaching forward with your arms.
- Keep your feet on the ground.
- Start the upward movement from the top of your spine and head. Begin the lowering phase from the bottom of your spine, ending with your neck.

# EXERCISE: LEG RAISE

DIFFICULTY: **2** LOWER BACK: **HIGH RISK**

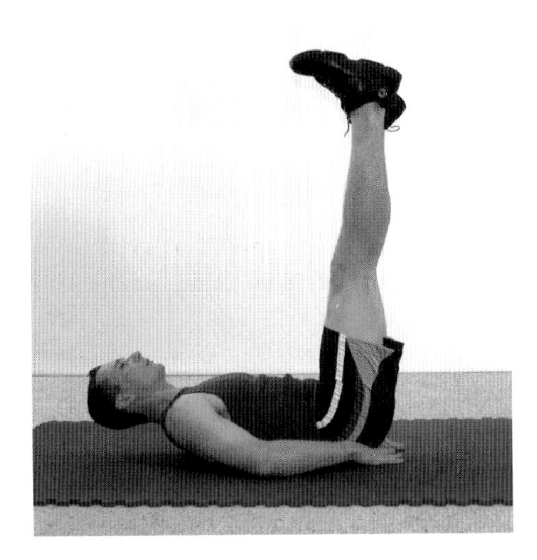

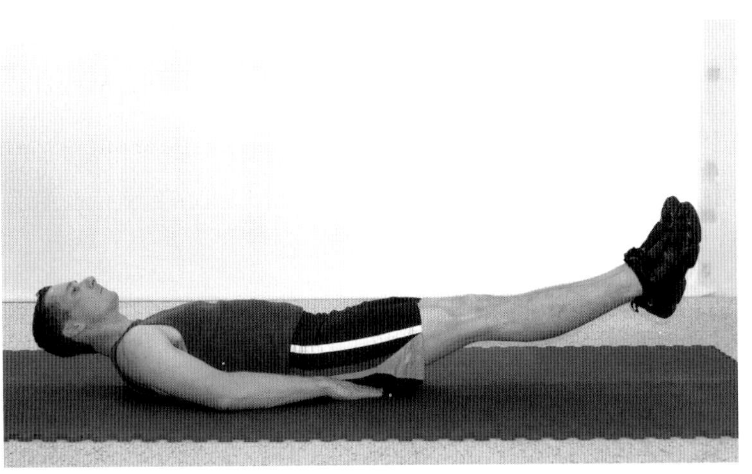

**STARTING POSITION:** Lie on your back, legs raised perpendicular to your upper body. Place your hands at your sides (or under your butt for support), neutral spine, neck lengthened.

**THE MOVE:** Lower your legs toward the floor. Lower your legs, only to a distance that will enable you to maintain a neutral spine. This is your range of motion. Then raise your legs back to the starting position in a controlled motion. Repeat. This move can also be done with one leg at a time. Alternate legs with each rep.

### TRAINING TIPS

- Don't allow your spine to move out of neutral, creating an exaggerated arch in your lower back.
- Keep your inner core activated.
- Move from the center of your body.

# MOVEMENT SEQUENCES

DIFFICULTY: **3** LOWER BACK: **HIGH RISK**

**SCISSORS:** Using your core muscles, lower your right leg as far as you can while maintaining a neutral spine. Then raise it back to the starting position as you simultaneously lower your left leg. Your legs will pass each other midway.

**FIGURE EIGHTS:** Within your range of motion, draw imaginary figure eight with your feet. Switch directions after each figure is drawn. Continue until you complete your set.

**CIRCLES:** Within your range of motion, draw circles with your feet; switch directions with the completion of each circle. Continue movement until you complete your set.

**CRISSCROSSES.** Within your range of motion, crisscross your legs back and forth, alternating top and bottom positions with your legs. Each cross counts as a rep.

# EXERCISE: SWIMMING ON BACK

DIFFICULTY: **2** LOWER BACK: **MODERATE RISK**

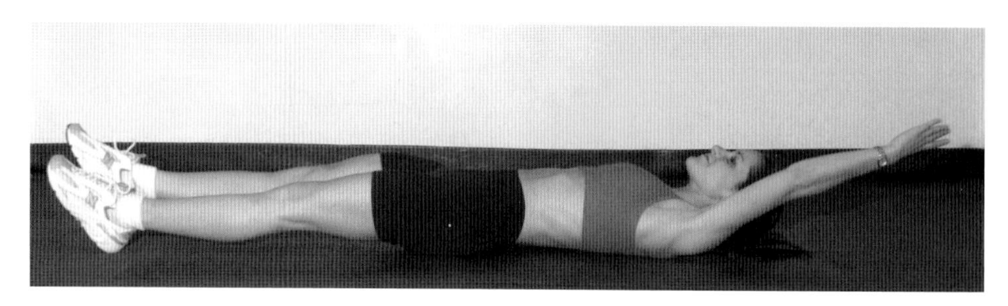

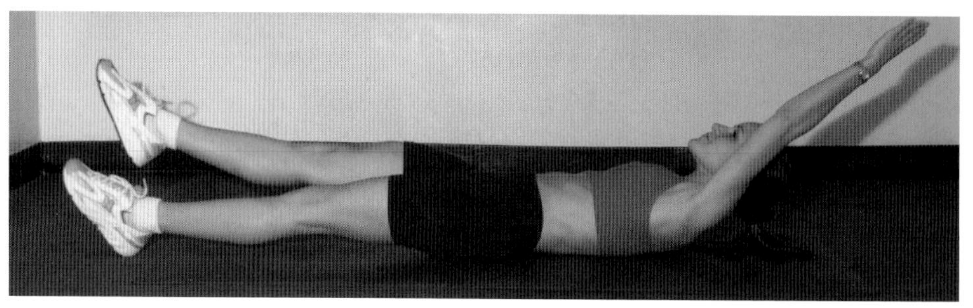

**STARTING POSITION:** Lie on your back with your legs fully extended on the floor and your arms extended over your head.

**THE MOVE:** Simultaneously raise your left arm, torso, and right leg. Hold the contraction at the top of the movement. Lower the arm and leg until they lightly touch the floor. Then repeat with the other arm and leg.

### TRAINING TIPS

- Before you raise your arm, extend the spine by lengthening the arm and leg you are going to raise.
- Feel the movement initiating from the center of your body.
- Control both the up and down phases of the movement.

# EXERCISE: DOUBLE SIDE JACKKNIFE

DIFFICULTY: **3**   LOWER BACK: **MODERATE RISK**

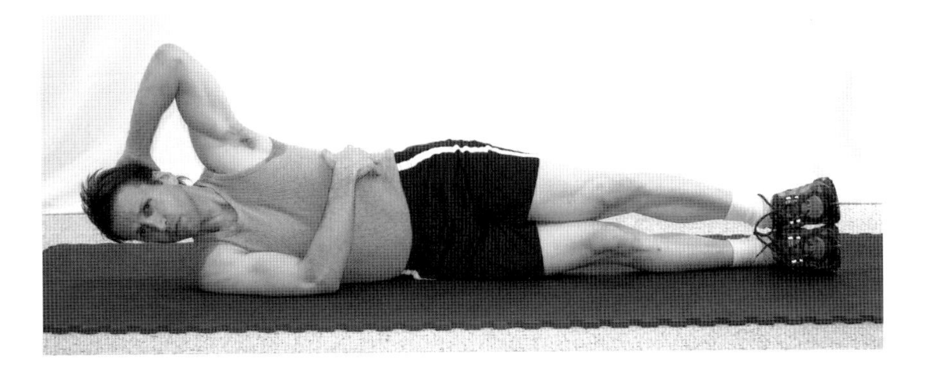

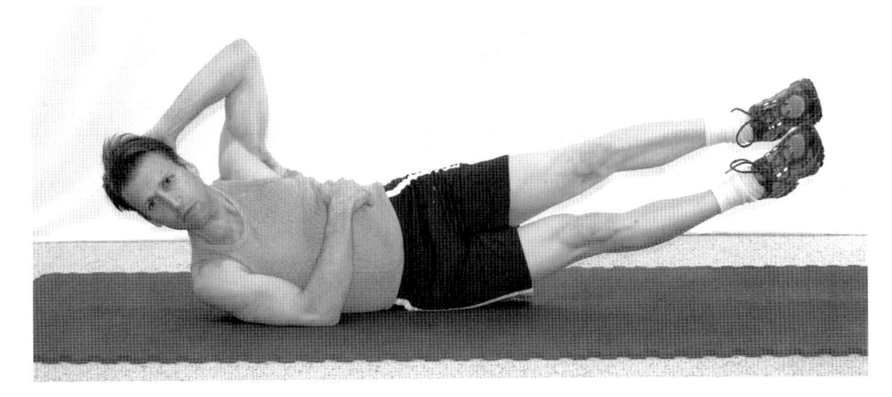

**STARTING POSITION:** Lie on your right hip, legs together and fully extended. Place your right hand on your hip and your left hand behind your ear.

**THE MOVE:** Simultaneously raise your torso and legs. Lower your body in a controlled motion and repeat. Then execute the movement on the other side.

### TRAINING TIPS

- Bring your legs slightly forward to increase your range of motion.
- Focus on moving from the center of your body.
- Make sure your upper body moves off the floor. Don't move just your head.

# EXERCISE: INCHWORM

DIFFICULTY: **2** LOWER BACK: **MODERATE RISK**

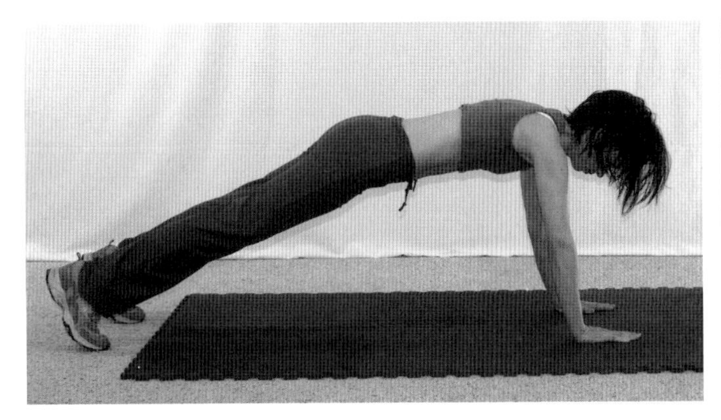

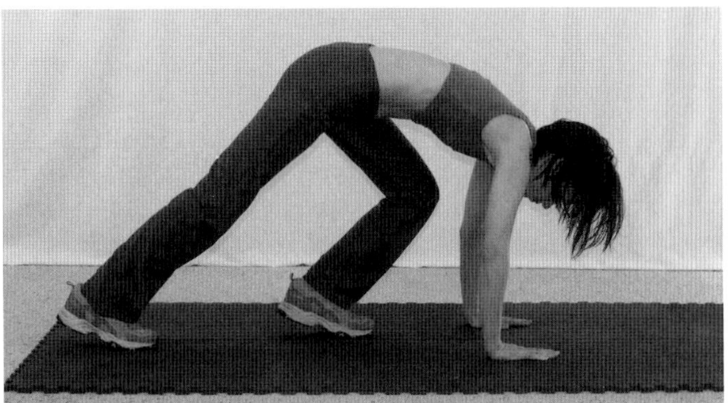

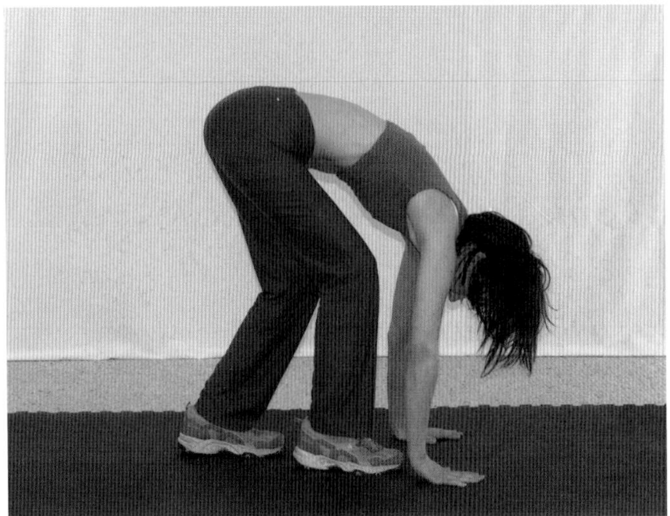

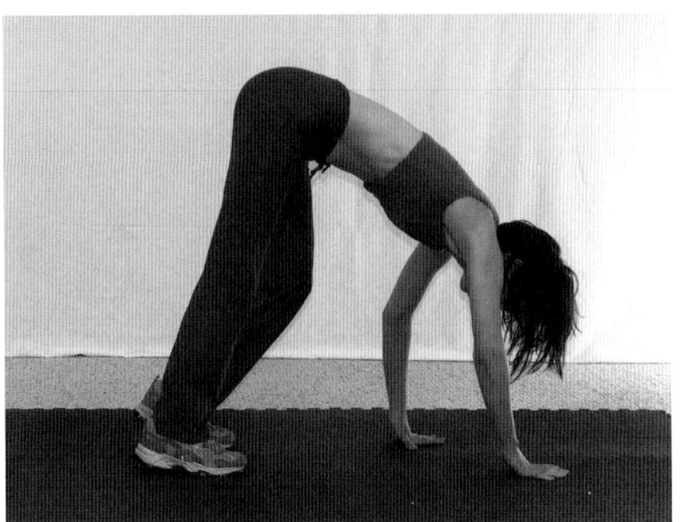

**STARTING POSITION:** Begin in a push-up position.

**THE MOVE:** Walk your feet up toward your hands as far as you can. Then walk your hands out to the plank push-up position. Continue to repeat the move, like an inch-worm moving across the floor.

**VARIATION:** This exercise can also be done moving backward.

### TRAINING TIPS

- Focus on keeping your body aligned and straight.
- Keep your neck lengthened and in line with your spine.
- Maintain a steady balance.
- Keep the motion fluid.
- Since you will move forward with each repetition, give yourself room to crawl. If you are in a limited space, move forward and backward.

## EXERCISE: SIDE DOUBLE CRUNCH

DIFFICULTY: **2** LOWER BACK: **MODERATE RISK**

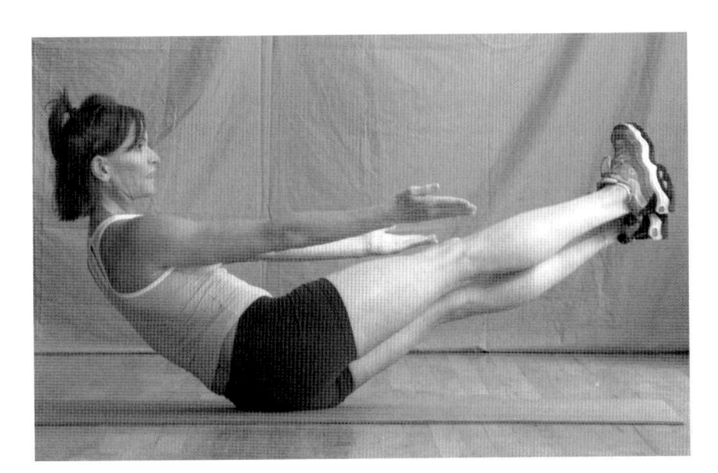

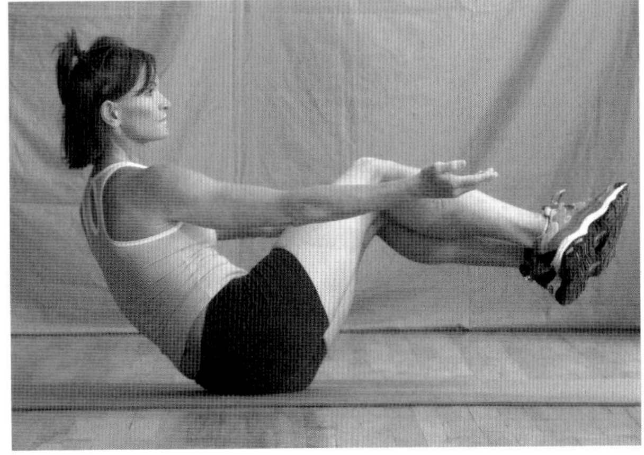

**STARTING POSITION:** Balance on your left buttock, legs and arms fully extended (knees unlocked).

**THE MOVE:** Simultaneously bring your knees and torso toward each other. Then return to the starting position. Repeat, then switch sides.

### TRAINING TIPS

- Don't let your legs and torso rest on the floor at the bottom of the movement.
- Focus your mind on feeling your core do the work.
- Keep your inner core activated.

# EXERCISE: SIDE SUPERMAN

DIFFICULTY: **3** LOWER BACK: **MODERATE RISK**

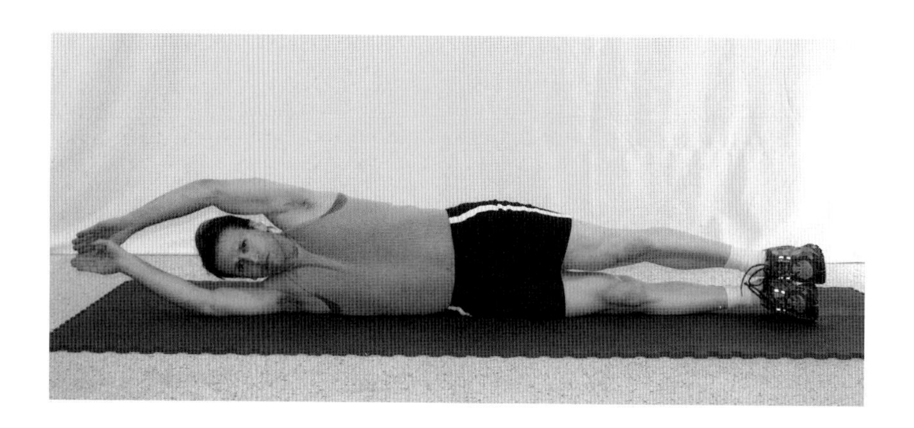

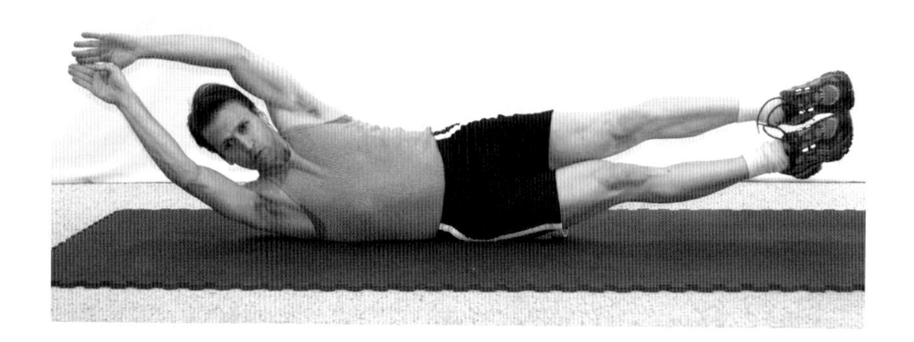

**STARTING POSITION:** Lie on your right side with your legs and arms fully extended (arms above your head).

**THE MOVE:** Simultaneously raise your arms, torso, and legs, as if you were flying on your side. Hold the contraction at the top of the movement. Lower your right arm and leg until they lightly touch the floor. Repeat.

### TRAINING TIPS

- Before you raise your arms and legs, lengthen your spine by stretching your arms and legs in opposite directions, as if someone was pulling on them.
- Feel the movement initiating from the center of your body.
- Try to keep your elbows in line with your ears.
- Control both the up and down phases of the movement.

# EXERCISE: ON THE BALL—JACKKNIFE

DIFFICULTY: **2** LOWER BACK: **MODERATE RISK**

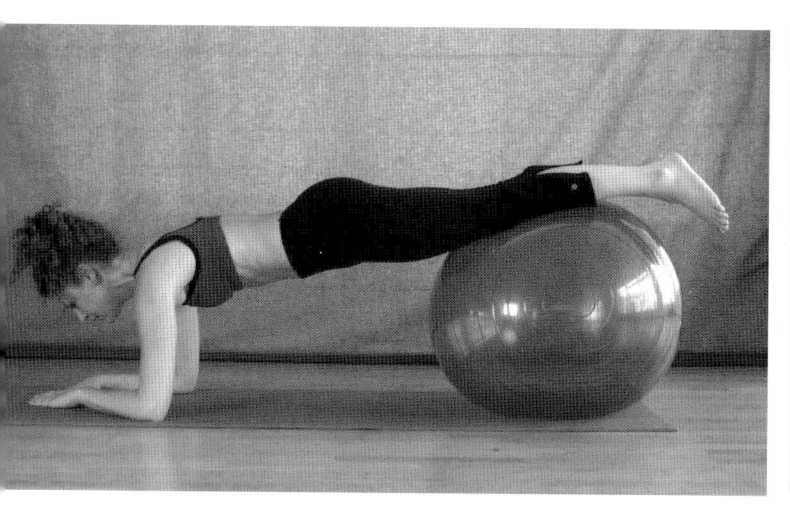

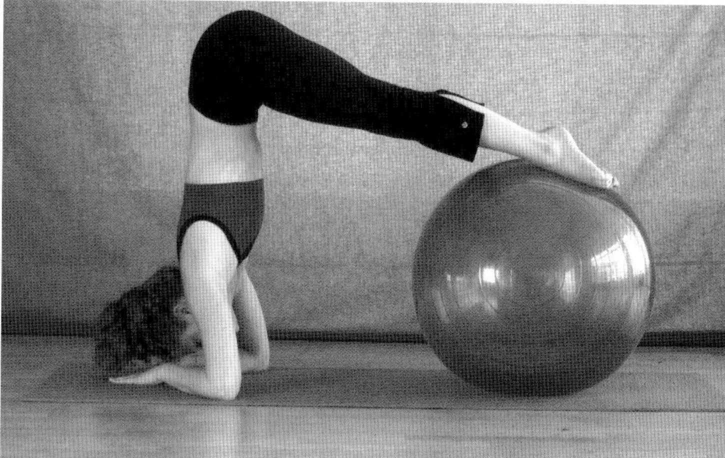

**STARTING POSITION:** From a push-up position, place your shins on top of the exercise ball, and place your elbows under your shoulders. Your body should form a straight line.

**THE MOVE:** Use your legs to pull the ball toward your hands as you raise your hips high. Roll the ball back to the starting position and repeat.

### TRAINING TIPS

- Keep the ball's movement under control.
- Focus your mind on feeling your core do the work.
- Keep your neck lengthened and in alignment with your spine.
- Keep your hands under your shoulders for the entire movement.
- To make this exercise more difficult, place the balls of your feet on top of the ball.

# EXERCISE: ON THE BALL—ROLL IN

DIFFICULTY: **3** LOWER BACK: **MODERATE RISK**

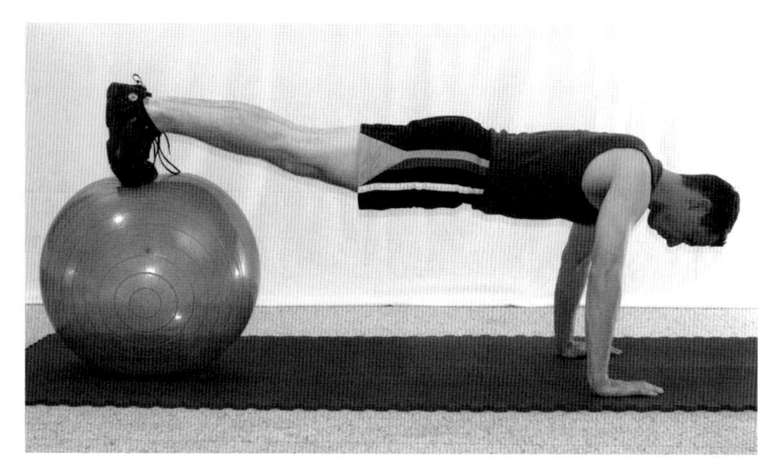

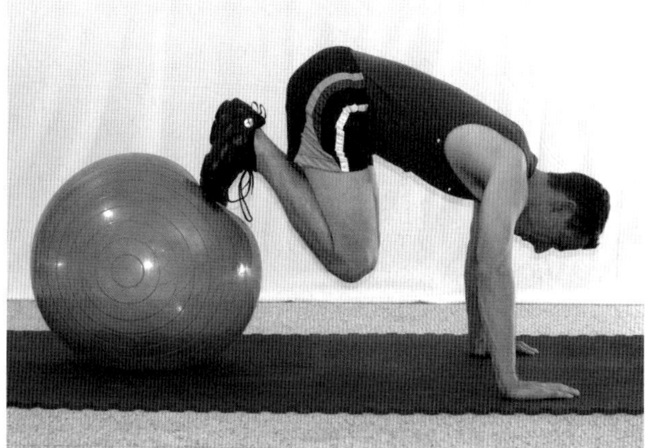

**STARTING POSITION:** From a push-up position, place the balls of your feet on top of the ball, your hands directly under your shoulders.

**THE MOVE:** Bring your knees toward your chest as you slowly roll the ball forward with your feet. Then straighten your legs, rolling the ball back out to the starting position.

### TRAINING TIPS

- Keep the ball's movement under control.
- Focus your mind on feeling your core do the work.
- Look straight down and keep your neck lengthened.
- Keep your hands under your shoulders for the entire movement.

# EXERCISE: ON THE BALL—ROLL OUT

DIFFICULTY: **2** LOWER BACK: **MODERATE TO HIGH RISK**

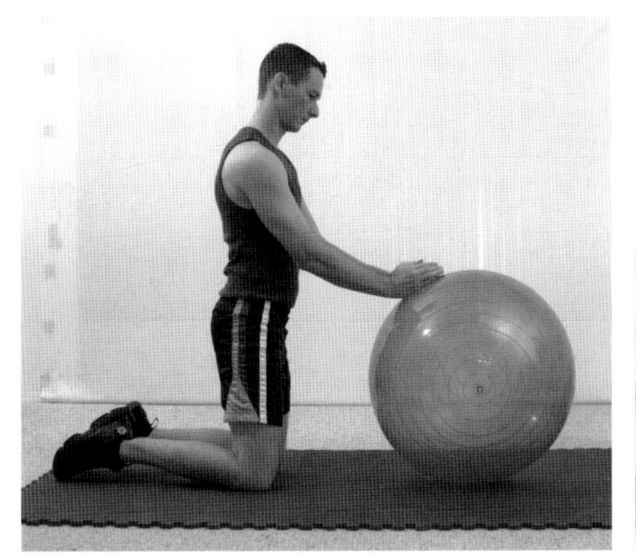

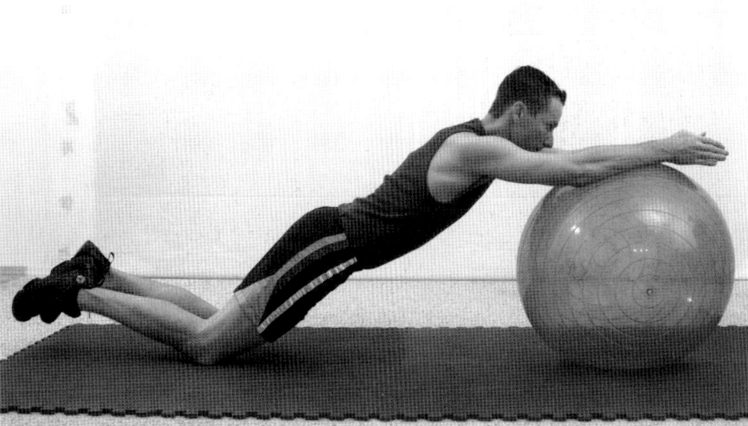

**STARTING POSITION:** Kneel in front of the ball, placing your hands in prayer position on the ball.

**THE MOVE:** Roll the ball forward until your arms are fully extended. Then roll the ball back to the starting position. Extending your hips and legs forward will make the exercise more difficult.

### TRAINING TIPS

- Focus your mind on your core.
- Keep your neck lengthened and look straight down.
- Keep your buttocks contracted and your hips stable to protect your lower back.
- Placing your hands lower on the ball will increase the difficulty.

# EXERCISE: ON THE BALL—SINGLE-LEG CRUNCH

DIFFICULTY: **3** LOWER BACK: **MODERATE RISK**

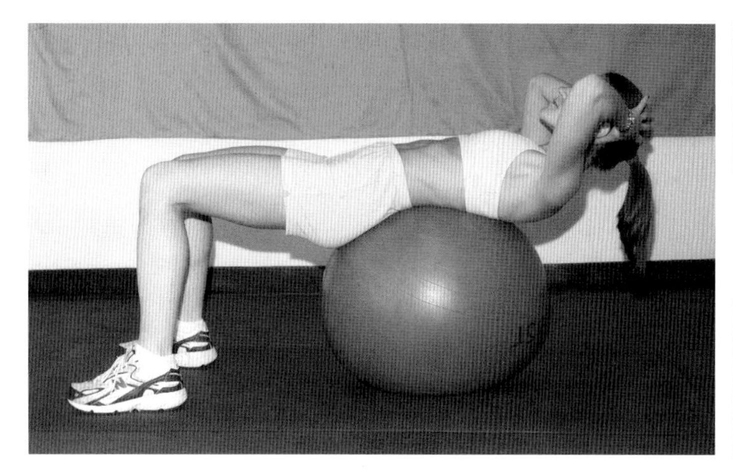

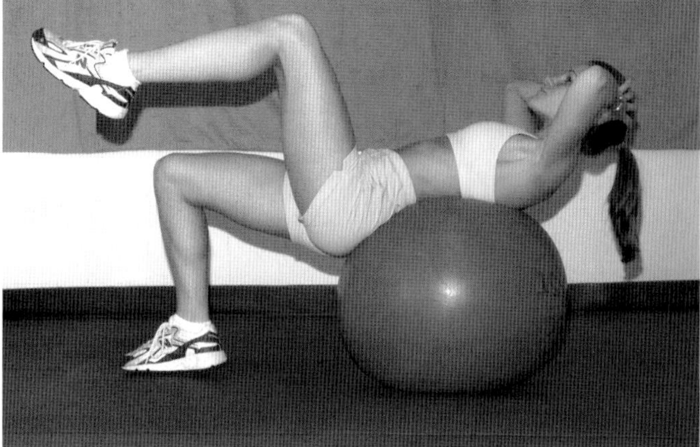

**STARTING POSITION:** Sit on top of the ball, your feet flat on the floor for support. Then slide forward so your shoulder blades drop behind the highest part of the ball.

**THE MOVE:** Curl your upper body forward over the peak of the ball as you raise your left leg, knee bent. Lower both your torso and leg, then repeat the movement, raising your other leg.

### TRAINING TIPS

- Don't let the ball move.
- Focus your mind on feeling your core do the work.
- Make sure you are far enough back on the ball, so you have to overcome the angle of the ball as you raise your torso.

# EXERCISE: STANDING KNEE FLEXION

DIFFICULTY: **1** LOWER BACK: **LOW RISK**

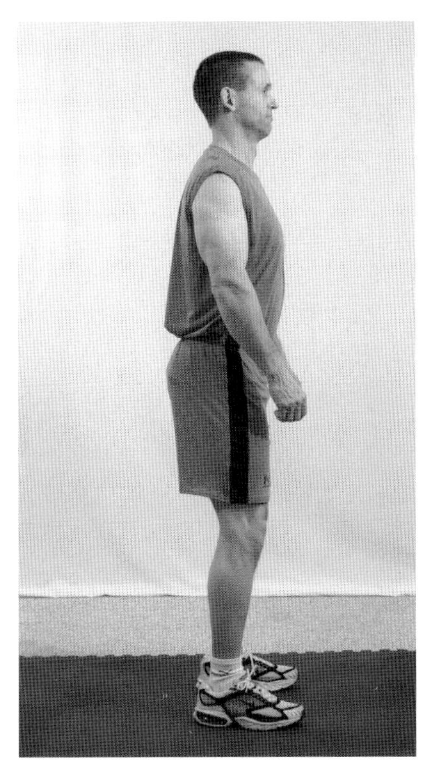

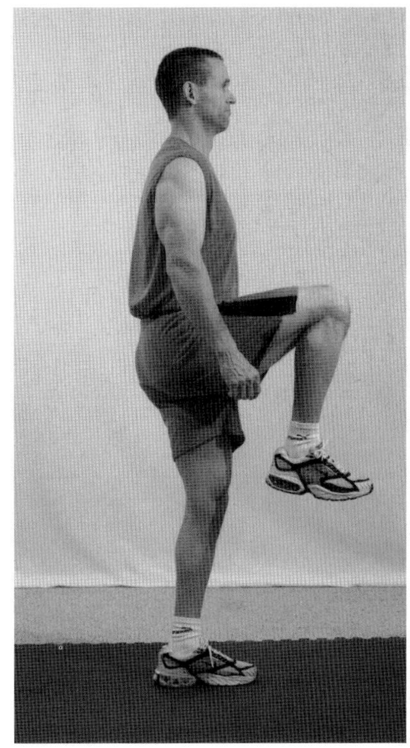

**STARTING POSITION:** Stand in ready position, arms at your sides.

**THE MOVE:** Bring your knee up so your thigh is perpendicular to your upper body. Hold this position stable.

### TRAINING TIPS

- Keep your inner core activated.
- Keep a neutral spine.
- Initiate the movement from the center of your body, not your arms and legs.
- Maintain spinal alignment.

# EXERCISE: STANDING KNEE FLEXION WITH ARMS

DIFFICULTY: **1** LOWER BACK: **LOW RISK**

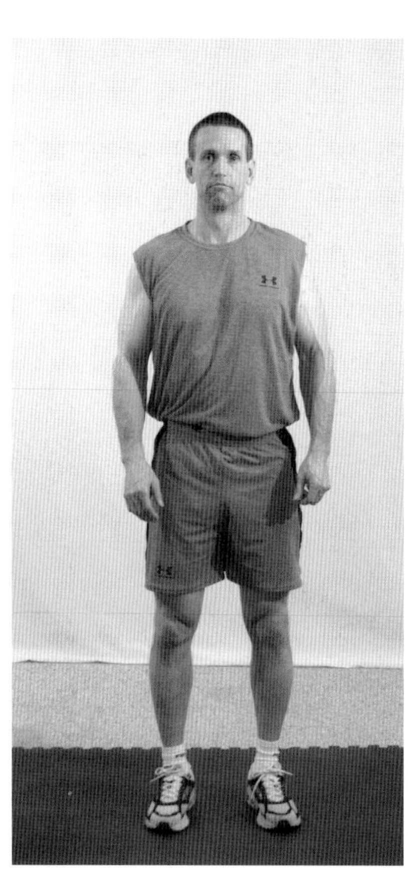

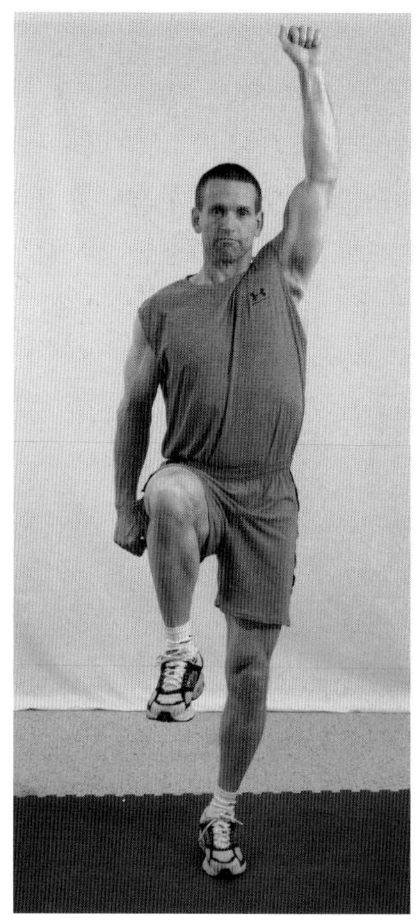

**STARTING POSITION:** Stand in ready position, arms at your sides.

**THE MOVE:** As you raise your left hand, bring your right knee up so your thigh is perpendicular to your upper body. Repeat to the other side, raising your left knee and your right hand.

### TRAINING TIPS

- Keep your inner core activated.
- Keep a neutral spine.
- Initiate the movement from the center of your body, not your arms and legs.
- Maintain spinal alignment.

# 25

# EXTENSION MOVES

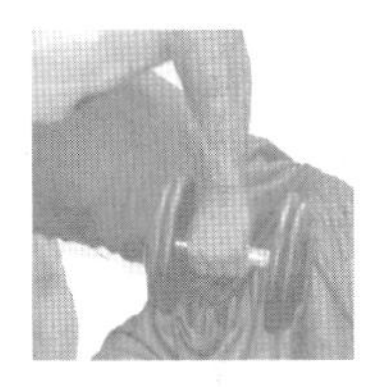

# EXERCISE: BASIC TRUNK EXTENSION

DIFFICULTY: **1** LOWER BACK: **MODERATE RISK**

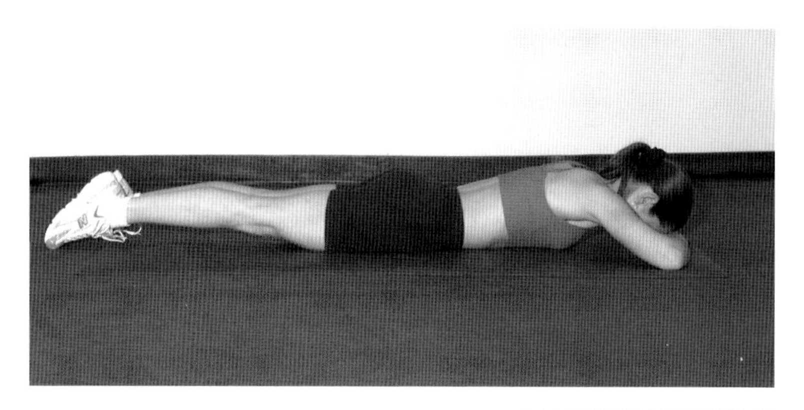

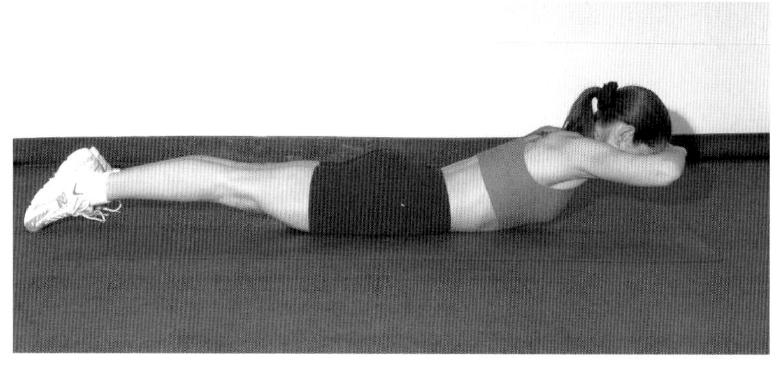

**STARTING POSITION:** Lie on your stomach and rest your forehead on your hands, which are placed palms down on top of each other.

**THE MOVE:** Lengthening your spine, raise your torso and your head off the floor as high as you can while keeping your hips and feet on the ground. Lower your body back to the starting position. Repeat the movement.

### TRAINING TIPS

- Throughout the movement think of lengthening the spine, so the exercise is making you longer and taller.
- Keep your butt and leg muscles tight to protect your lower back.
- Focus on feeling and isolating your lower back muscles as you raise your torso.

# EXERCISE: OPPOSITE ARM AND LEG—ALL FOURS

DIFFICULTY: **2** LOWER BACK: **MODERATE RISK**

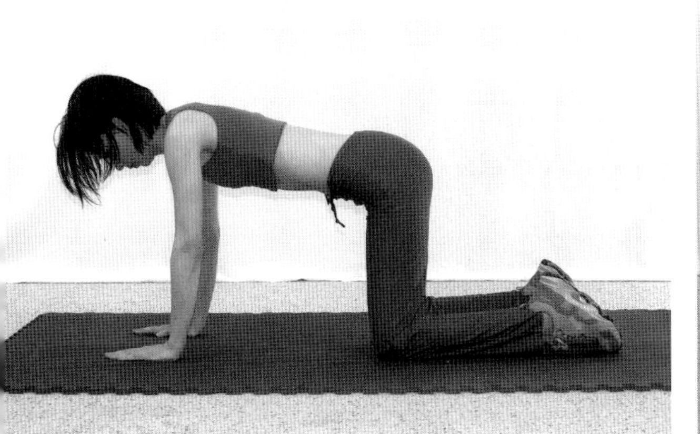

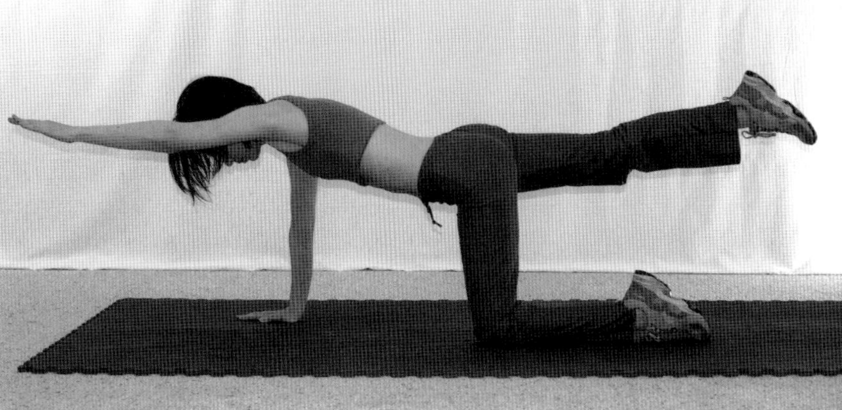

**STARTING POSITION:** Assume an all-fours position, arms aligned under shoulders and knees under hips. Look straight down.

**THE MOVEMENT:** Simultaneously raise and straighten your left arm and right leg until they are parallel to the ground. Repeat with right arm and left leg.

### TRAINING TIPS

- Don't use momentum to complete your exercise.
- Even if you can't reach parallel, get as close as you can.
- Initiate the movement from the center of your body.

# EXERCISE: SWIMMING—ON YOUR BELLY

DIFFICULTY: **2** LOWER BACK RISK: **MODERATE RISK**

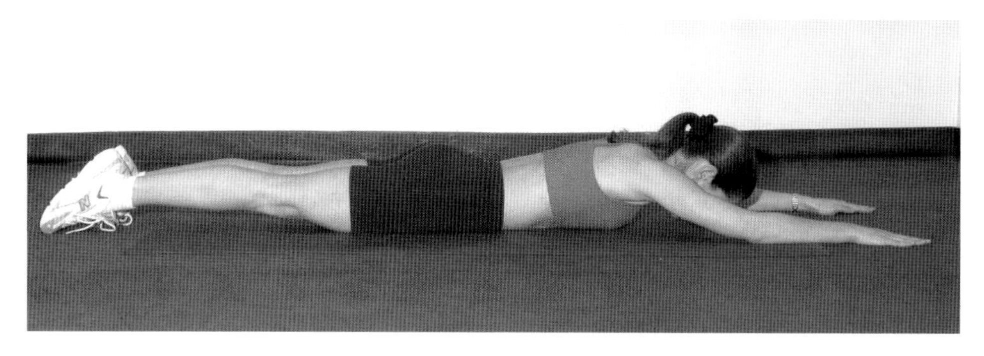

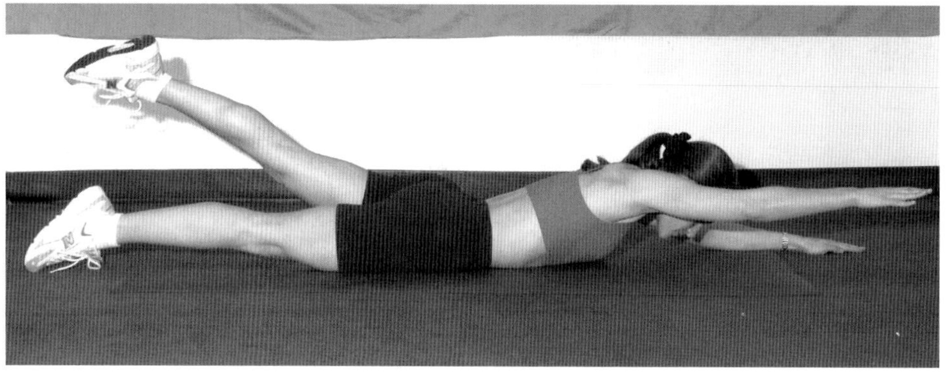

**STARTING POSITION:** Lie on your stomach with your legs on the floor and arms fully extended, your head facing straight down.

**THE MOVE:** Simultaneously raise your right arm, torso, and left leg. Hold the contraction at the top of the movement. Lower the arm and leg until they lightly touch the floor. Then repeat with the other arm and leg.

## TRAINING TIPS

- Before you raise your arm, extend the spine by lengthening the arm and leg you are going to raise.
- Feel the movement initiating from the center of your body.
- Control both the up and down phases of the movement.
- Keep your neck lengthened and not arched up.

# EXERCISE: SUPERMAN

DIFFICULTY: **2** LOWER BACK RISK: **MODERATE RISK**

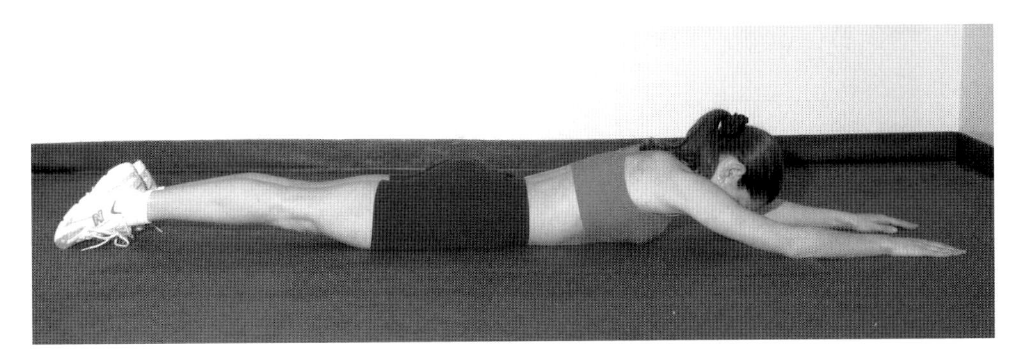

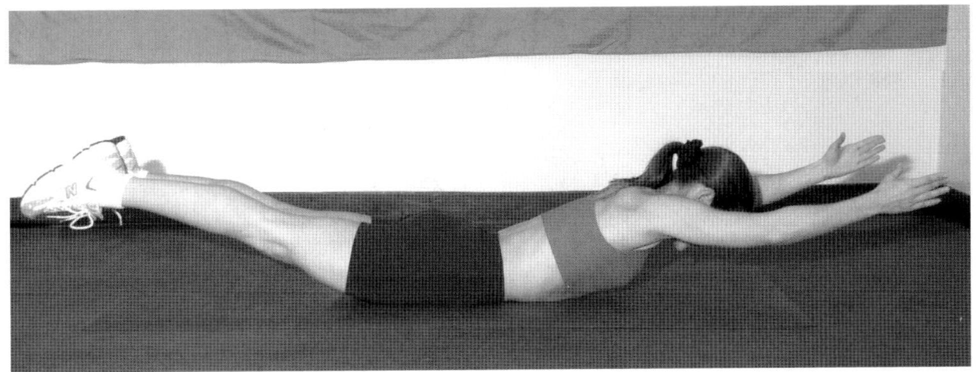

**STARTING POSITION:** Lie on your stomach with your legs and arms fully extended. Your head faces straight down.

**THE MOVE:** Simultaneously raise your arms, torso, and legs as if you were flying. Hold the contraction at the top of the movement. Lower your arms and legs until they lightly touch the floor. Repeat.

### TRAINING TIPS

- Before you raise your arms and legs, lengthen your spine by stretching your arms. and legs in opposite directions, as if someone was pulling on them.
- Feel the movement initiating from the center of your body.
- Control both the up and down phases of the movement.
- Don't arch your neck up.

# EXERCISE: ANKLE REACH

DIFFICULTY: **2** LOWER BACK RISK: **MODERATE RISK**

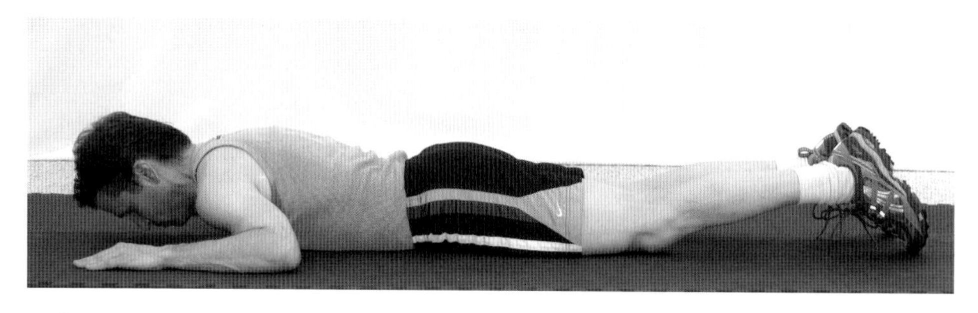

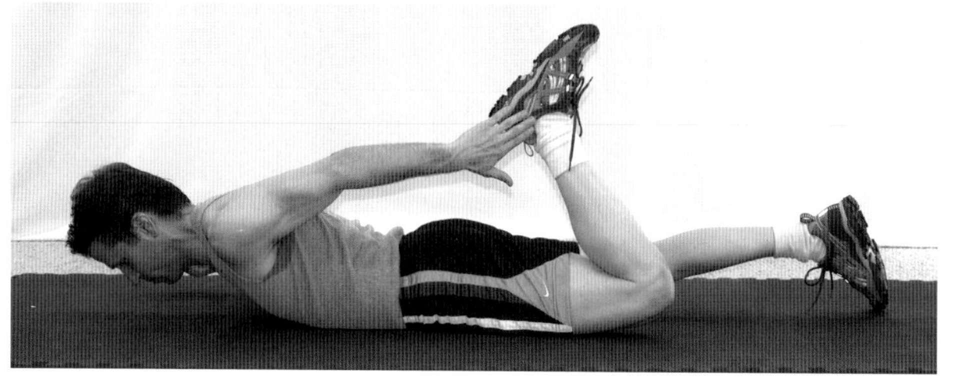

**STARTING POSITION:** Lie on your stomach, legs extended and arms bent so your hands are even with the top of your head.

**THE MOVE:** Reach your arm back and up, bending your lower leg up toward your butt as you touch your hand to your ankle.

**VARIATIONS:** You can also do a double touch move, reaching back with both arms, as you bring both legs up. An advanced variation is a cross touch, reaching back with your right hand to touch your left ankle.

### TRAINING TIPS

- Keep your neck lengthened and in line with your spine.
- Maintain a steady balance.
- Keep the motion fluid.
- Initiate the movement from the center of your body.
- If you can't reach your ankles, get as close as you can.

# EXERCISE: GOOD MORNINGS

DIFFICULTY: **3** LOWER BACK: **HIGH RISK**

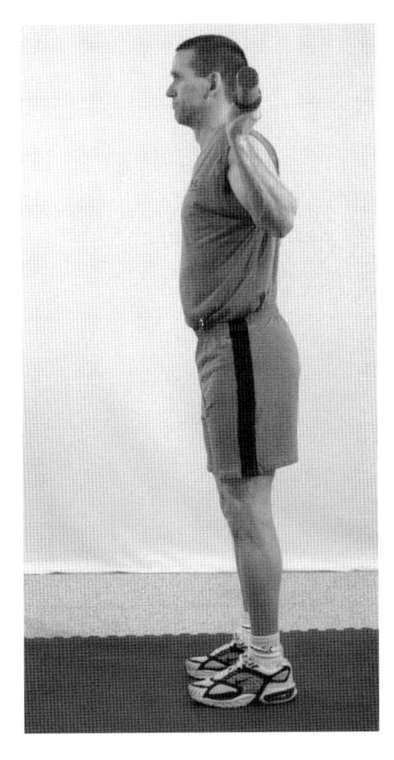

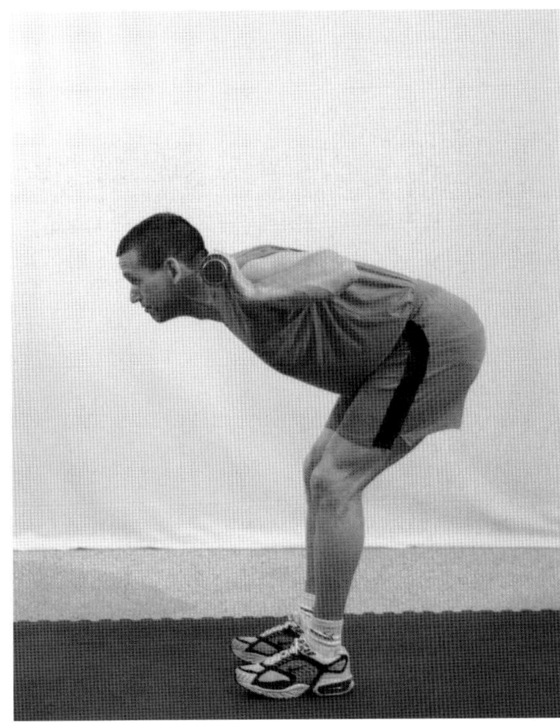

**STARTING POSITION:** Stand in ready position with your feet slightly wider than shoulder-width apart. Hold a bar behind your neck or your trapezius muscles or place your hands behind your ears.

**THE MOVE:** Bend forward at the hip, keeping your back flat and your knees slightly bent throughout the movement. Bend until your torso is parallel to the ground, maintaining a straight line with your torso, neck, and head (don't allow your chin to drop forward or your shoulders to hunch). Raise torso back up to starting position.

## TRAINING TIPS

- Keep your inner core activated.
- Keep your knees unlocked.
- Contract your butt.
- Keep your shoulders down and together.
- Make sure the bar doesn't put pressure on your neck.

# EXERCISE: BACK EXTENSION—ROMAN CHAIR

DIFFICULTY: **2** LOWER BACK RISK: **MODERATE RISK**

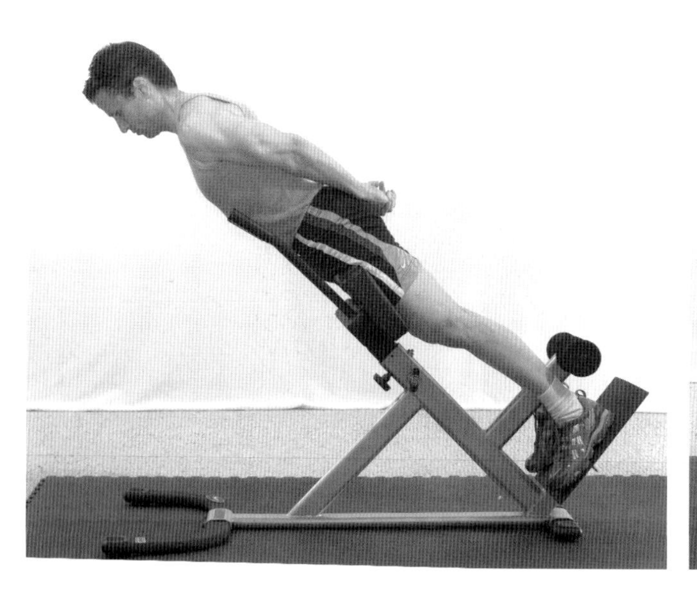

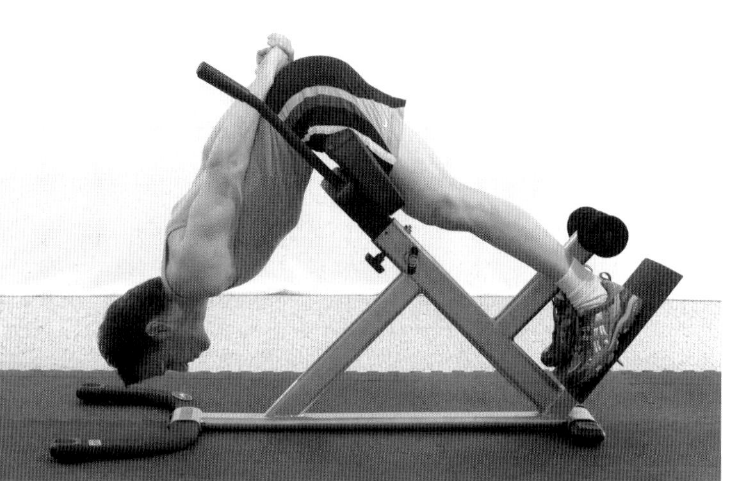

**STARTING POSITION:** Secure yourself in a Roman chair, your feet under supports. Make sure the chair is adjusted so your waist can bend completely forward.

**THE MOVE:** Bend forward through a full range of motion, making sure your spine and neck stay in alignment. Raise your torso back to the starting position with your spine neutral, not arched or rounded.

### TRAINING TIPS

- Keep your neck lengthened and in line with your spine.
- Place your hands behind your head, across your chest, behind your back, or hold a weight plate.
- Keep the motion fluid.
- Don't hyperextend (bring your torso up and back beyond your spine's natural alignment).

# EXERCISE: SUN SALUTE

DIFFICULTY: **2** LOWER BACK RISK: **MODERATE RISK**

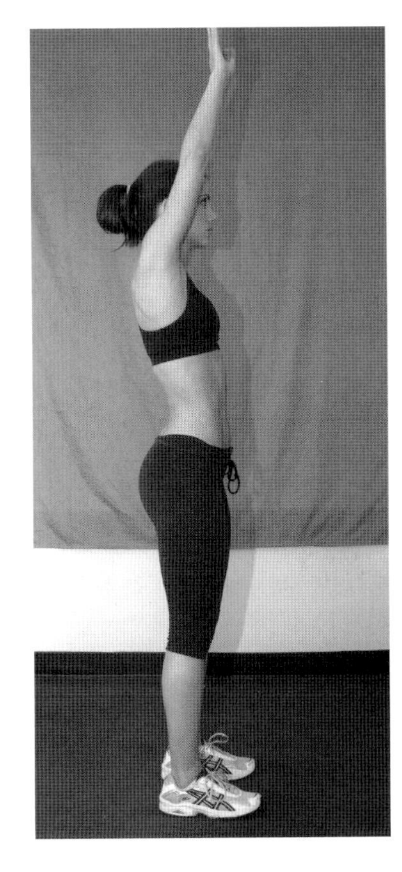

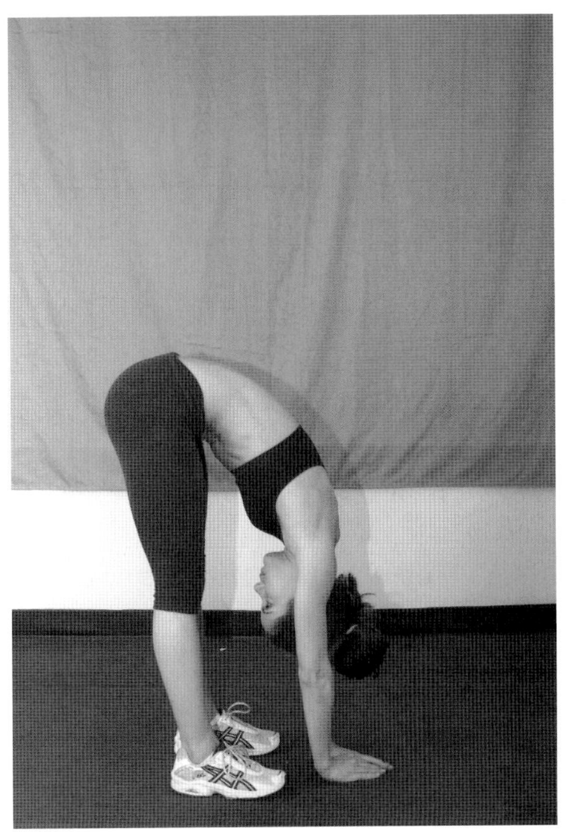

**STARTING POSITION:** Stand with your legs shoulder-width apart and your arms extended above your head.

**THE MOVE:** Bend at the waist and reach down and touch the floor (or go down as far as you can), extending your torso and moving as one unit. Straighten back to the starting position. Maintain a straight spine. Repeat.

### TRAINING TIPS

- Focus on keeping your body as straight as a board.
- Keep your neck lengthened and in line with your spine.
- Maintain a steady balance.
- Initiate the movement from your core.
- Keep your inner core activated throughout the exercise.
- Contract your butt muscles as you rise up.

# EXERCISE: ON THE BALL—BACK EXTENSION

DIFFICULTY: **2** LOWER BACK RISK: **MODERATE RISK**

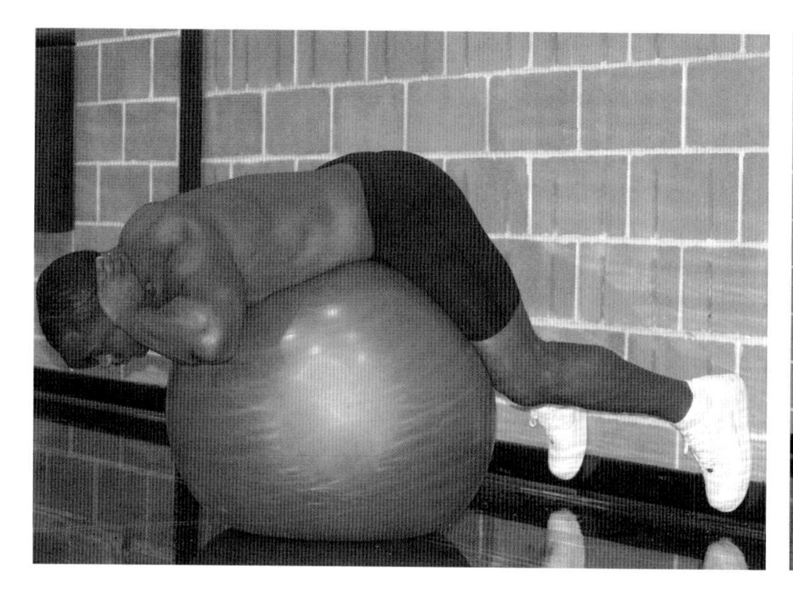

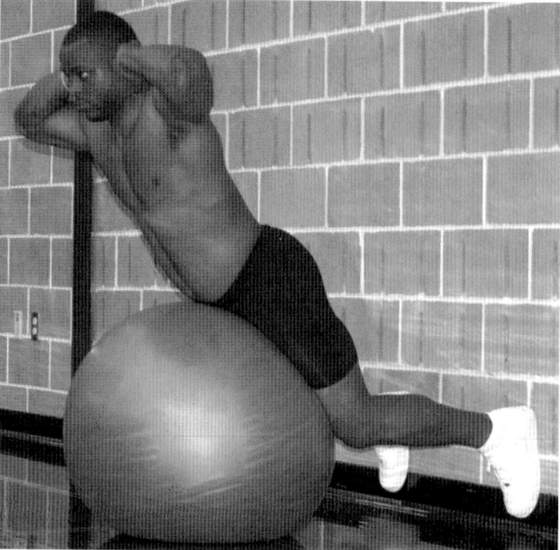

**STARTING POSITION:** Lie on your belly across an exercise ball, brace your feet against the wall for support, drape your torso over the peak of the ball, placing your hands behind your ears.

**THE MOVE:** Lengthen your spine as you raise your torso off the ball, making a straight line with your body. Return to the starting position and repeat.

**TRAINING TIPS**

- Keep your butt muscles contracted to protect your lower back.
- Kep your inner core activated throughout the movement.
- Throughout the movement continue to lengthen your spine, making your torso longer.
- You can also do this exercise by simply placing your feet on the floor.

# 26

# ROTATION AND CROSSING MOVES

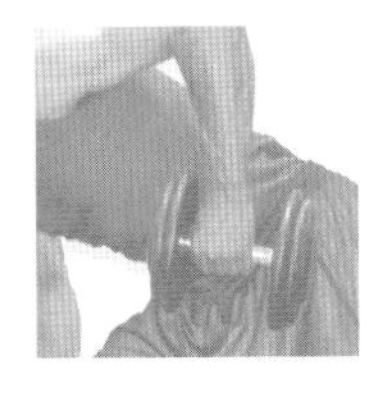

# EXERCISE: CATCHES

DIFFICULTY: **1** LOWER BACK: **LOW RISK**

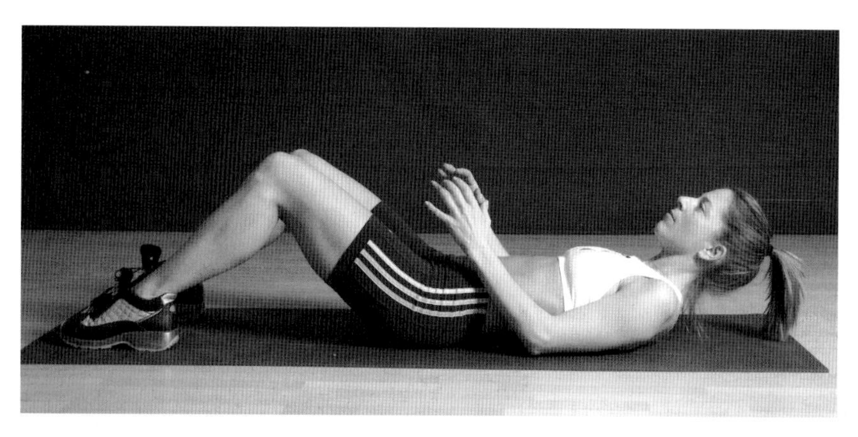

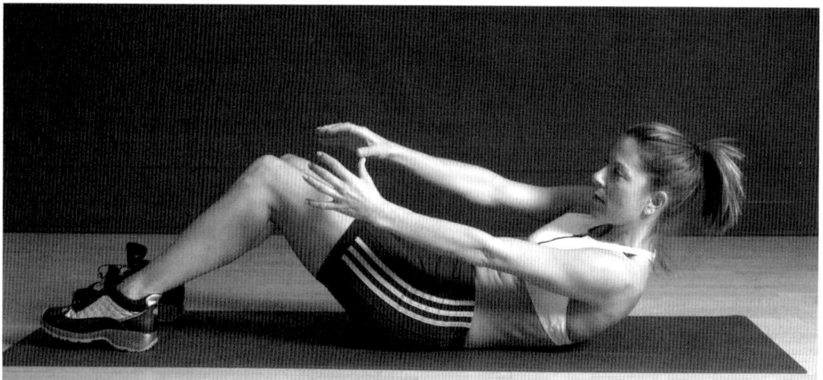

**STARTING POSITION:** Lie on your back with your knees bent, feet flat on the floor, and arms in front of your body.

**THE MOVE:** Raise your torso diagonally, bringing your right shoulder across the center line of your body and both hands outside and above your left knee, as if you were going to catch a ball. Lower your torso back to the starting position and repeat to the other side.

### TRAINING TIPS

- Make sure you get both arms outside the knees and slightly above knee level.
- Focus your mind on your core as you cross from side to side.
- Pretend you're catching a ball.
- Initiate the movement from the center of your body.

# EXERCISE: HEEL TOUCH 1

DIFFICULTY: **1** LOWER BACK: **LOW RISK**

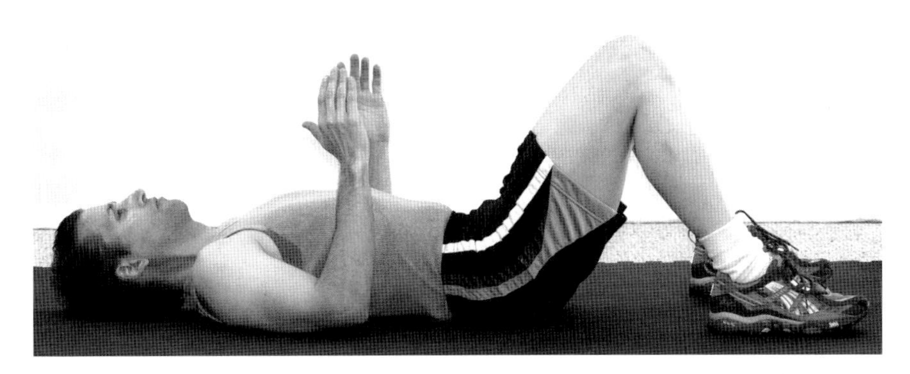

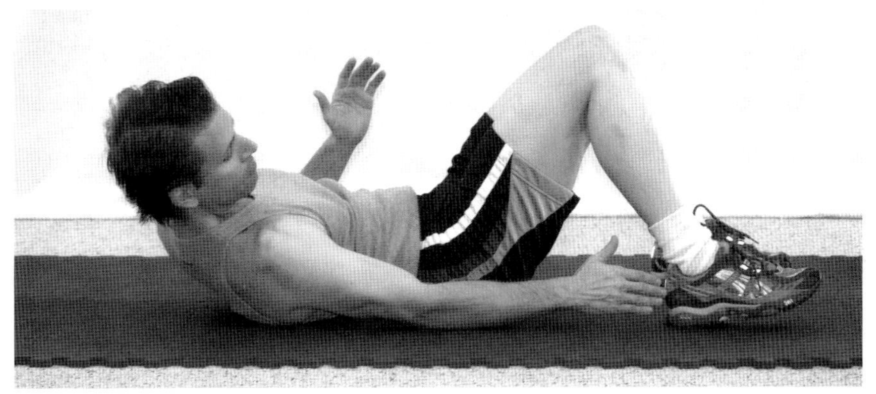

**STARTING POSITION:** Lie flat on your back, knees bent, feet flat on the floor, and hands pointing up.

**THE MOVE:** Moving to your side, touch your right heel with your right hand. Repeat to the other side.

### TRAINING TIPS

- Keep your inner core activated.
- Keep a neutral spine.
- Initiate the movement from the center of your body, not your arms and legs.
- Keep the motion fluid.

# EXERCISE: HEEL TOUCH 2

DIFFICULTY: **2** LOWER BACK: **LOW RISK**

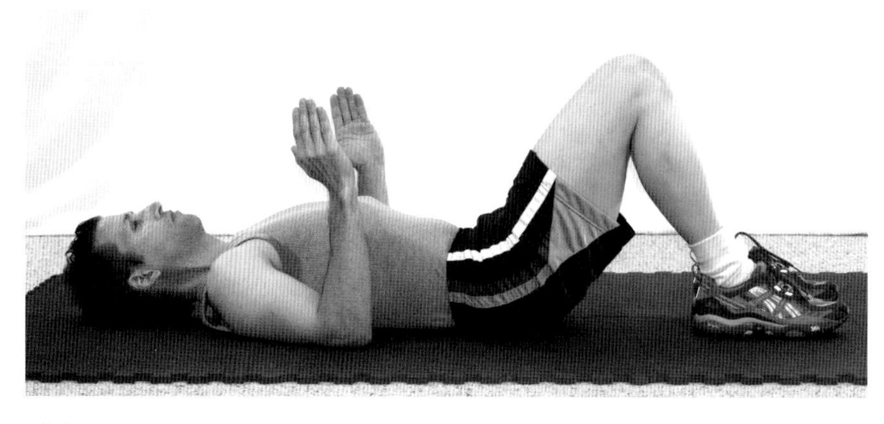

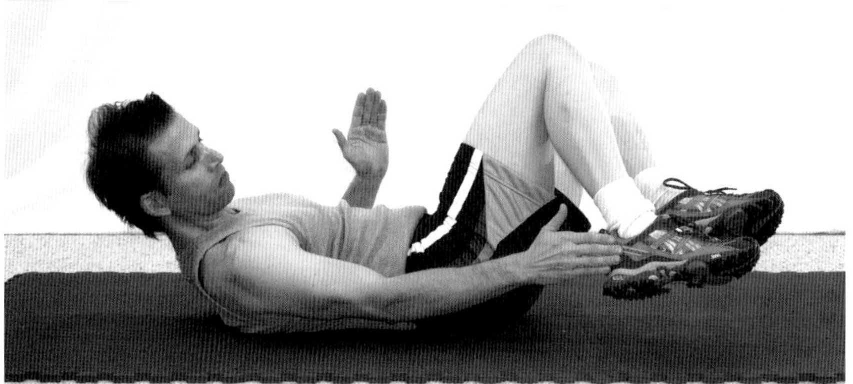

**STARTING POSITION:** Lie flat on your back, knees bent, feet flat on the floor, and hands pointing up.

**THE MOVE:** Moving to your side, touch your right heel with your right hand as you bring both feet off the floor. Repeat to the other side.

**TRAINING TIPS**

- Keep your inner core activated.
- Keep a neutral spine.
- Initiate the movement from the center of your body, not your arms and legs.
- Don't rest at the bottom of the movement.

# EXERCISE: HEEL TOUCH 3

DIFFICULTY: **3** LOWER BACK: **MODERATE RISK**

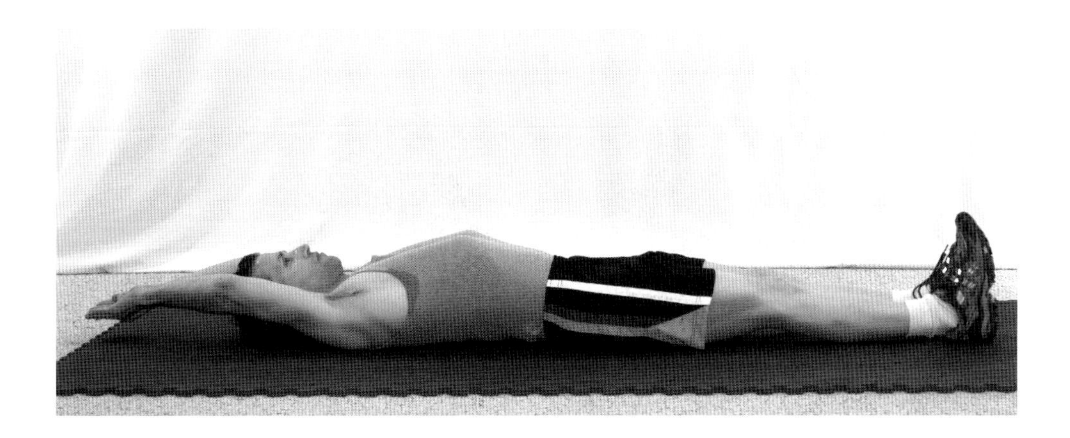

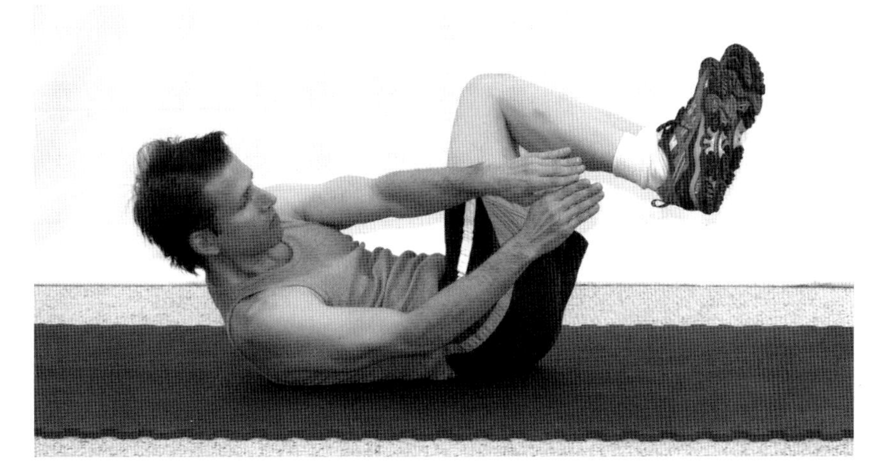

**STARTING POSITION:** Lie flat on your back with your legs fully extended and hands extended over your head.

**THE MOVE:** Move both hands and both feet to your right side, touching your heels with your hands. Repeat to the other side.

### TRAINING TIPS

- Keep your inner core activated.
- Keep a neutral spine.
- Initiate the movement from the center of your body, not your arms and legs.
- Don't rest at the end of the movement.

# EXERCISE: LEG OVERS—BENT-KNEE, SINGLE LEG

DIFFICULTY: **1** LOWER BACK: **LOW RISK**

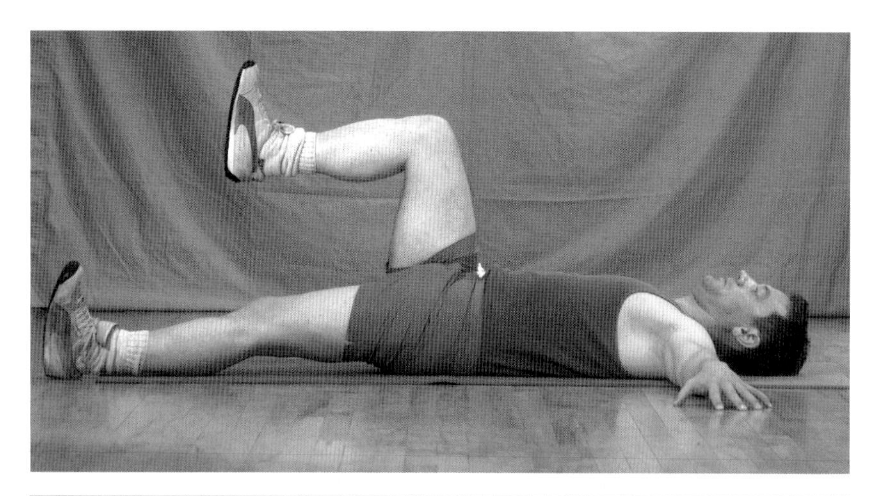

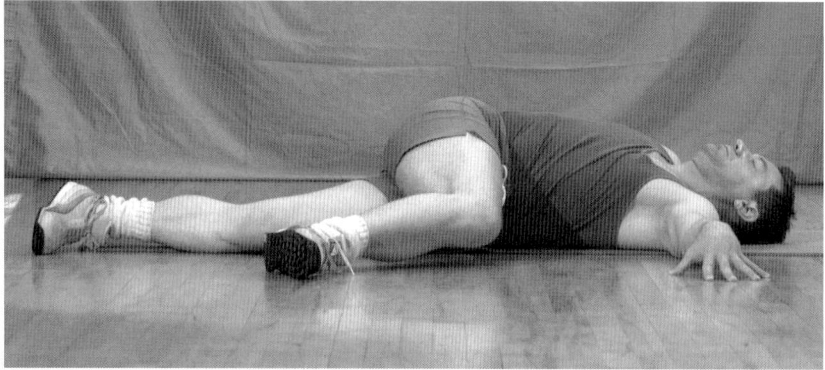

**STARTING POSITION:** Lie flat on your back, hands spread out perpendicular to your body at shoulder level, left leg fully extended on the floor and right leg raised with a bent knee at a 90 degree angle with your upper body.

**THE MOVE:** Cross your right knee over your body, lightly touching the floor on the opposite side. Then cross it back over to the starting position. Repeat. Work both legs.

**TRAINING TIPS**

- As you cross your leg over, allow your hip to roll with the motion.
- Concentrate on feeling your core do the work.
- Keep both shoulder blades on the floor throughout the movement.
- Initiate the movement from your center.

# EXERCISE: LEG OVERS—SINGLE LEG

DIFFICULTY: **1** LOWER BACK: **LOW RISK**

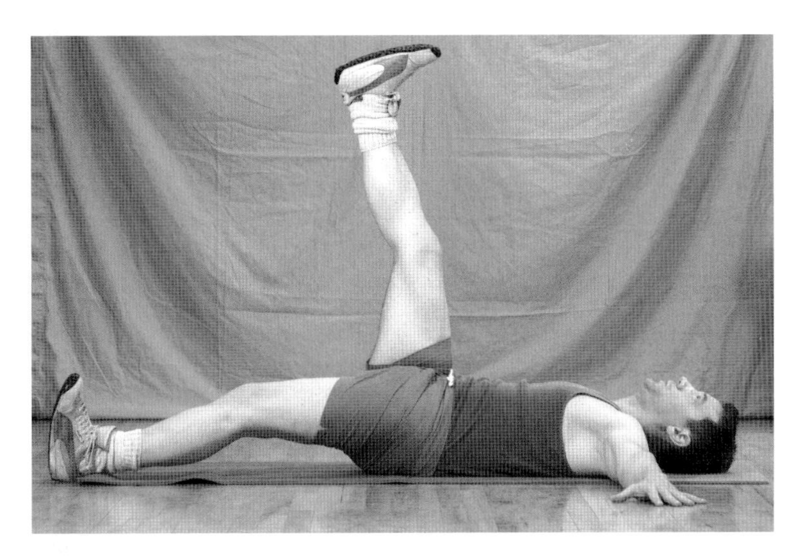

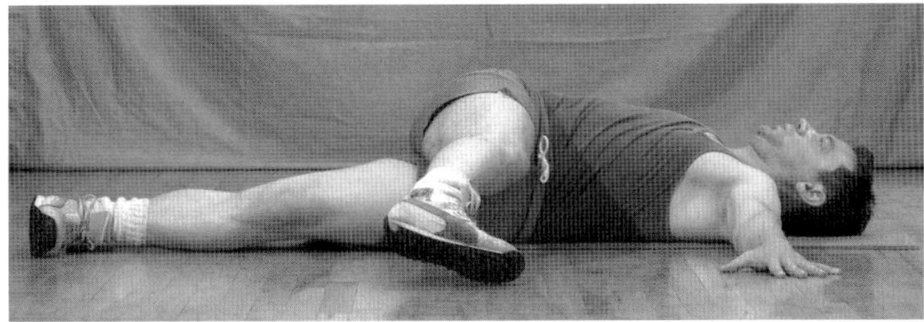

**STARTING POSITION:** Lie flat on your back, hands spread out perpendicular to your body at shoulder level, left leg fully extended, right leg straight up.

**THE MOVE:** Use your oblique muscles to cross your right leg toward your left hand. Lightly touch the floor with your foot, then cross the leg back to the straight-up starting position. Repeat. Then switch legs.

### TRAINING TIPS

- As you cross your leg over, allow your hip to roll with the motion.
- Concentrate on feeling your core do the work.
- If you can't raise your leg to a 90 degree angle, keep it at a position that is comfortable. Your flexibility will improve.
- Keep both shoulder blades on the floor throughout the movement.
- Initiate the movement from your center.

# EXERCISE: LEG OVERS—DOUBLE LEG

DIFFICULTY: **3** LOWER BACK: **MODERATE RISK**

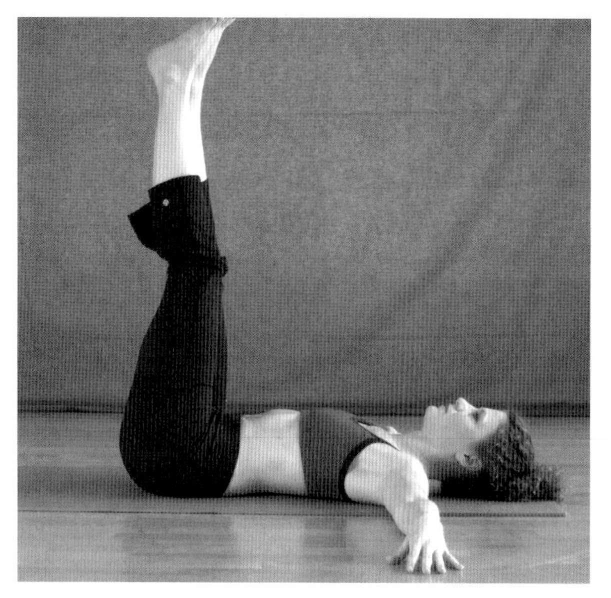

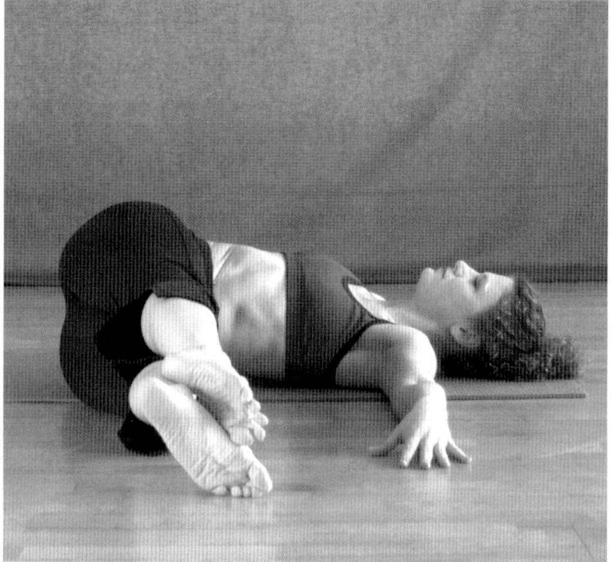

**STARTING POSITION:** Lie flat on your back, hands spread out perpendicular to your body at shoulder level, with both legs extended straight up.

**THE MOVE:** Lower both legs to your left side until your feet lightly touch the floor, then raise them back to the starting position. Repeat the movement to the opposite side.

### TRAINING TIPS

- As you lower both legs to the side, let your hips roll in that direction with the motion.
- Try to lower your legs at a 90 degree angle from your upper body.
- If you can't move your legs to the straight-up position or lower them at a 90 degree angle, take them to an angle that is comfortable.
- Keep your shoulders on the floor throughout the entire movement.
- Concentrate on feeling your core do the work.
- Initiate the movement from the center of your body.

# EXERCISE: PRONE CROSSOVER

DIFFICULTY: **2** LOWER BACK: **MODERATE RISK**

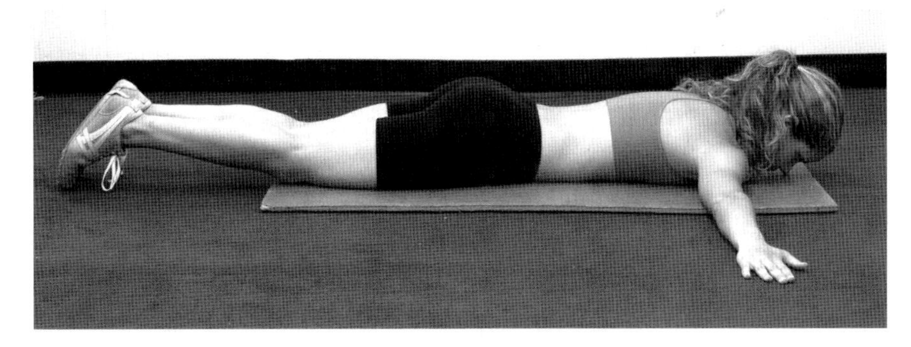

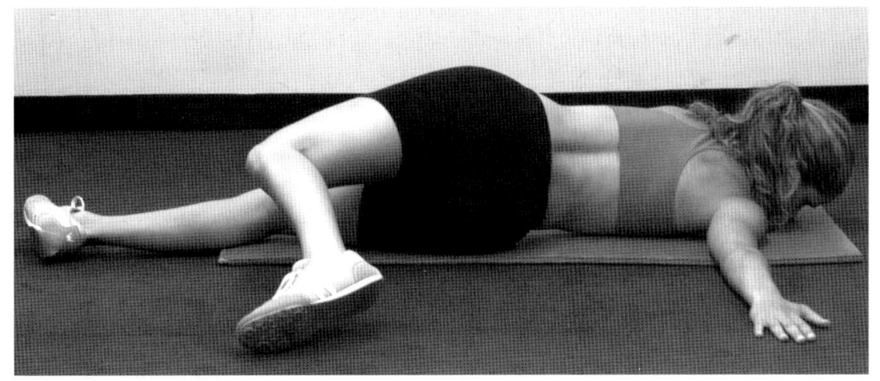

**STARTING POSITION:** Lie on your stomach with your arms spread out to the sides at shoulder level.

**THE MOVEMENT:** Activate your left glute and bring your left heel over and up toward your right hand, touching the floor with your foot. Alternate legs.

### TRAINING TIPS

- The movement should be powerful but controlled.
- Squeeze your glute as you thrust your heel.
- Keep your inner core activated.
- Initiate the movement from the center of your body.

# EXERCISE: PRONE DOUBLE LEG CROSSOVER

DIFFICULTY: **2**    LOWER BACK: **MODERATE RISK**

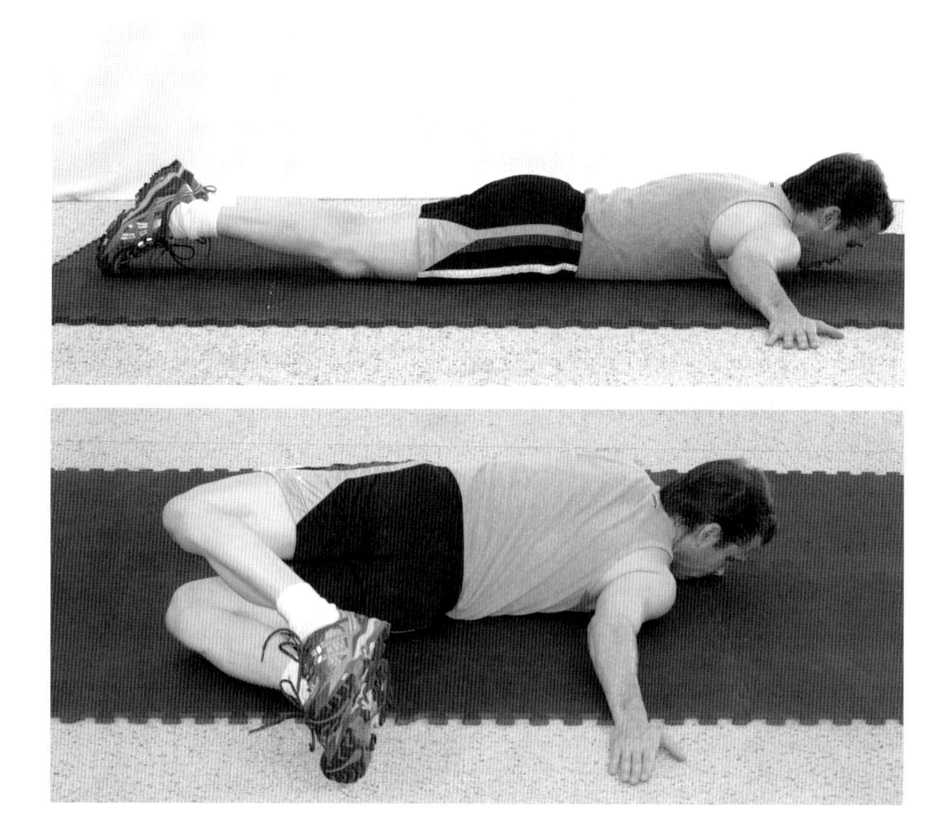

**STARTING POSITION:** Lie on the floor on your belly, with your arms spread out to your sides at shoulder level.

**THE MOVE:** Activate your glutes, bringing both heels over and up toward your right hand. Repeat to the other side.

**TRAINING TIPS**

- Keep your inner core activated.
- Initiate the movement from the center of your body, not your legs.
- Extending your arms straight above your head makes the move more difficult.

# EXERCISE: RUSSIAN TWISTS

DIFFICULTY: **3** LOWER BACK: **HIGH RISK**

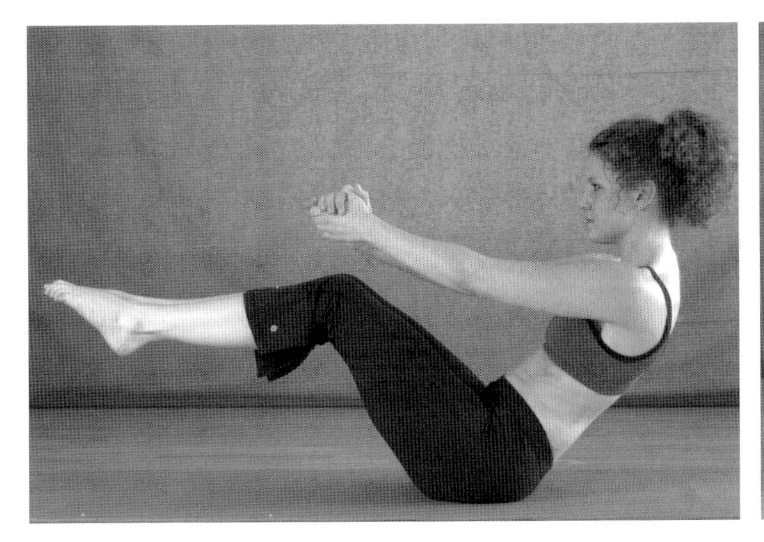

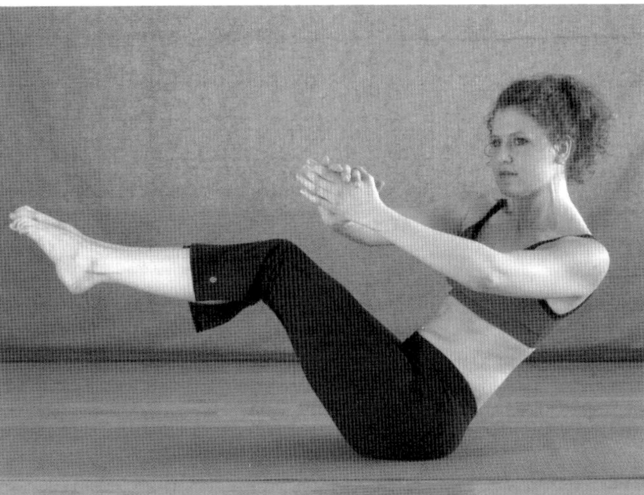

**STARTING POSITION:** Find a position of balance on your buttocks, feet in the air with legs extended halfway out, hands clasped and extended out in front of you.

**THE MOVE:** From this position, begin to twist from your right to left while maintaining balance on your buttocks, keeping constant tension on your core.

### TRAINING TIPS

- Don't crunch your body together. Keep good posture.
- Twist through a full range of motion, twisting as far to the right as you can and then as far to the left as you can.
- Head and neck should remain lengthened and aligned with rest of the spine.
- Don't move your head from side to side.
- Maintain a stable position on your buttocks.

# EXERCISE: SIDE JACKKNIFE

DIFFICULTY: **2** LOWER BACK: **LOW RISK**

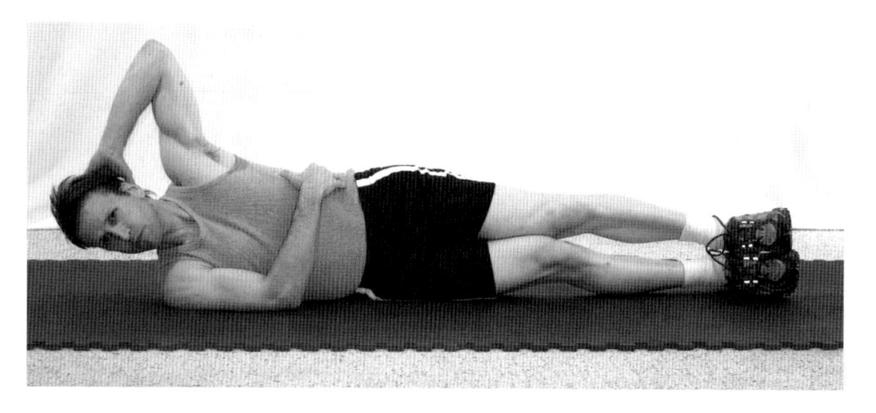

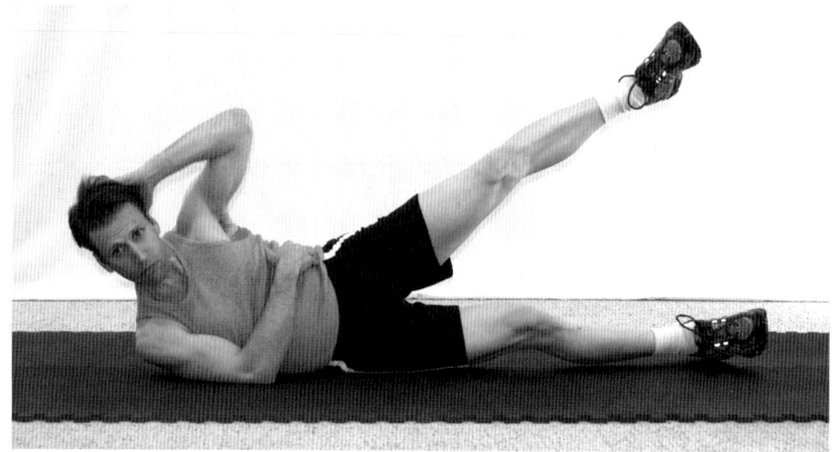

**STARTING POSITION:** Lie on your right hip, legs together. Place your left hand behind your ear and your right hand on your left side.

**THE MOVE:** Simultaneously raise your top leg and your torso, bringing them together. Repeat. Reverse the procedure for the opposite side.

### TRAINING TIPS

- Bring your leg slightly forward to increase your range of motion.
- Make sure your upper body moves off the floor. Don't move just your head.
- Don't rest your leg and torso at the bottom of the movement.
- Keep your inner core activated.
- Initiate the movement from the center of your body.

# EXERCISE: ON THE BALL—RUSSIAN TWISTS

DIFFICULTY: **2**   LOWER BACK: **MODERATE RISK**

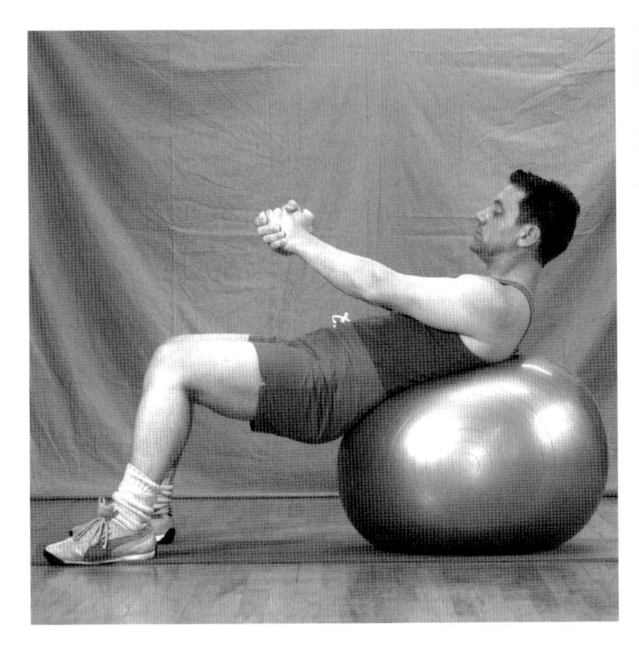

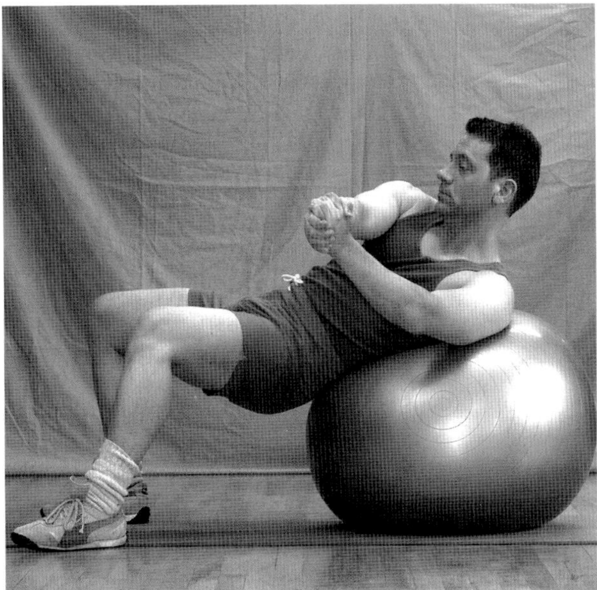

**STARTING POSITION:** Lie on the ball so your shoulder blades rest on the highest part of the ball. Keep your feet in front and flat on the floor for support. Extend your arms straight out and clasp your hands together by interlacing your fingers.

**THE MOVE:** Slightly raise your torso so your shoulder blades come off the ball. Twist your torso and arms to the left, then twist them to the right.

### TRAINING TIPS

- Try to keep the ball from moving.
- Initiate the movement form the center of your body.
- Keep your neck lengthened.
- Keep your hips and legs stable, so only your upper body moves.
- To make the movement more difficult, bring your feet closer together.

**VARIATIONS:** This exercise can also be done holding a medicine ball, weight plate, or dumbbell.

# EXERCISE: ON THE BALL—PLANK TWIST

DIFFICULTY: **2** LOWER BACK: **MODERATE RISK**

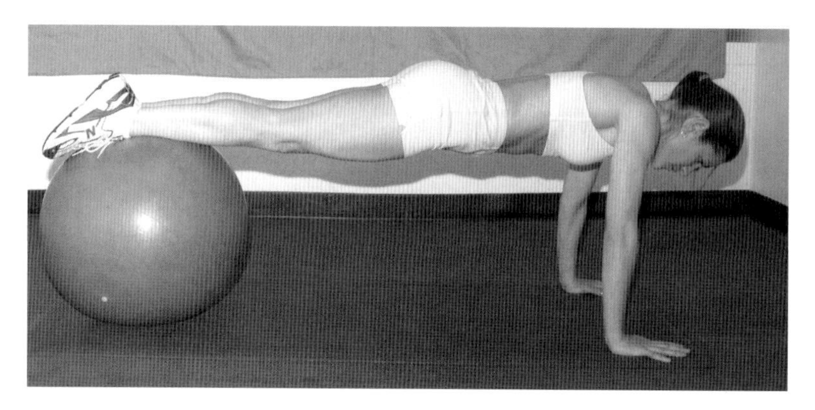

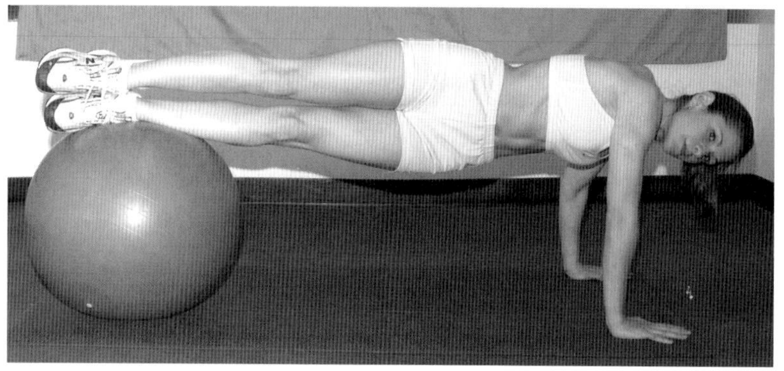

**STARTING POSITION:** From a plank push-up position, place your feet on the ball. Place your hands directly under your shoulders.

**THE MOVE:** Keeping your legs on top of the ball, rotate your right hip up to the 12 o'clock position. Return to the starting position. Then rotate your left hip up to the 12 o'clock position.

**TRAINING TIPS**

- Try to keep the ball from moving.
- Look straight down and keep your neck lengthened.
- Keep your hands under your shoulders for the entire movement.
- Initiate the movement from the center of your body.
- Keep your upper body stationary.

# EXERCISE: ON THE BALL—SHOULDER ROLL

DIFFICULTY: **2** LOWER BACK: **MODERATE RISK**

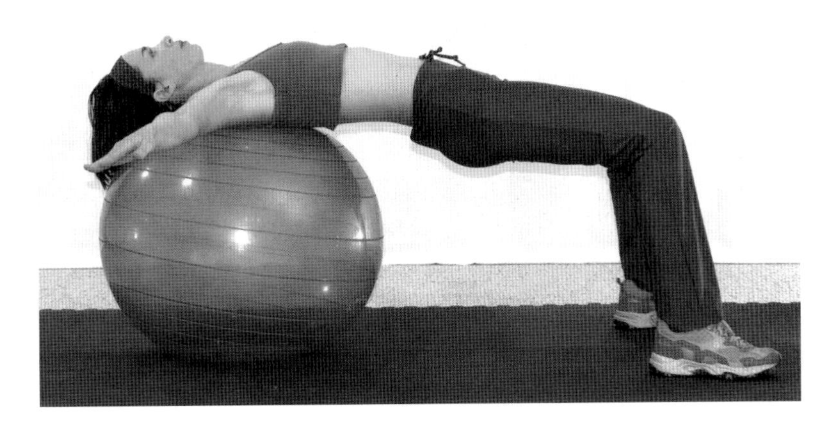

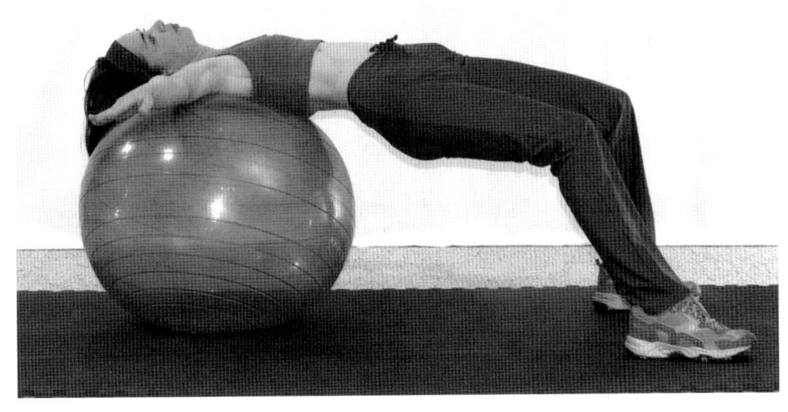

**STARTING POSITION:** Lie with the ball between your shoulders in the reverse bridge position and your feet shoulder-width apart.

**THE MOVEMENT:** Hold your arms out horizontally at your sides or across your chest and slowly roll the ball sideways from one shoulder blade to the other, then back in the opposite direction.

### TRAINER'S TIPS

- Don't allow your hips to sag.
- Initiate the sliding movement from the center of your body.
- Keep your inner core activated.

# EXERCISE: LATERAL CORE FLEXION

DIFFICULTY: **2** LOWER BACK RISK: **MODERATE RISK**

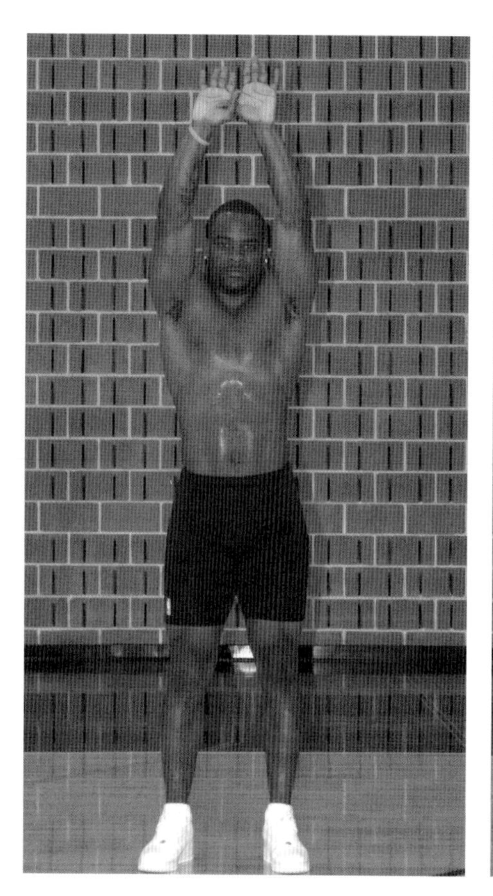

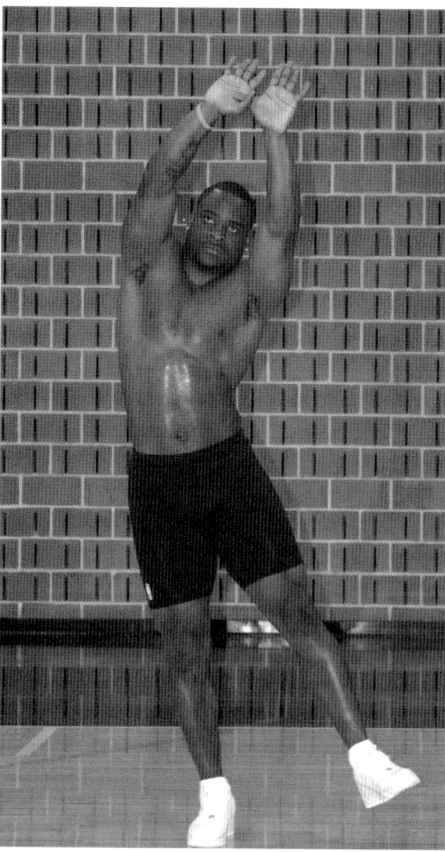

**STARTING POSITION:** Standing in the ready position, raise your arms above your head.

**THE MOVE:** Simultaneously move your right leg directly out to your right side, as you bend your upper body in the same direction. Return to the starting position and repeat.

### TRAINING TIPS

- As you bend to the right, create a C-like curve with your body.
- Feel the movement initiating from the center of your body.
- Keep your inner core activated throughout the movement.
- You can do all the repetitions on one side, then switch. Or alternate sides with each rep.

# EXERCISE: LATERAL CROSS CORE FLEXION

DIFFICULTY: **2** LOWER BACK RISK: **MODERATE RISK**

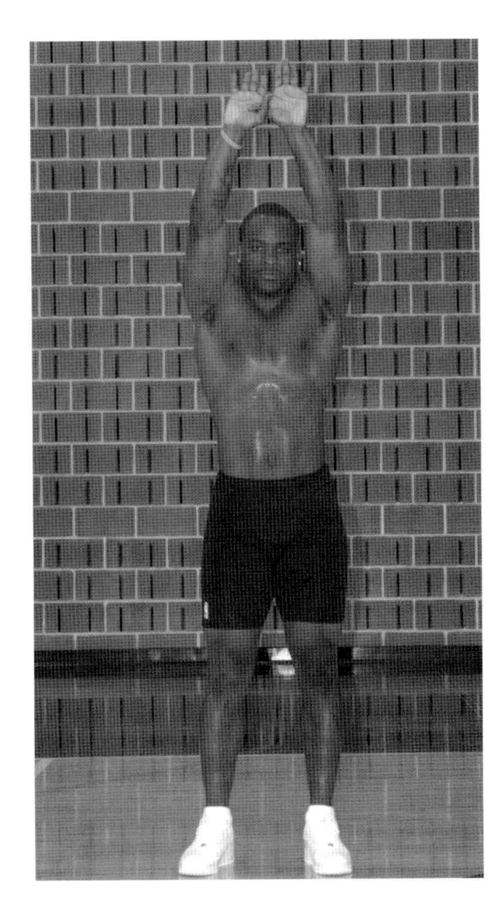

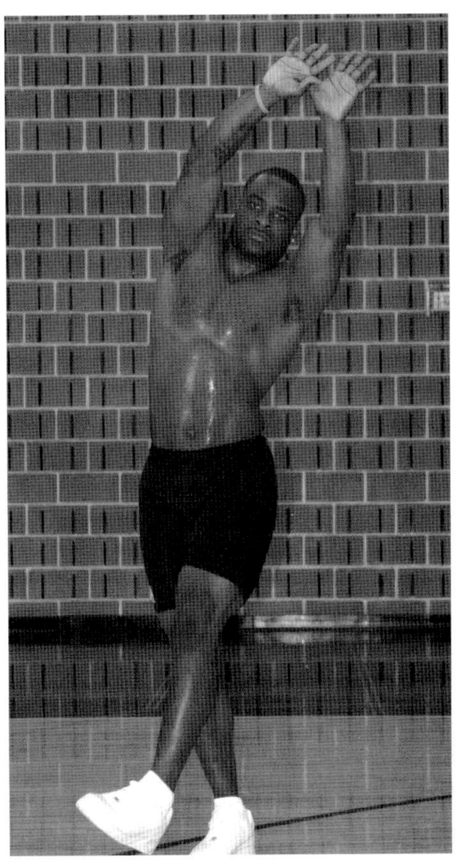

**STARTING POSITION:** Standing in the ready position, raise your arms above your head.

**THE MOVE:** Simultaneously move your left leg to your right across your body as you bend your upper body to the left. Return to the starting position and repeat.

### TRAINING TIPS

- As you bend to the left, create a C-like curve with your upper body.
- Feel the movement initiating from the center of your body.
- Keep your inner core activated throughout the movement.
- You can do all the repetitions on one side, then switch. Or alternate sides with each rep.

# 27

# BUTT AND HIP MOVES

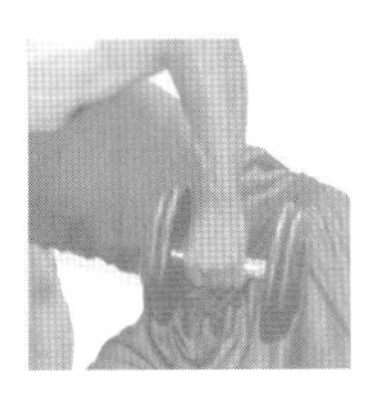

# EXERCISE: ON THE BALL—
# GLUTE BRIDGE WITH HIP ROTATION

DIFFICULTY: **3** LOWER BACK: **MODERATE RISK**

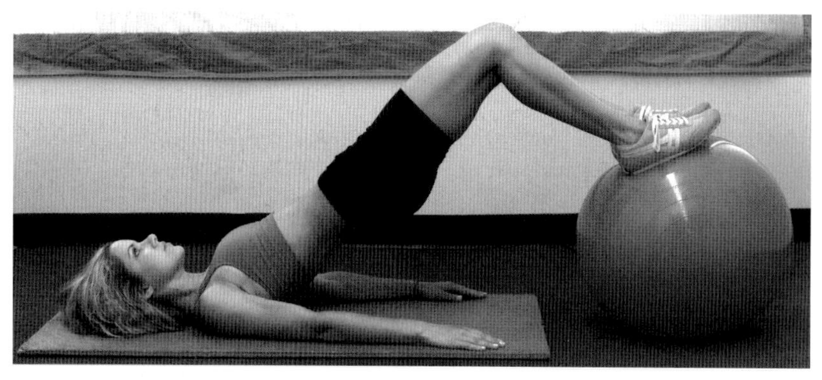

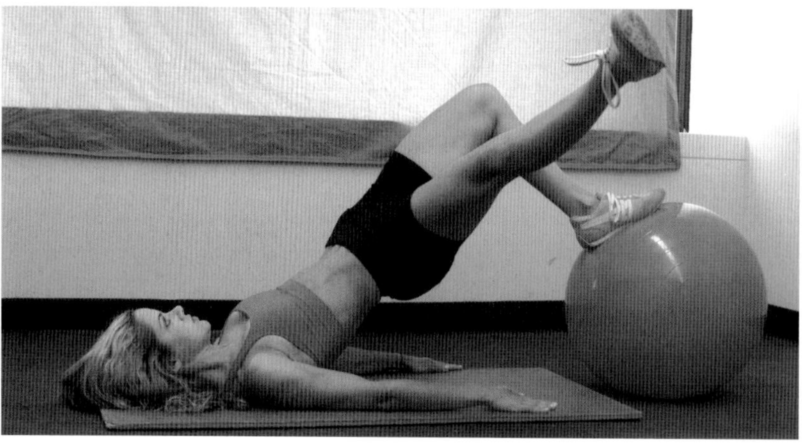

**STARTING POSITION:** Lie on the floor, feet on top of the exercise ball, hands at your sides.

**THE MOVE:** Elevate your hips, then raise your right leg from the ball, sticking it out at about a 45 degree angle. Rotate your hip outward, then draw circles with your leg. Reverse circular directions with each rep. Switch legs.

### TRAINING TIPS

- Don't let your hips sag.
- Keep your entire body still, except for your hip.
- Keep your inner core activated.
- Initiate the movement from the center of your body.

# EXERCISE: PELVIC ROCK

DIFFICULTY: **1** LOWER BACK: **LOW RISK** AREA: **CORE MUSCLES**

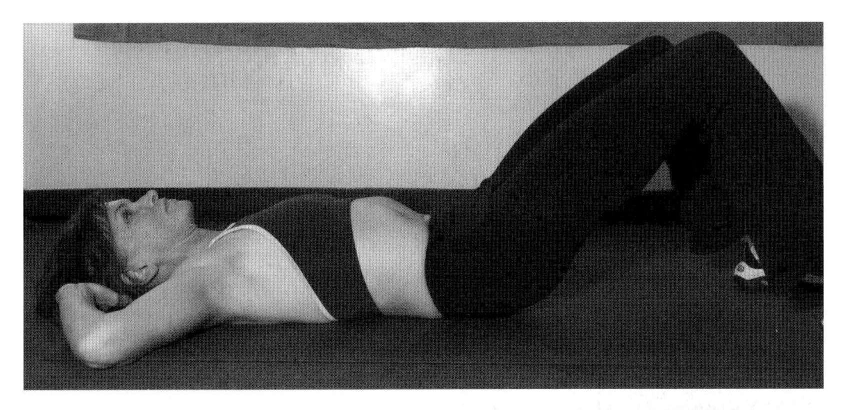

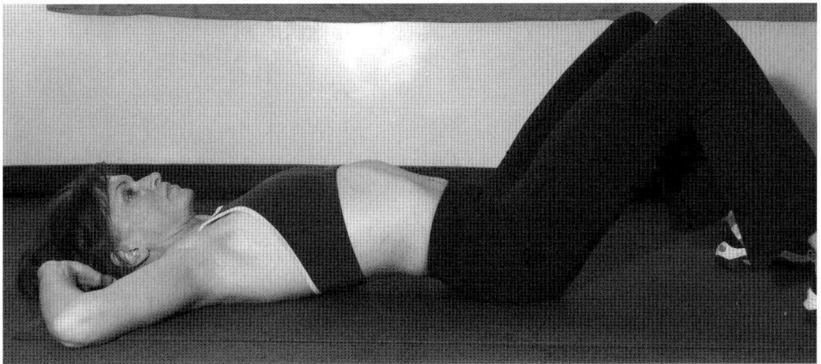

**STARTING POSITION:** Lie on your back, knees bent, feet flat on the floor, hands behind your head.

**THE MOVE:** Rotate your pelvis backward toward your rib cage, pushing the small of your back against the floor. Then rock the pelvis forward, so your lower back gently arches. Rock back and forth until you complete your set.

### TRAINING TIPS

- Feel your inner muscles initiate the movement.
- Move fluidly between positions.
- Don't hold your breath.

# EXERCISE: PELVIC CLOCK

DIFFICULTY: **2**    LOWER BACK: **LOW RISK**

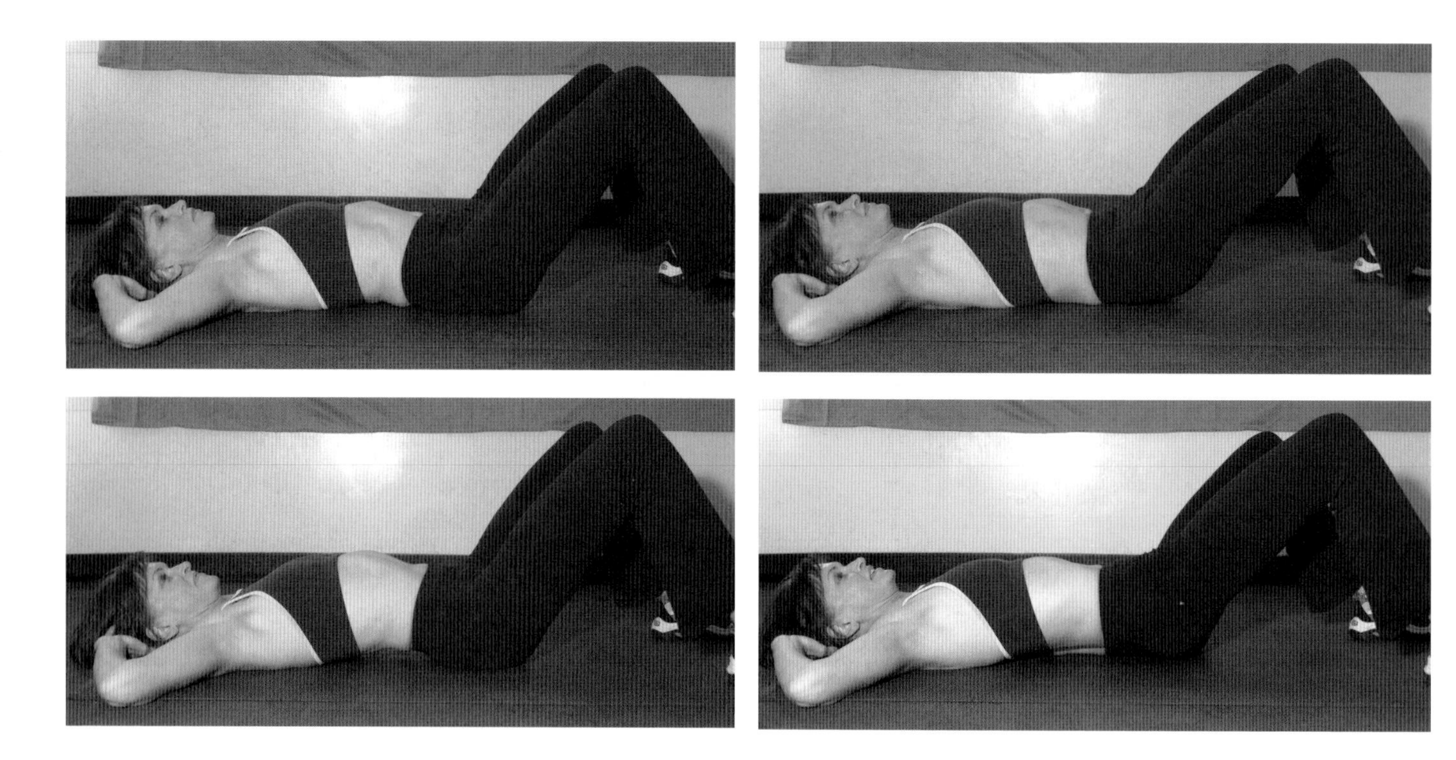

**STARTING POSITION:** Lie on your back, knees bent, feet flat on the floor, hands behind your head.

**THE MOVE:** Imagine your pelvis is a clock with 12 o'clock toward your feet, 6 toward your chest, 3 to your right side, and 9 to your left side. Work your way around the clock, gently hitting all twelve numbers; then repeat in the opposite direction.

### TRAINING TIPS

- Don't lift your buttocks off the floor instead of rotating the hips.
- Be precise with each number. This may be frustrating at first, but you will gain better control with practice.
- Breathe. When the movements are small, it is easy to forget to breathe.

# EXERCISE: GLUTE BRIDGE

DIFFICULTY: **1** LOWER BACK: **LOW RISK**

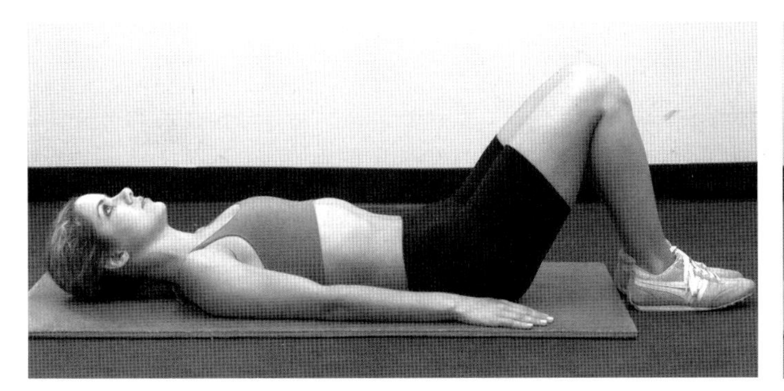

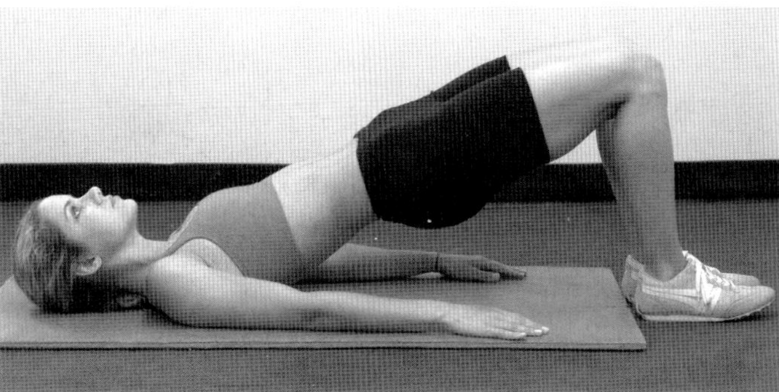

**STARTING POSITION:** Lie on your back with your knees bent and feet flat on the floor.

**THE MOVE:** Using your glutes, move your hips toward the ceiling. Only your shoulders and heels should remain on the ground. Hold this position, then lower your hips toward the floor. Repeat.

### TRAINING TIPS

- Initiate movement with your glutes.
- Don't let your glutes rest on the floor after each repetition.
- Keep your inner core activated.
- Don't let your hips sag.
- Don't let your hips rest on the floor between sets.

# EXERCISE: SIDE LEG RAISE: ALL FOURS

DIFFICULTY: **1** LOWER BACK: **MODERATE RISK**

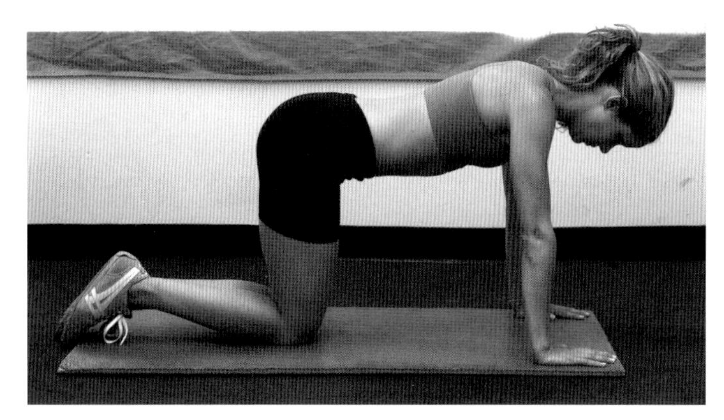

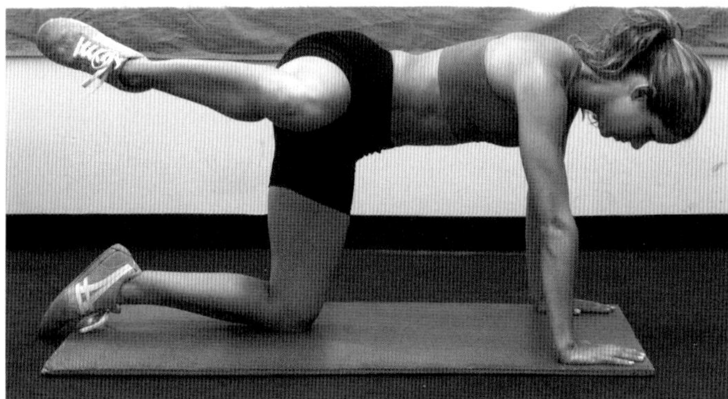

**STARTING POSITION:** Get on all fours, hands directly underneath your shoulders and knees underneath your hips.

**THE MOVE:** Keeping your working leg bent at a 90 degree angle, raise it to the side parallel to the ground or as high as possible without twisting your upper torso. Return to starting position. Repeat.

### TRAINING TIPS

- Control your return to the starting position.
- Focus your mind on the outer part of the hip throughout the exercise.
- Look straight down, keeping your neck aligned.
- Keep your back flat.

# EXERCISE: BENT-LEG KICKBACKS

DIFFICULTY: **2**   LOWER BACK: **MODERATE RISK**

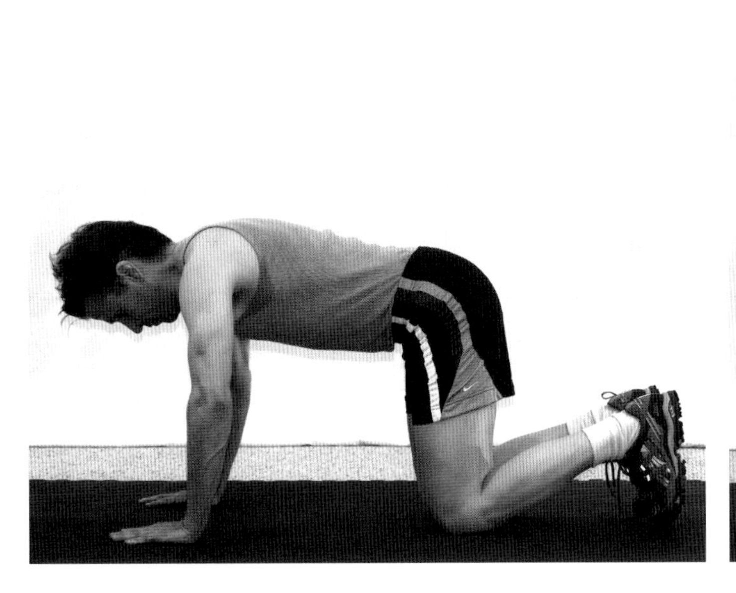

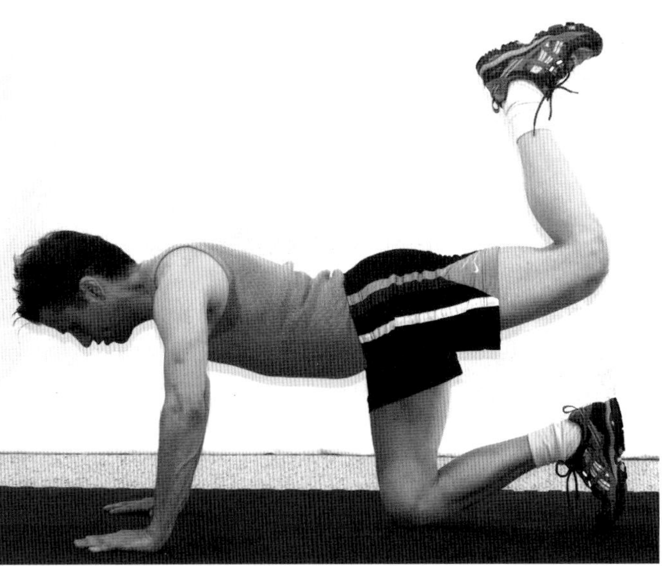

**STARTING POSITION:** Get on all fours on the floor, back flat, hands directly under your shoulders, and knees under your hips.

**THE MOVE:** Keeping your exercising leg bent at a 90 degree angle throughout the exercise, raise the leg back and up until you feel tightness in the butt (raise the sole of your foot toward the ceiling). Return your knee even or slightly in front of the nonworking leg. Repeat.

### TRAINING TIPS

- Do not overpush. Your thigh should be parallel to or slightly above the ground at the top of the motion.
- Keep motion controlled so you can feel constant tension in the butt.
- Overkicking or jerky motions can make the exercise potentially dangerous and ineffective.

# EXERCISE: HIP CIRCLES—ALL FOURS

DIFFICULTY: **2**    LOWER BACK: **LOW RISK**

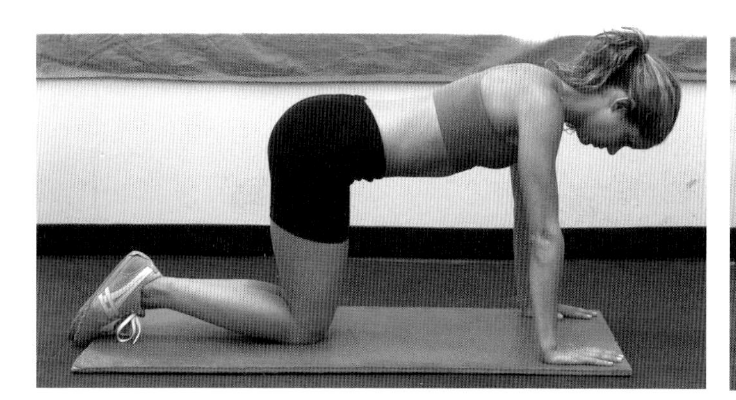
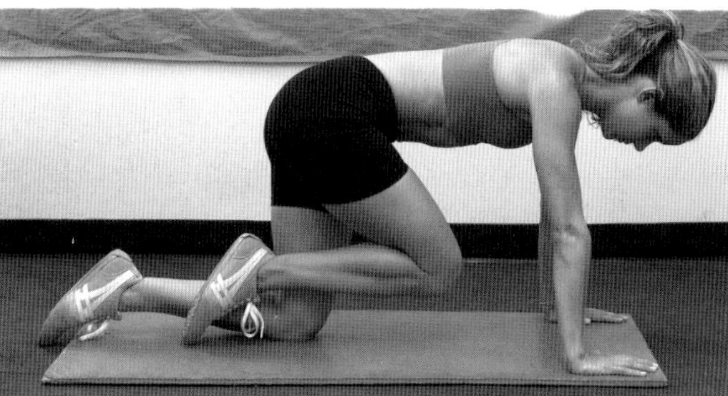
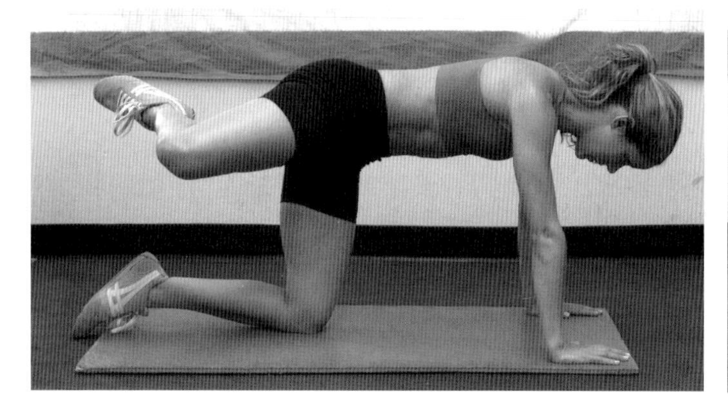
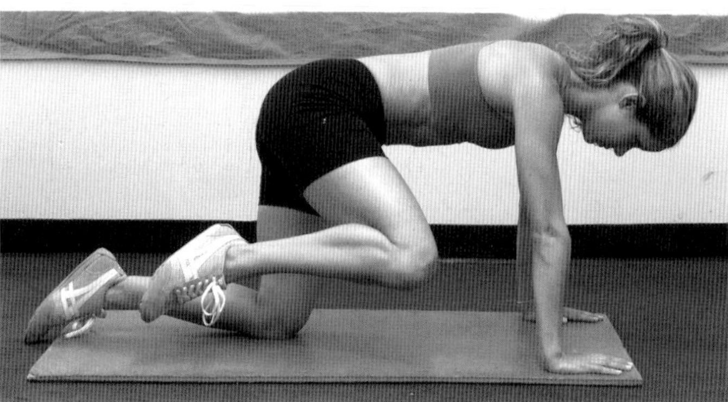

**STARTING POSITION:** Get on all fours, hands directly underneath your shoulders and knees underneath your hips.

**THE MOVEMENT:** Tuck your right knee to your chest. Then lift the leg out to the side of your hip, and rotate your hip in a circle until your leg is again tucked back into your chest. Reverse the motion for the same number of reps. Then repeat with your other leg.

### TRAINING TIPS

- Keep your back flat and head looking down.
- Take the hip through a full circle.
- Keep your inner core activated.

# EXERCISE: PRONE SINGLE-LEG RAISES

DIFFICULTY: 1 LOWER BACK: **MODERATE RISK**

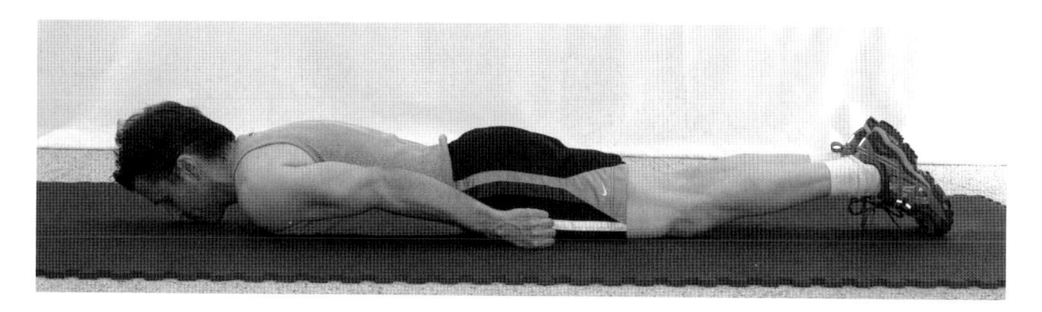

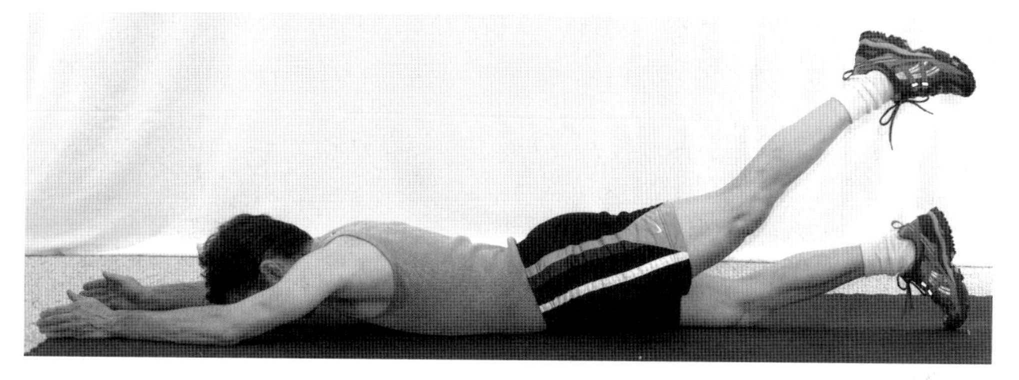

**STARTING POSITION:** Lie on your stomach with your legs extended, hands at your side, thumbs down.

**THE MOVE:** Raise working leg (keeping it slightly bent at the knee) until you feel tightness in your butt. Return to starting position. Your leg should remain extended throughout the exercise.

**VARIATION:** This move can also be done by bending your working leg to a 90 degree angle.

### TRAINING TIPS

- Do not raise leg so high that you feel pain in the lower back.
- Keep motion controlled so you can feel constant tension in the butt.
- Initiate the movement from the center of your body, not your leg.
- Keep your inner core activated.
- Your arms can be placed at your sides, extended above your head, or placed underneath your forehead. Picture two shows an alternative arm position.

# EXERCISE: BALL BRIDGE WITH LEG RAISE

DIFFICULTY: **2** LOWER BACK: **MODERATE RISK**

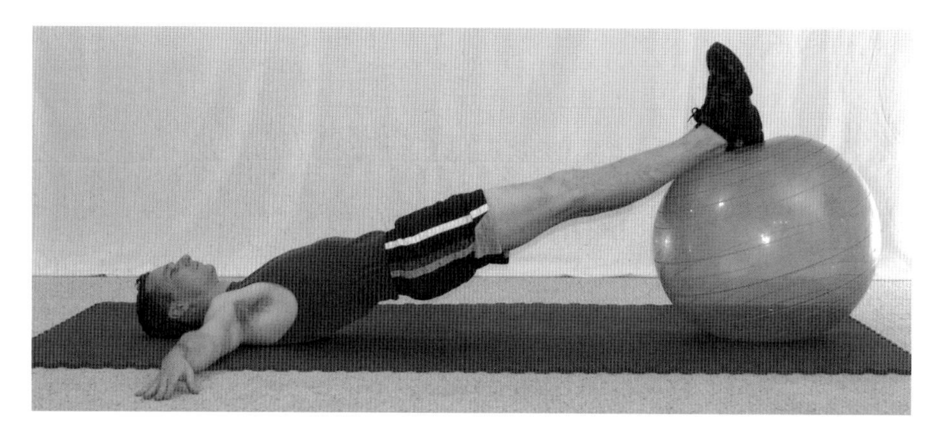

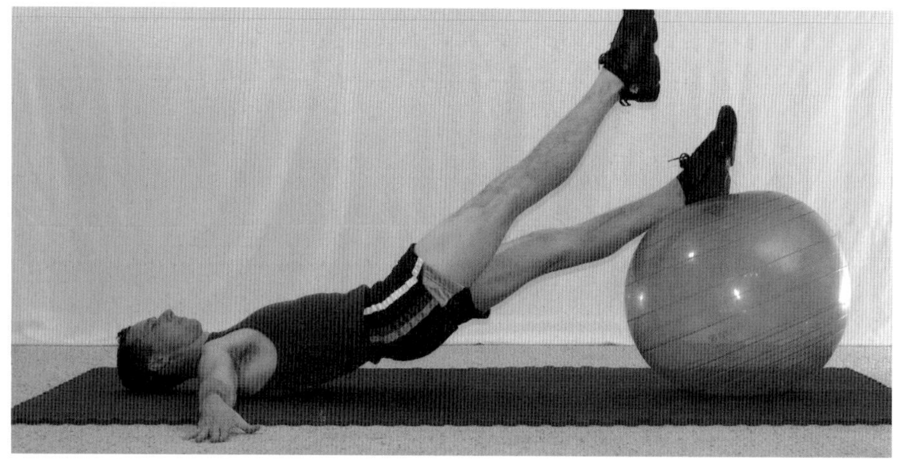

**STARTING POSITION:** Lie on the floor, arms extended out to your sides, and feet and lower legs on top of the exercise ball.

**THE MOVE:** Raise your pelvis and body from the floor so that your body is diagonal from shoulders to feet. Slowly raise one leg from the ball and hold. Return to starting position and repeat with the other leg.

### TRAINING TIPS

- Keep the ball still.
- Keep your inner core activated.
- Don't let your hips sag down toward the floor.
- Initiate the movement from the center of your body.

# EXERCISE: ON THE BALL—GLUTE BRIDGE

DIFFICULTY: **2**  LOWER BACK: **LOW RISK**

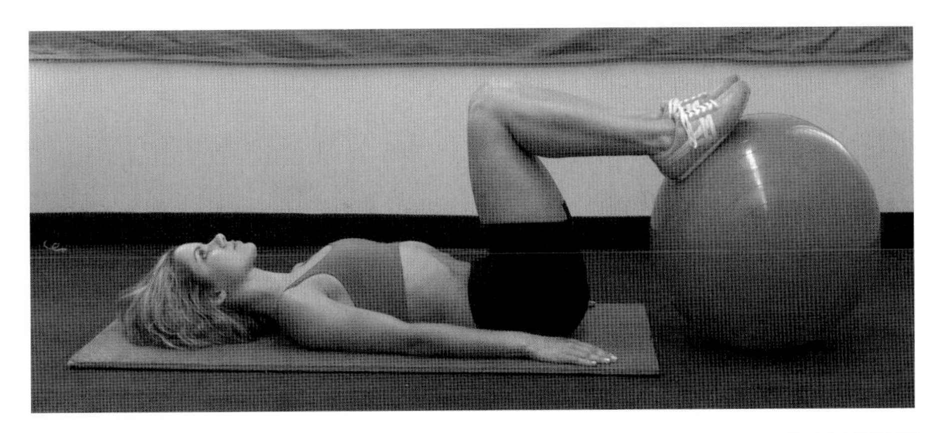

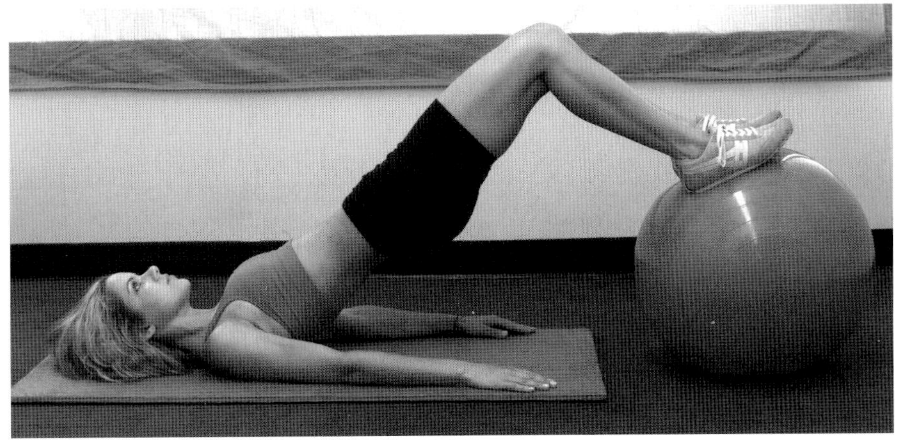

**STARTING POSITION:** Lie on the floor with your feet planted flat on top of the ball, your arms placed by your sides.

**THE MOVE:** Slowly raise your pelvis from the floor until your body is diagonal from feet to shoulders. Slowly return to the starting position and repeat.

**TRAINING TIPS**

- Keep your inner core activated.
- Keep the ball stable.
- Initiate the movement from your butt.

# EXERCISE: ON THE BALL—REVERSE HYPEREXTENSION

DIFFICULTY: **1** LOWER BACK: **LOW RISK**

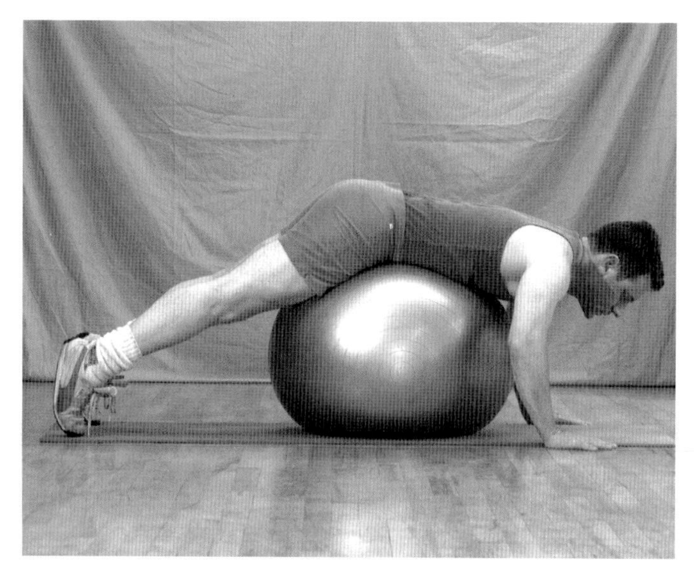

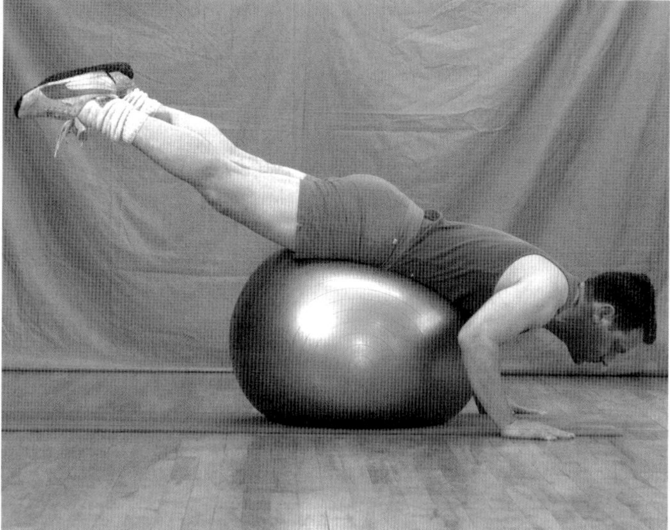

**STARTING POSITION:** Lie on your stomach over the top of an exercise ball with your hands on the ground and your legs extended straight.

**THE MOVE:** Keeping your upper body stable, use your glutes to lift your legs and create a straight diagonal line with your upper body.

### TRAINING TIPS

- Keep shoulder blades back and down as you squeeze the glutes.
- Initiate the movement from your center; not your feet.
- Keep your inner core activated.

**VARIATION:** You can do one leg at a time, alternating legs with each rep.

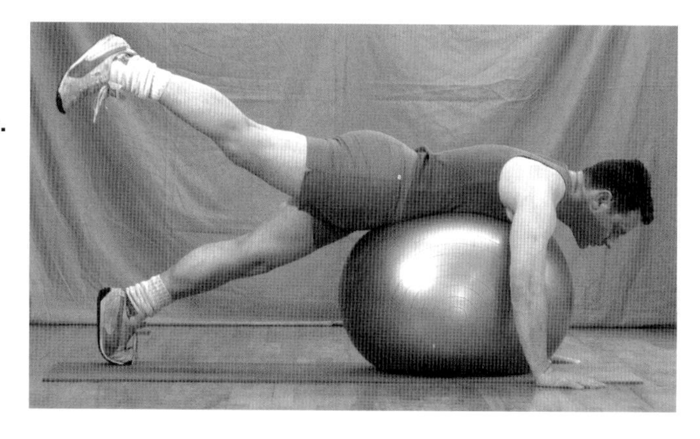

# EXERCISE: ON THE BALL—STRAIGHT LEG BRIDGING

DIFFICULTY: **2** LOWER BACK: **LOW RISK**

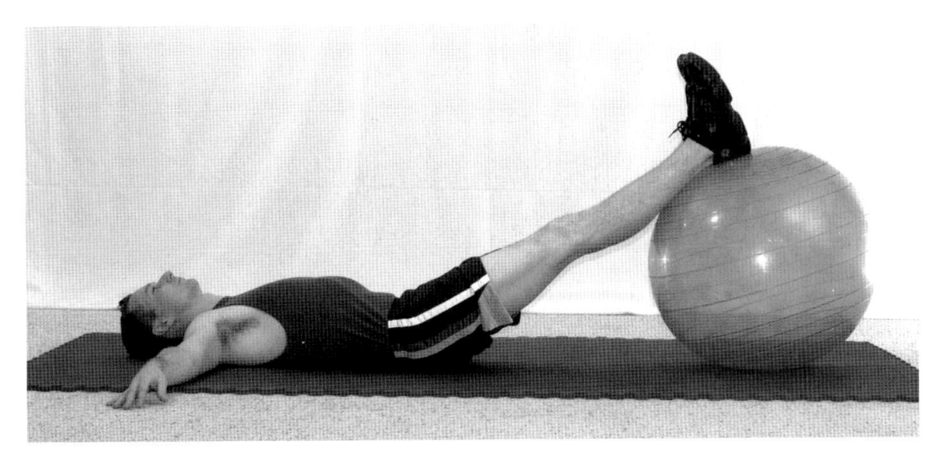

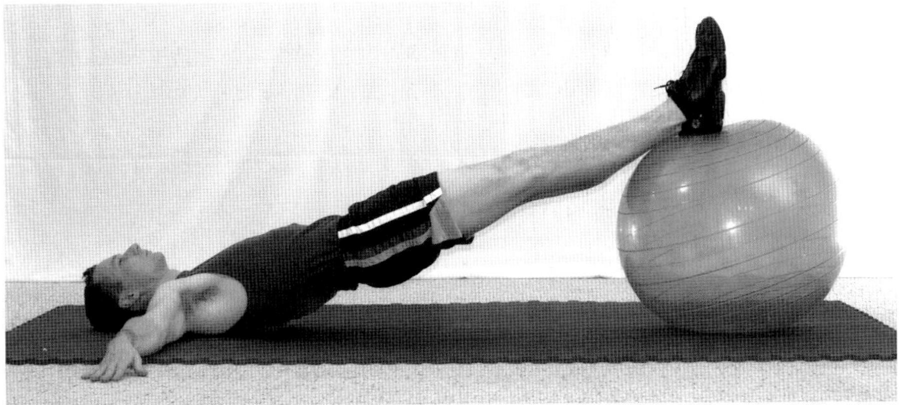

**STARTING POSITION:** Lie on your back with your feet on the ball, arms at shoulder level, and shoulder blades pulled back and down.

**THE MOVE:** Raise your hips so that only your head, shoulders, and arms are touching the floor. There should be a straight line between your ankles and shoulders.

### TRAINING TIPS

- Initiate the movement from the center of your body.
- Don't let your hips sag.
- Keep your inner core activated.

# EXERCISE: STRAIGHT-LEG ROTATIONS

DIFFICULTY: **2** LOWER BACK: **MODERATE RISK**

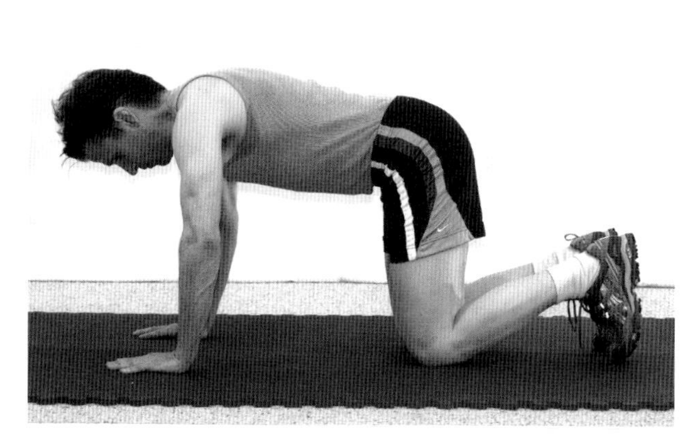

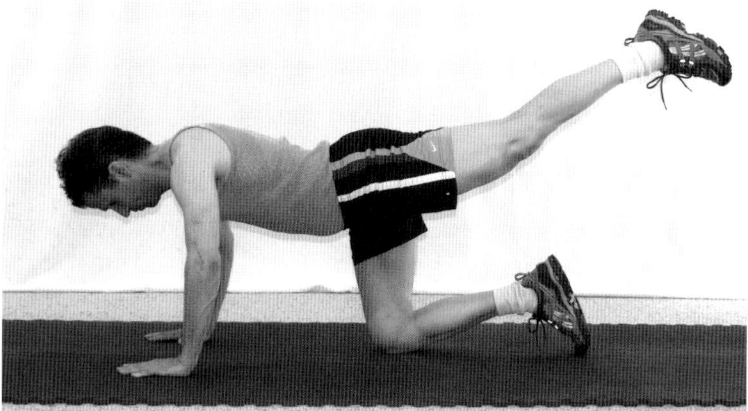

**STARTING POSITION:** Get on all fours, hands underneath your shoulders and knees under your hips. Extend working leg back and parallel to the ground. Your head and neck should be aligned with the spine, head looking straight down.

**THE MOVE:** Keeping your working leg straight, make a small circular clockwise motion. Alternate directions with each repetition. Repeat with other leg.

### TRAINING TIPS

- Avoid making too big a circle. Keep circles small to avoid stress on the lower back.
- Keep the rest of your body stationary throughout the exercise.
- This exercise can be performed using ankle weights.
- Initiate the movement from the center of your body, not from the leg.
- Keep your inner core activated.

# EXERCISE: ON THE BALL—GLUTE RAISE HIP ROTATION

DIFFICULTY: **2** LOWER BACK: **MODERATE RISK**

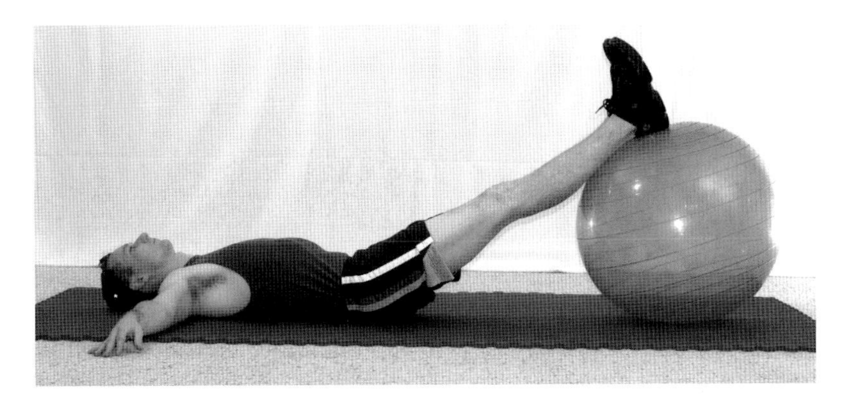

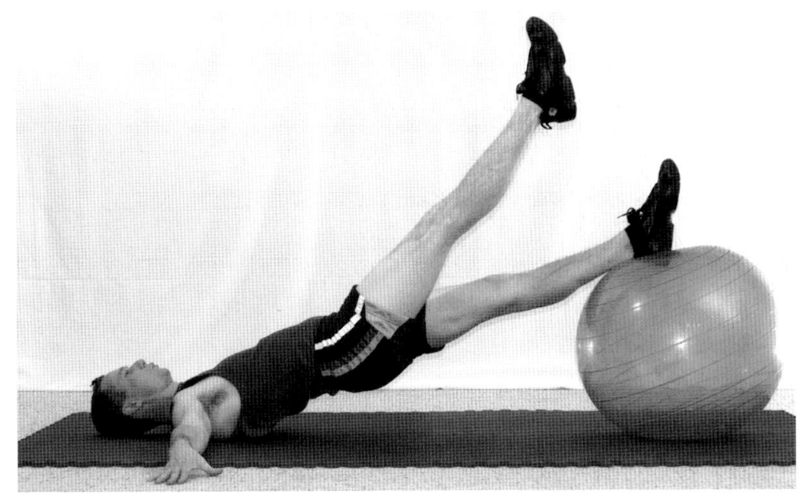

**STARTING POSITION:** Lie on the floor, feet on top of an exercise ball, hands at your sides.

**THE MOVE:** Raise your body off the floor into a plank position. Raise your right leg from the ball about 45 degrees, slowly turn the leg outward from the hip, then draw circles, alternating directions with each repetition. Return the leg to the ball and repeat with the left leg.

**TRAINING TIPS**

- Keep your inner core activated.
- Initiate the movement from your hip, not your leg.
- Keep your spine long and aligned.

# EXERCISE: LATERAL LUNGE

DIFFICULTY: **2** LOWER BACK: **MODERATE RISK**

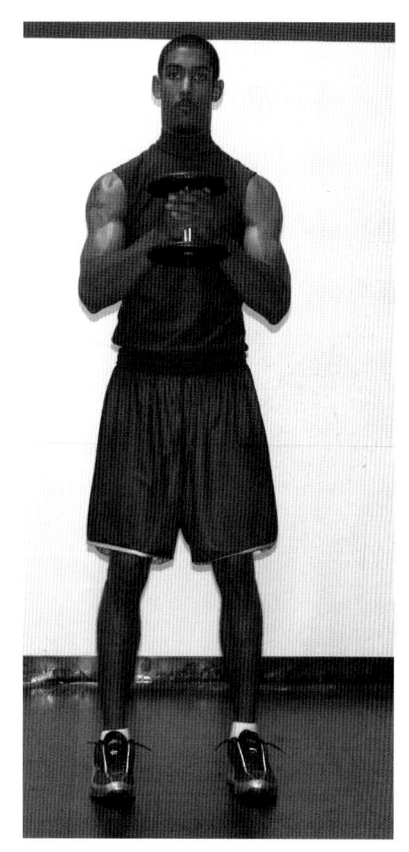

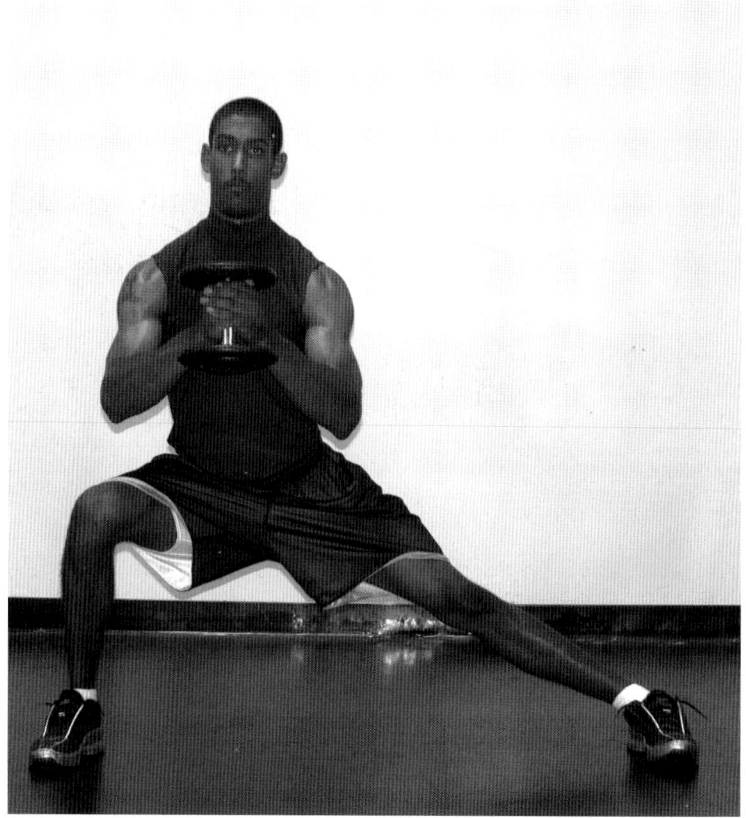

**STARTING POSITION:** Stand in ready position with hands at your sides or holding a weight.

**THE MOVEMENT:** Step out to side and lower your body down over your right leg. Keeping your left leg at a diagonal and straight, return to standing position and repeat.

### TRAINING TIPS

- Keep both feet flat and pointed forward.
- Keep your upper body straight and aligned.
- Keep your inner core activated.
- Using the weight increases the difficulty.

# EXERCISE: ON THE BALL: REVERSE GLUTE BRIDGE

DIFFICULTY: **2** LOWER BACK RISK: **MODERATE RISK**

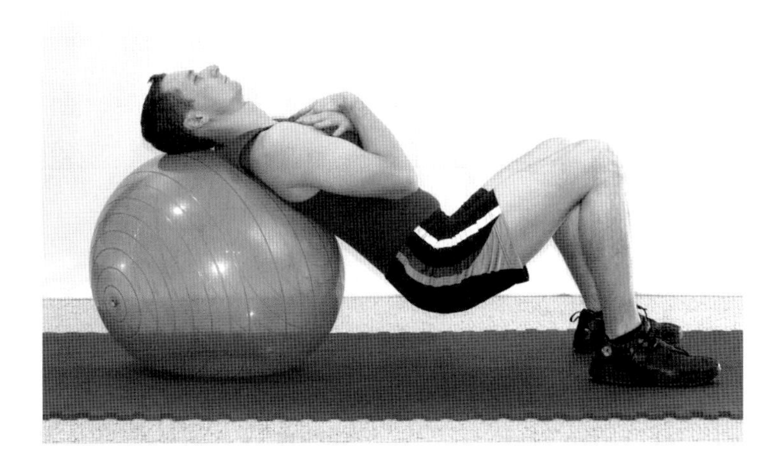

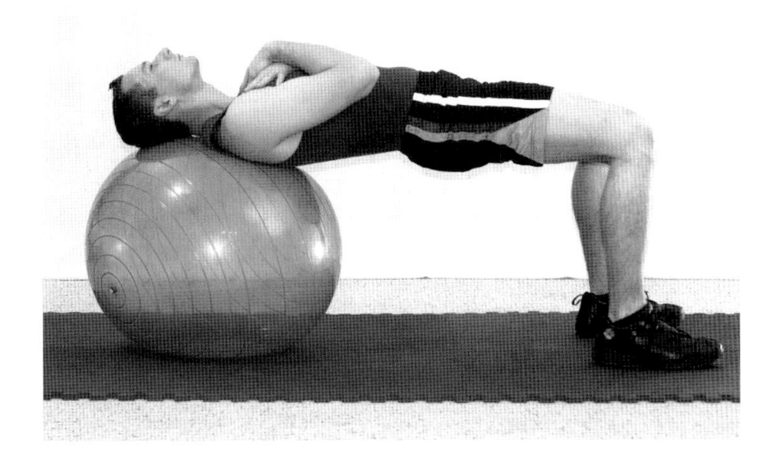

**STARTING POSITION:** Sit with your upper back resting against an exercise ball and your butt dropped down a few inches above the floor.

**THE MOVE:** Raise your hips up, creating a straight line from your knees to your shoulders.

### TRAINING TIPS

- Keep your inner core activated throughout the movement.
- Your ankles should be directly below your knees.
- Initiate the movement from your buttocks.

# EXERCISE: LYING SIDE LEG RAISE

DIFFICULTY: **1** LOWER BACK RISK: **LOW RISK**

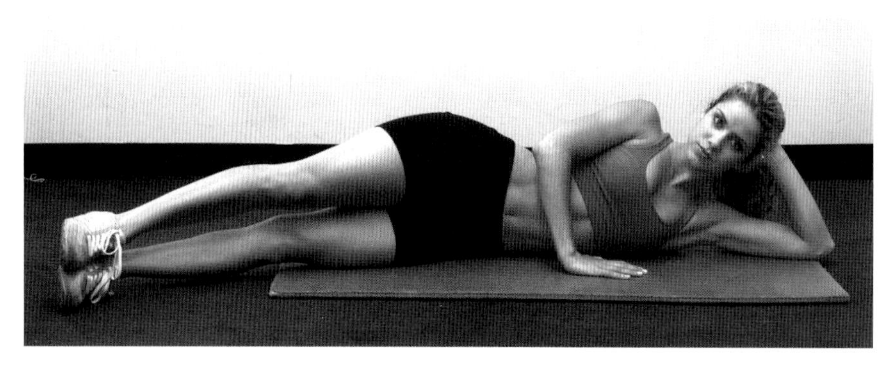

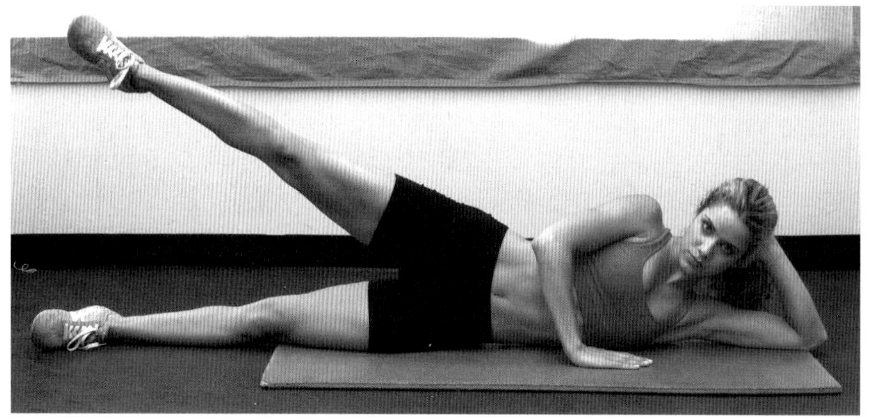

**STARTING POSITION:** Lie on your left side, supporting your head with your left arm, stabilizing your body with your right arm, and extending your legs.

**THE MOVE:** Raise your top leg straight up, then return to the starting position and repeat.

### TRAINING TIPS

- Keep your inner core activated throughout the movement.
- Let your hip socket determine the range of motion of the raise.
- Initiate the movement from your hips.

# EXERCISE: LYING INSIDE LEG RAISE

DIFFICULTY: **1** LOWER BACK RISK: **LOW RISK**

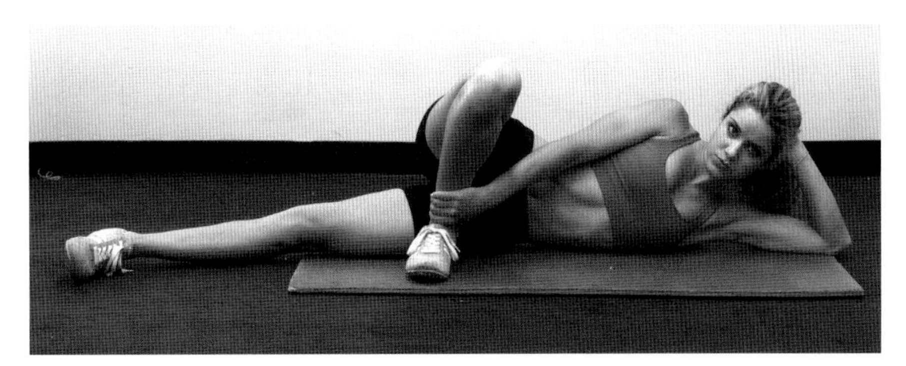

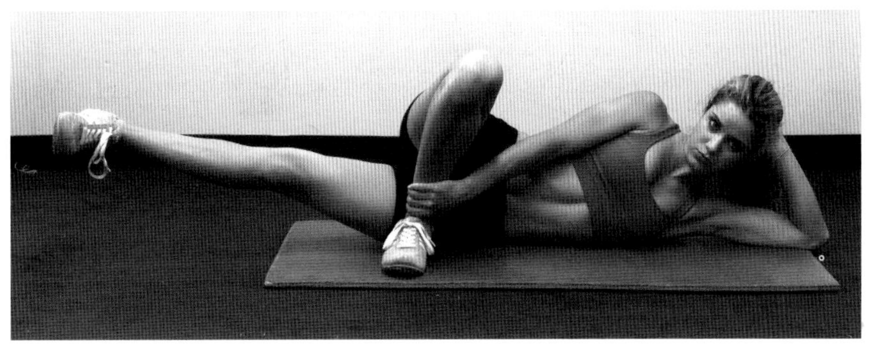

**STARTING POSITION:** Lie on your left side, supporting your head with your left arm, and extending your legs. Take your top foot and cross it over the outside of your bottom leg.

**THE MOVE:** Raise your bottom leg straight, then return to the starting position. Repeat.

### TRAINING TIPS

- Keep your inner core activated throughout the movement.
- Initiate the movement from your hip and inner thigh.
- Keep your body stable during the movement.
- Use your right arm for support or to secure your leg.

# EXERCISE: LYING HIP ROTATION

DIFFICULTY: **2** LOWER BACK RISK: **LOW RISK**

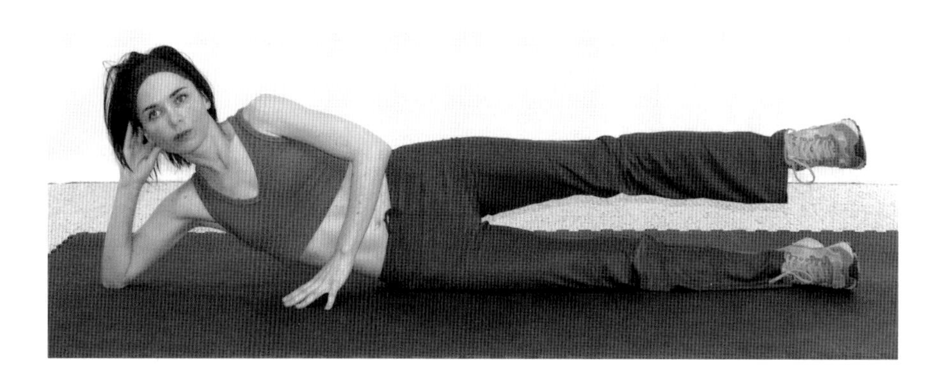

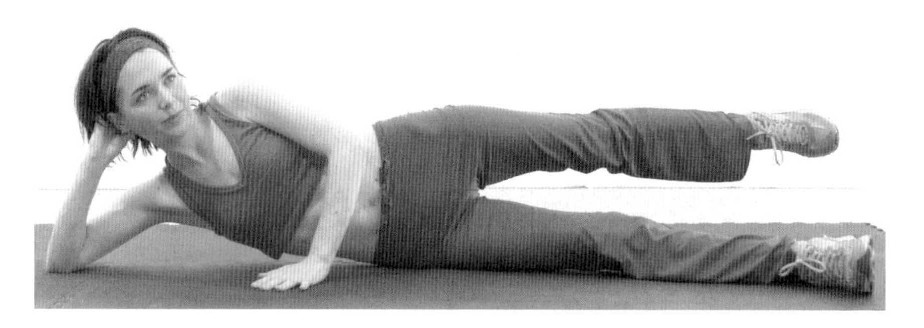

**STARTING POSITION:** Lie on your right side, supporting your head with your right arm, and extending your legs.

**THE MOVE:** Make a small circle with your upper leg. Change directions after each completed circle.

### TRAINING TIPS

- Keep your inner core activated throughout the movement.
- Initiate the movement from your hip.
- Keep the motion controlled and isolated to the hip area.

# EXERCISE: LYING HIP SWINGS

DIFFICULTY: **2** LOWER BACK RISK: **LOW RISK**

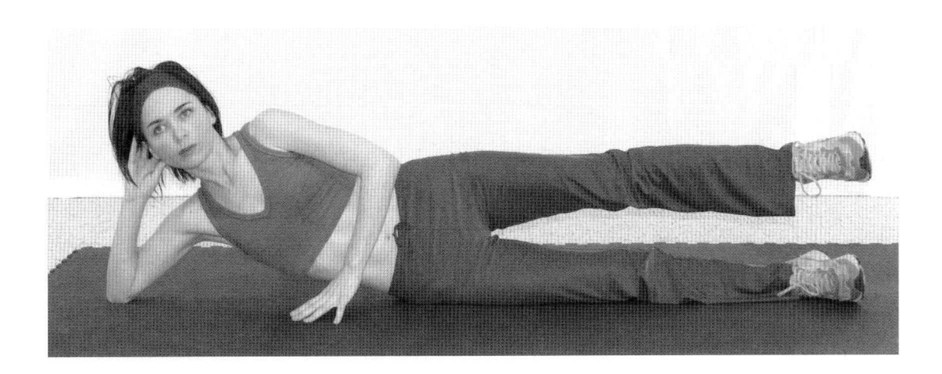

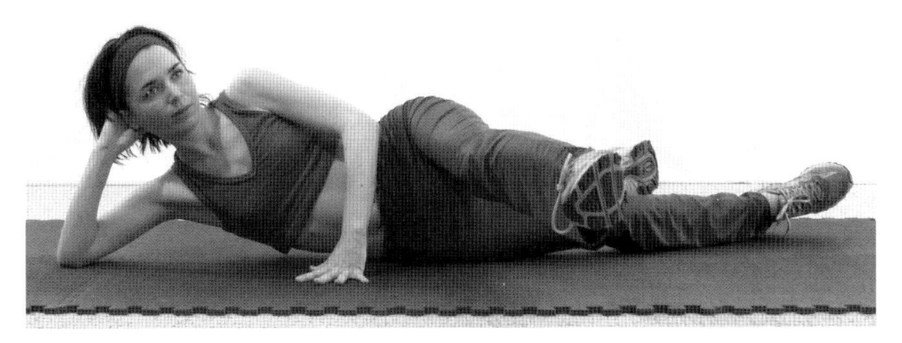

**STARTING POSITION:** Lie on your right side, supporting your head with your right arm, and extending your legs.

**THE MOVE:** Raise your upper leg a couple of inches above your bottom leg, then in a controlled motion swing the upper leg forward in front of your body, then backward behind your body. Repeat.

### TRAINING TIPS

- Keep your inner core activated throughout the movement.
- Initiate the movement from your hip.
- Keep the motion controlled and isolated to the hip area.
- Keep the swinging leg on a level plane in the forward and backward motion.

# EXERCISE: GLUTE BRIDGE, SINGLE LEG

DIFFICULTY: **3** LOWER BACK RISK: **MODERATE RISK**

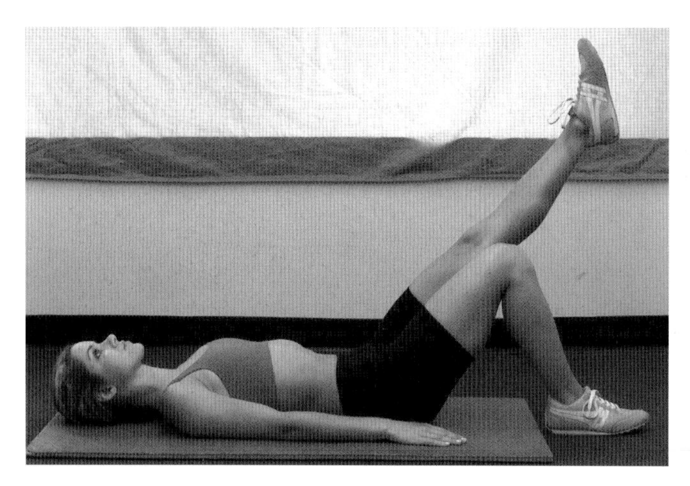

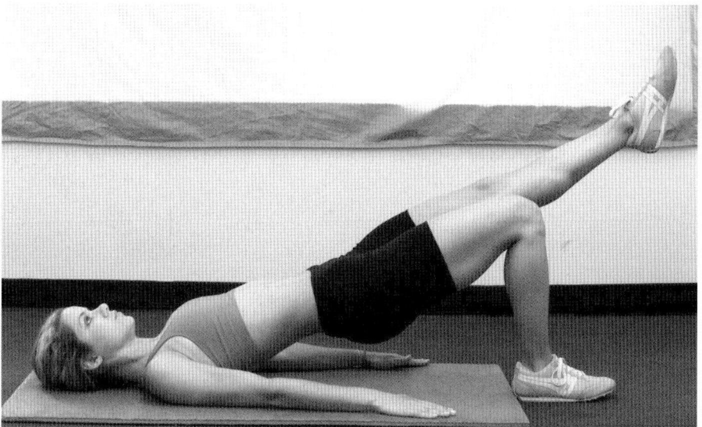

**STARTING POSITION:** Lie on your back with your knees bent and your feet flat on the floor. Then extend and raise one leg until it is level with the knee of the bent leg.

**THE MOVE:** Using your glute muscles, raise your hips up toward the ceiling. Only your shoulders and heels should remain on the ground. Pause, then lower your hips back to the floor. Repeat without resting your hips on the ground.

**VARIATION:** This move can also be done on an exercise ball.

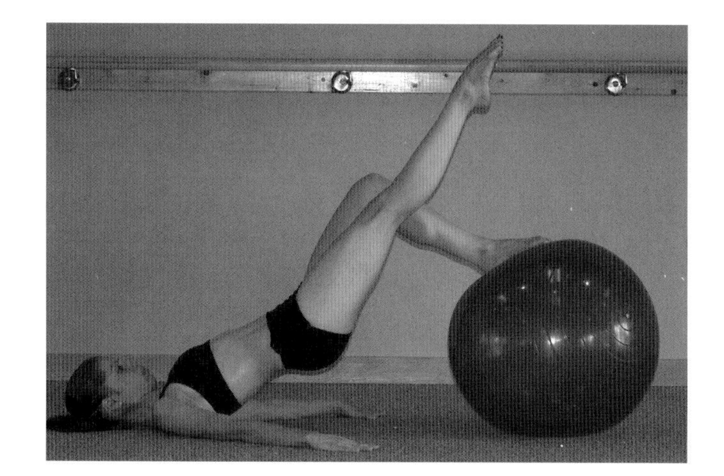

**TRAINING TIPS**

- Keep your leg extended and up throughout the exercise.
- Initiate the movement with your glutes.
- Don't rest at the bottom of the movement.
- Keep your inner core activated throughout the movement.
- Don't let your hips sag.

# EXERCISE: GLUTE BRIDGE, SINGLE-LEG ROTATION

DIFFICULTY: **3** LOWER BACK RISK: **HIGH RISK**

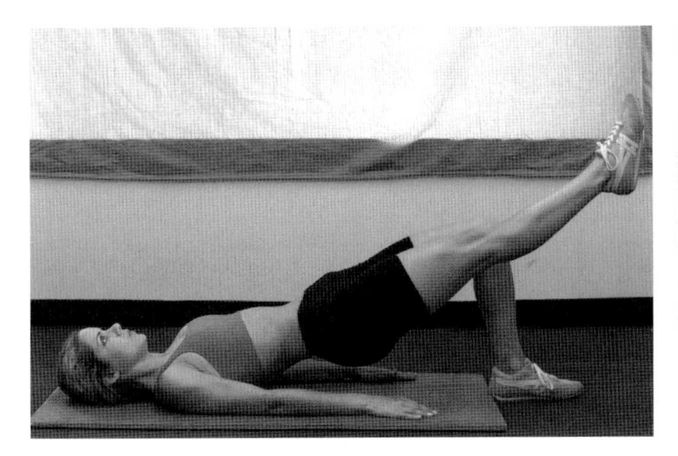

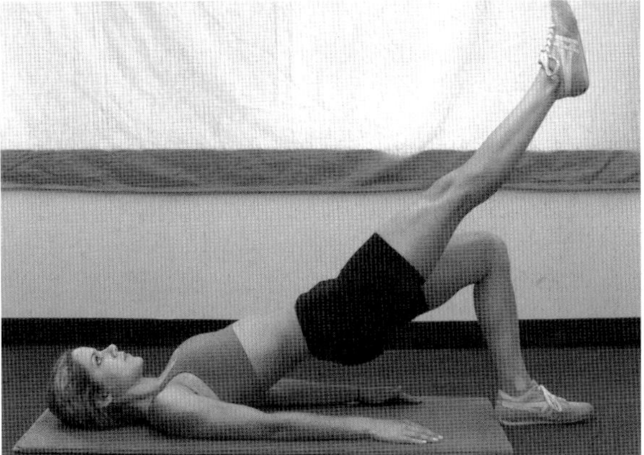

**STARTING POSITION:** Lie on your back with your knees bent and your feet flat on the floor. Extend and raise one leg until it is level with the knee of the bent leg.

**THE MOVE:** Using your glute muscles, raise your hips up toward the ceiling. Only your shoulders and heels should remain on the ground. With your leg extended, rotate your leg in a clockwise circle, and then in a counterclockwise circular motion, until you complete your prescribed number of repetitions.

**VARIATION:** This move can also be done on an exercise ball.

### TRAINING TIPS

- Keep your leg extended, up, and out throughout the exercise.
- On the bottom half of the rotation your leg will drop below knee level of the other leg.
- On the upward half of the movement the rotation of the leg will move above the knee of the other leg.
- Initiate the movement with your glutes and hip.
- Don't rest at the bottom of the movement.
- Keep your inner core activated throughout the movement.
- Don't let your hips sag.

# EXERCISE: GLUTE BRIDGE, SINGLE-LEG 45 DEGREE

DIFFICULTY: **3** LOWER BACK RISK: **HIGH RISK**

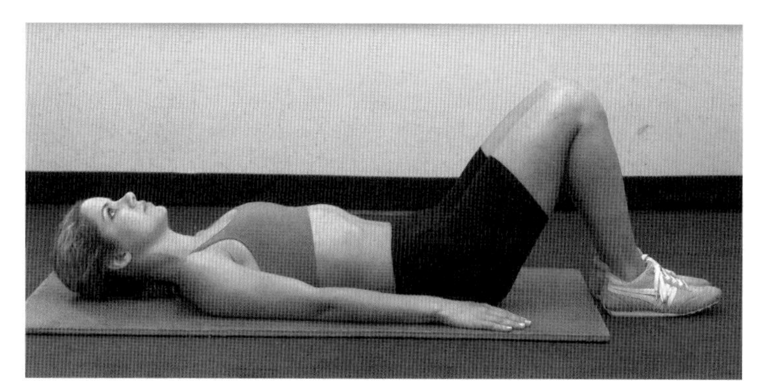

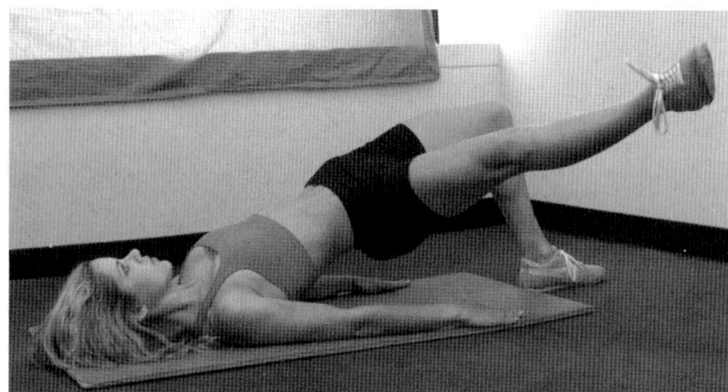

**STARTING POSITION:** Lie on your back with your knees bent and your feet flat on the floor. Extend and raise one leg until it is level with the knee of the bent leg, then move it away from the center of your body, making a 45 degree angle. If your leg was the hand on a clock it would be angled out at approximately between the 5 and the 10 on the clock face.

**THE MOVE:** Using your glute muscles, move your hips up toward the ceiling. Only your shoulders and heels should remain on the ground. Pause, then lower your hips back to the floor. Repeat.

**VARIATION:** This move can also be done on an exercise ball.

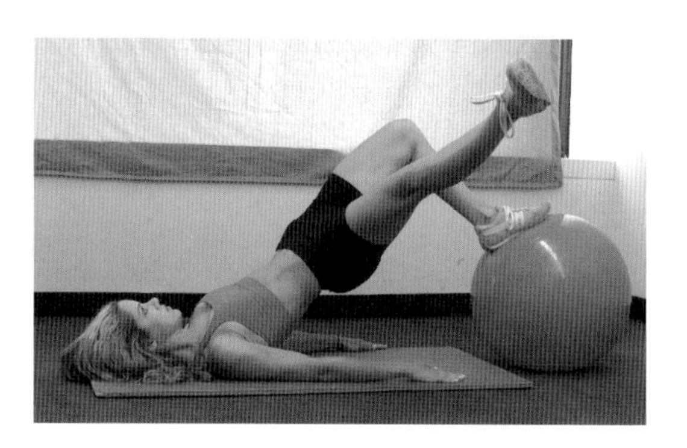

### TRAINING TIPS

- Keep your leg extended up and out at a 45 degree angle throughout the exercise.
- Initiate the movement with your glutes.
- Don't rest at the bottom of the movement.
- Keep your inner core activated throughout the movement.
- Don't let your hips sag.

# EXERCISE: HIP ABDUCTION

DIFFICULTY: **1** LOWER BACK: **LOW RISK**

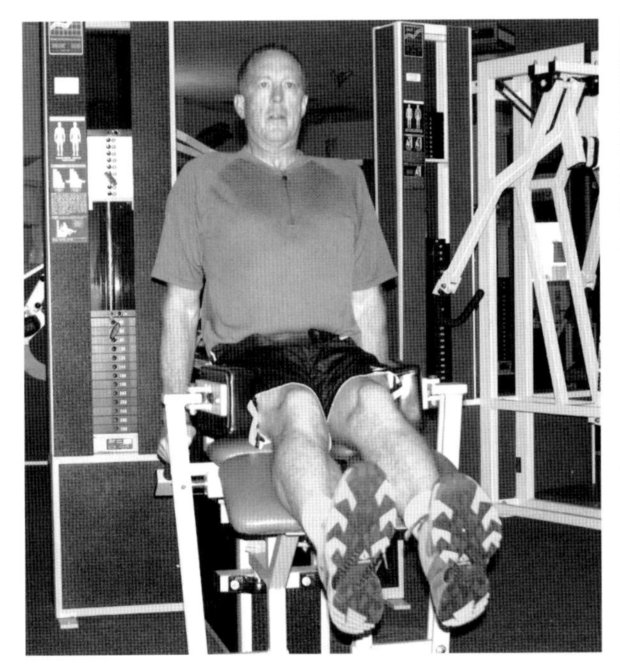

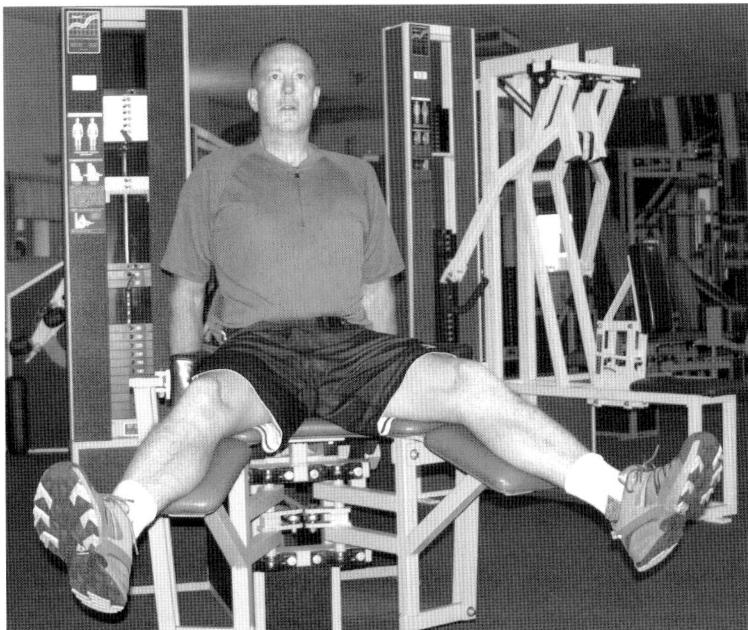

**STARTING POSITION:** Sit on the machine with your legs together, spine lengthened, and your hands lightly gripping the support handles.

**THE MOVE:** Using the abduction muscles of your hips, smoothly spread your legs apart. Return to the starting position and repeat.

### TRAINING TIPS

- Keep your inner core activated.
- Keep your hips stable as you move your legs apart.
- Keep your spine and neck in a lengthened position and in proper alignment; don't hunch.

# EXERCISE: HIP ADDUCTION

DIFFICULTY: **1** LOWER BACK: **LOW RISK**

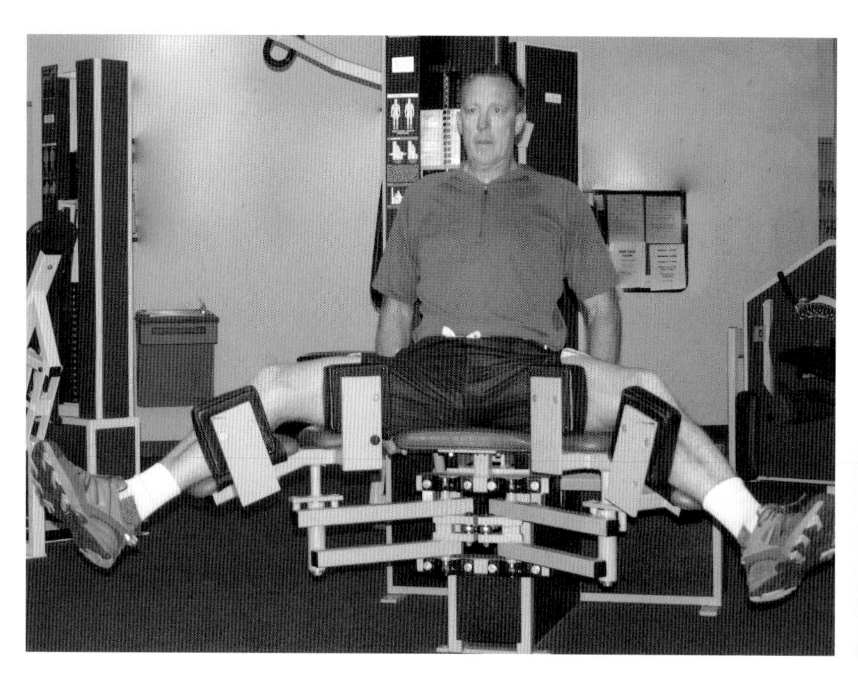

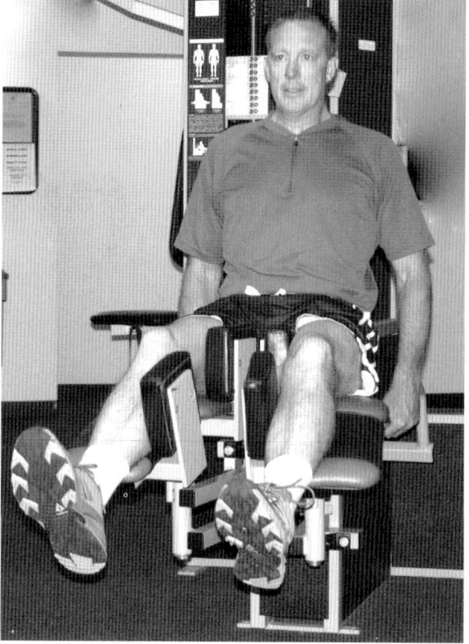

**STARTING POSITION:** Sit on the machine with your legs spread apart, spine lengthened, and your hands lightly gripping the support handles.

**THE MOVE:** Using the adduction muscles of your hips, smoothly bring your legs together. Return to the starting position and repeat.

### TRAINING TIPS

- Keep your inner core activated.
- Keep your hips stable as you move your legs apart.
- Keep your spine and neck in a lengthened position and in proper alignment; don't hunch.

# 28
# COMBO CORE MOVES

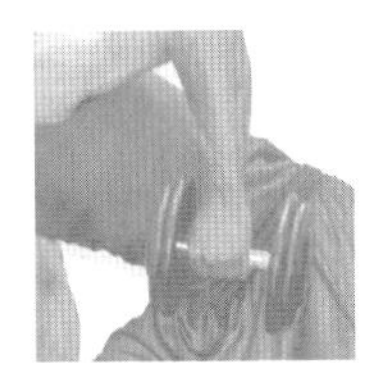

# EXERCISE: BICYCLES

DIFFICULTY: **2** LOWER BACK: **MODERATE RISK**

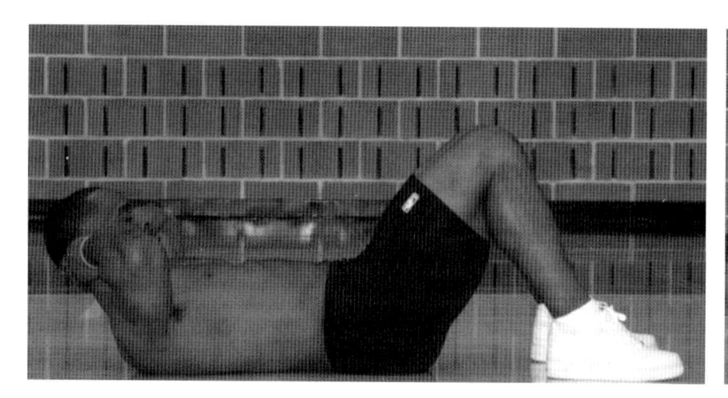

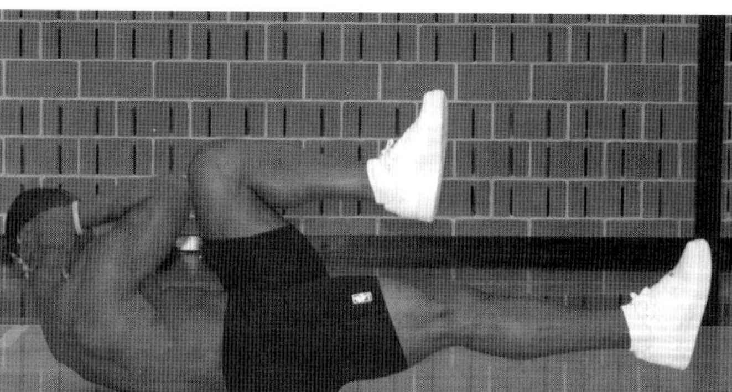

**STARTING POSITION:** Lie on your back, thighs perpendicular to your torso, feet on the floor, and hands behind your ears.

**THE MOVE:** Simultaneously bring your right shoulder and your left knee together toward each other, as you extend your left leg. Then repeat the motion to the other side. Keep the motion continuous, as if you were pedaling a bicycle.

**TRAINING TIPS**

- Keep the motion controlled; don't go too fast.
- Make sure your entire torso twists. Don't move just the elbow to the knee.
- Make sure your shoulder blades come off the floor each time.
- Don't let your legs touch the floor.
- Focus your mind on feeling the center of your body do the work.
- Keep the small of your back pressed against the floor and maintain a stable position. Do not rock.

# EXERCISE: CIRCLES

DIFFICULTY: **2** LOWER BACK: **MODERATE RISK**

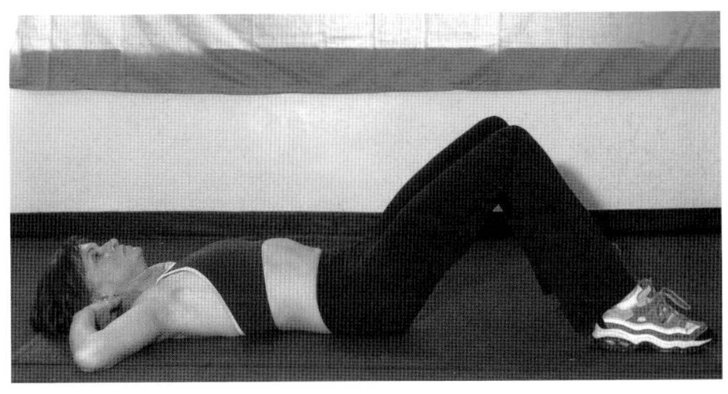

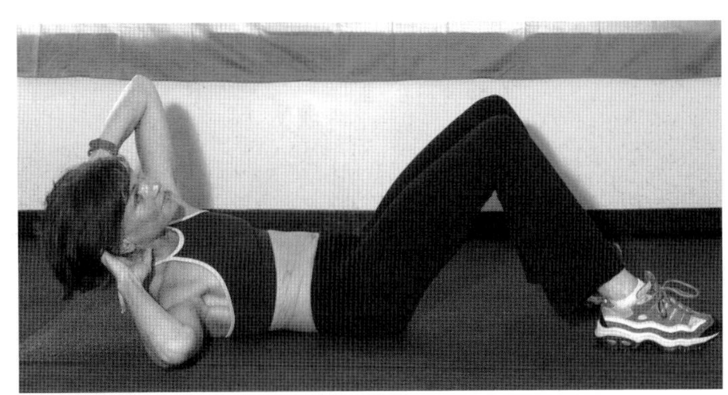

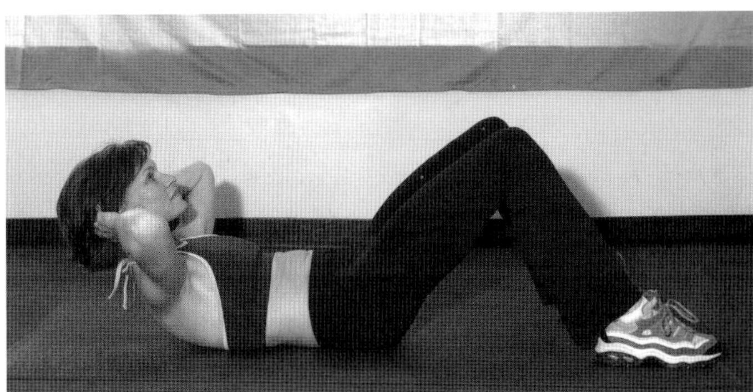

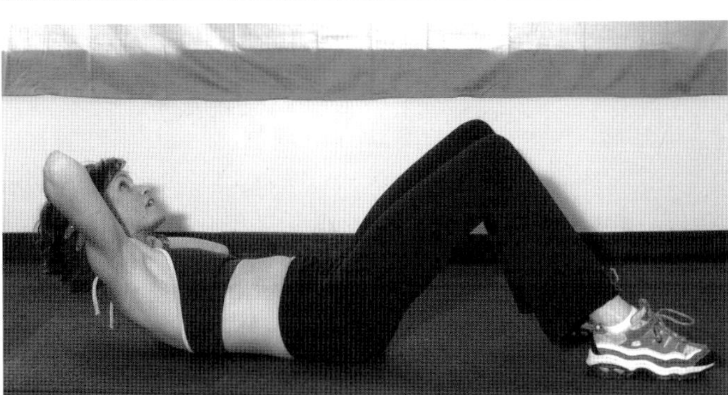

**STARTING POSITION:** Lie flat on your back, knees bent so your feet rest flat on the floor, with your hands in position of choice.

**THE MOVE:** Use your core to curl your torso toward your hip in a small circular motion. If your torso were a hand on a clock, the starting position would be 6 o'clock, moving up to the 3, then up to the 12 o'clock position. To finish, move down to the 9 and back to the 6 o'clock position, completing one repetition. Alternate directions with each repetition.

### TRAINING TIPS

- Keep constant tension on your muscles throughout the full range of motion (all directions).
- Raise your torso as high as you would on a normal crunch.
- Don't rest at the bottom of the movement.
- Focus your mind on your core.

# EXERCISE: TUMMY TUCKS

DIFFICULTY: **2** LOWER BACK: **LOW RISK**

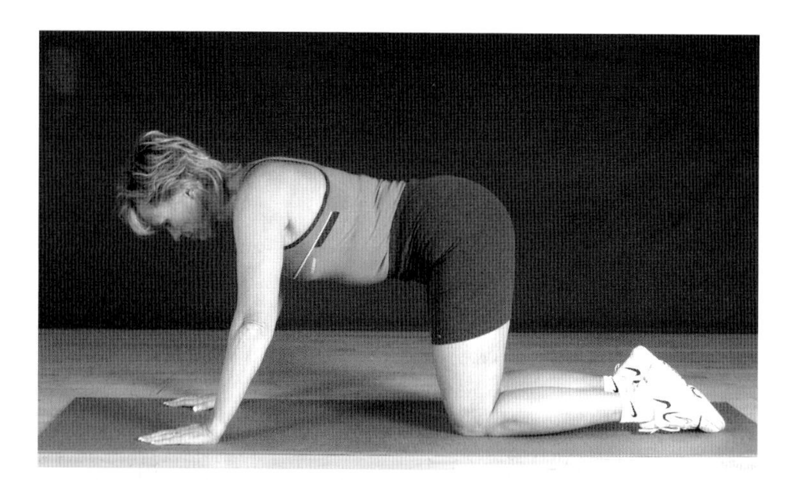

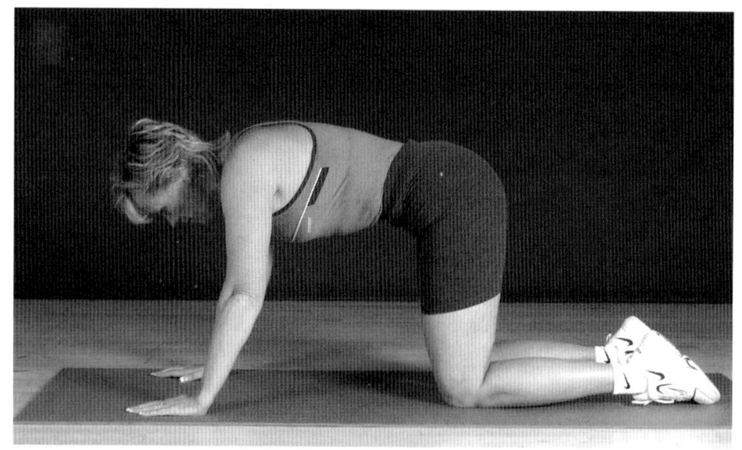

**STARTING POSITION:** On all fours, knees under your hips and hands under your shoulders.

**THE MOVE:** Inhale. Then, as you exhale, draw your belly button toward your spine. Inhale and repeat.

### TRAINING TIPS

- Focus on activating your inner core.
- Find a steady rhythm with your breathing.
- Keep your spine in neutral (neither arched nor rounded).

# EXERCISE: DYNAMIC V CRUNCH

DIFFICULTY: **3** LOWER BACK: **HIGH RISK**

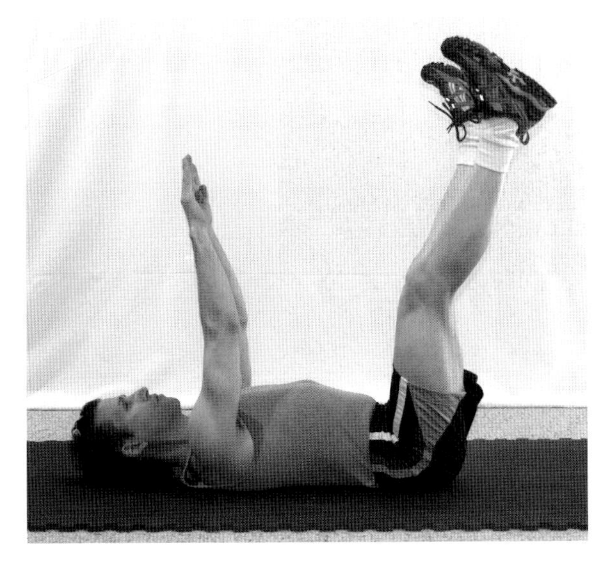

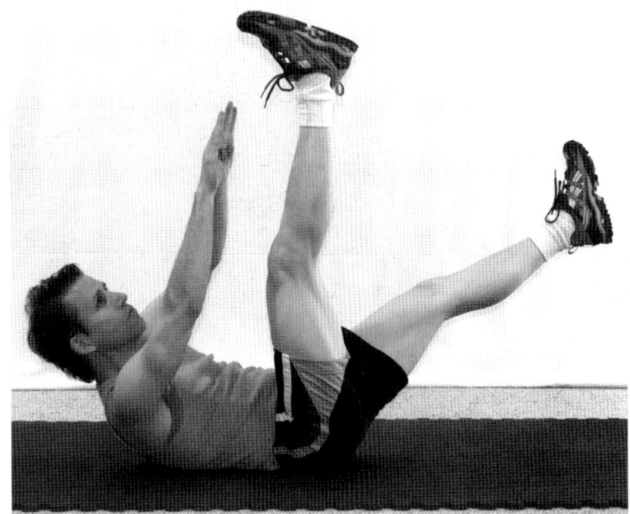

**STARTING POSITION:** Lie flat on your back, legs fully extended and raised perpendicular to your body, arms straight up.

**THE MOVE:** Lower your legs to about a 45 degree angle. Use your core to raise and cross your left shoulder toward your right leg, as you simultaneously raise your right leg, bringing it toward your hands. Simultaneously lower your leg and torso and repeat to the other side.

### TRAINING TIPS

- Keep your inner core activated.
- Keep a neutral spine.
- Initiate the movement from the center of your body, not your arms and legs.

# EXERCISE: V-UPS WITH A CROSS

DIFFICULTY: **3** LOWER BACK: **LOW RISK**

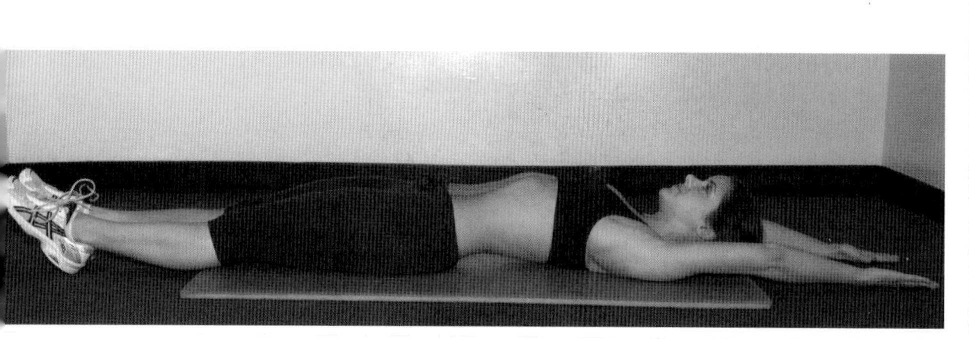

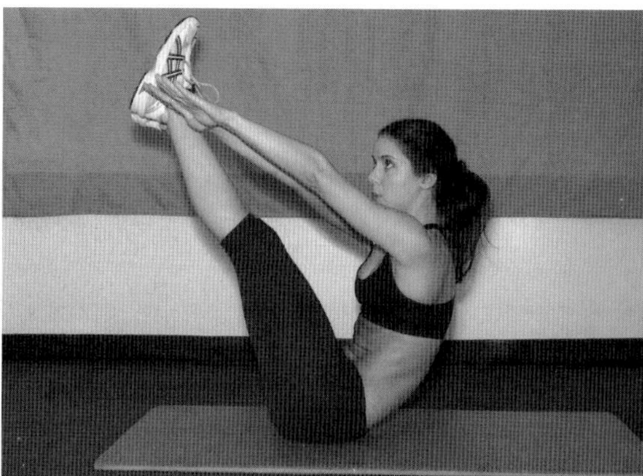

**STARTING POSITION:** Lie flat on your back, legs fully extended, heels resting on the floor, and arms extended over your head.

**THE MOVE:** Use your core to simultaneously bring your feet and hands together. As you raise your torso and legs, cross your right shoulder toward your left ankle and your left ankle toward your right shoulder. Then simultaneously lower your legs and torso. Repeat to the other side.

### TRAINING TIPS

- Think of raising your legs a split second after your torso.
- Keep your inner core activated.
- Don't rest at the bottom of the movement.
- Initiate the movement from the center of your body.

# EXERCISE: BASIC TRUNK EXTENSION WITH ROTATION

DIFFICULTY: **2** LOWER BACK: **MODERATE RISK**

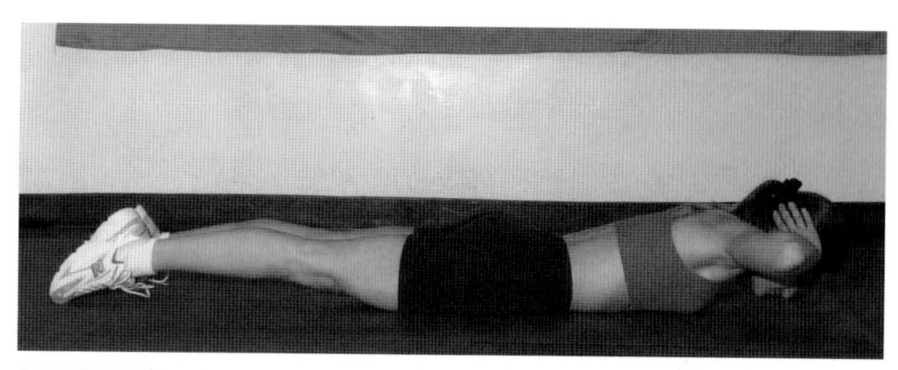

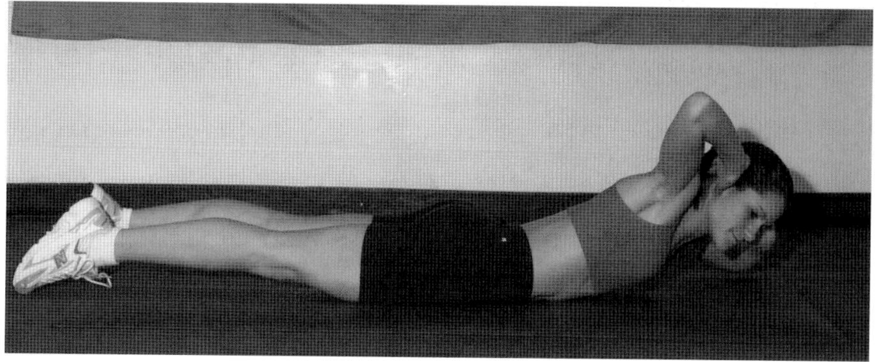

**STARTING POSITION:** Lie facedown on the floor. Place your hands behind your ears.

**THE MOVE:** Lengthening your spine, raise your torso off the floor and rotate your right shoulder up, turning your head in the same direction. Lower your torso back to the starting position and repeat to the opposite side, rotating up and to your left.

### TRAINING TIPS

- Throughout the movement, think of lengthening the spine so the exercise makes you longer and taller.
- Keep your butt muscles tight to protect your lower back.
- Focus on feeling and isolating your lower back muscles as your torso raises and turns.
- Keep your neck lengthened.

# EXERCISE: SUPERMAN WITH ROTATION

DIFFICULTY: **3** LOWER BACK RISK: **HIGH RISK**

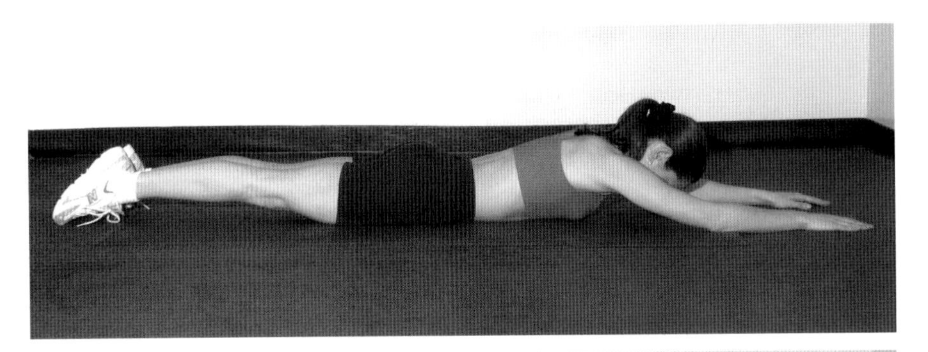

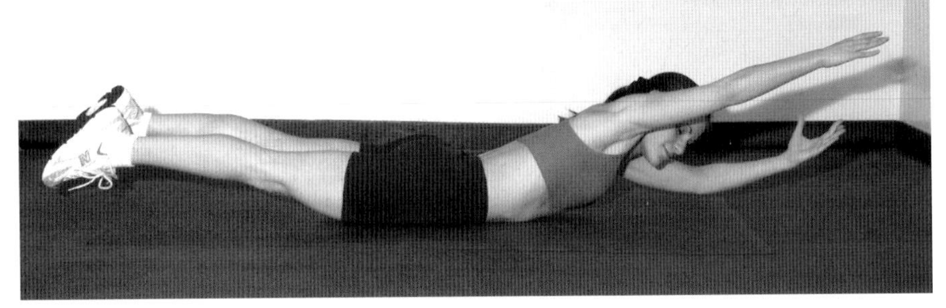

**STARTING POSITION:** Lie on your stomach with your legs fully extended on the floor and your arms extended over your head. Your head should look down.

**THE MOVE:** Simultaneously lengthen your spine and raise your arms, torso, and legs, as if you were flying. Then rotate your right shoulder up as you turn your head in the same direction. Lower your torso back to the starting position and repeat to the opposite side, rotating up and to your left. Return to the starting position and repeat.

### TRAINING TIPS

- Before you raise your arms and legs, lengthen your spine by stretching your arms and legs in opposite directions, as if someone was pulling on them.
- Feel the movement initiating from the center of your body.
- Control both the up and down phases of the movement.

# EXERCISE: ROMAN CHAIR—BACK EXTENSION WITH ROTATION

DIFFICULTY: **2** LOWER BACK RISK: **MODERATE RISK**

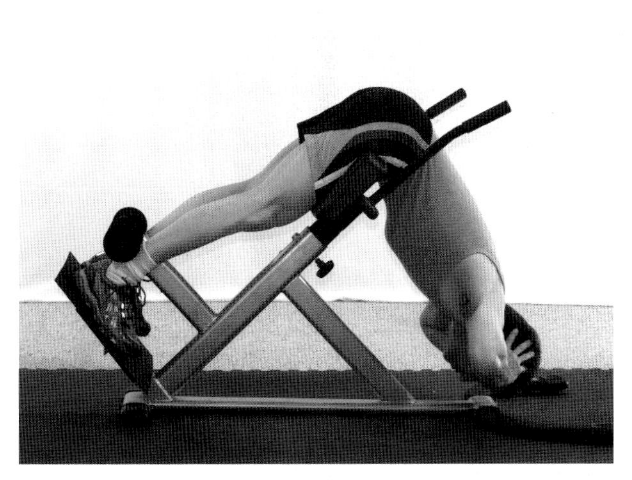

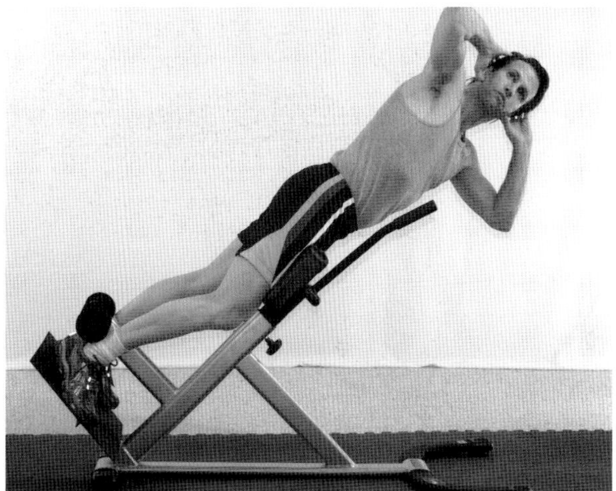

**STARTING POSITION:** Secure yourself in a Roman chair, feet under the supports. Align your body in a straight line. Make sure the chair is adjusted so your waist can bend completely forward.

**THE MOVE:** Bend forward through a full range of motion, making sure your spine and neck stay aligned. As you raise your torso back to the starting position, rotate your right shoulder up, twisting your torso in that direction. Alternate the direction of the twist with each repetition.

### TRAINING TIPS

- Let your head turn in the direction of the twist.
- Keep your neck lengthened and in line with your spine.
- Place your hands behind your head, across your chest, holding a weight plate.
- Keep the motion fluid.
- Don't hyperextend your back; return to a neutral spine.

# EXERCISE: ON THE BALL—45 DEGREE LEG EXTENSION

DIFFICULTY: **2** LOWER BACK: **MODERATE RISK**

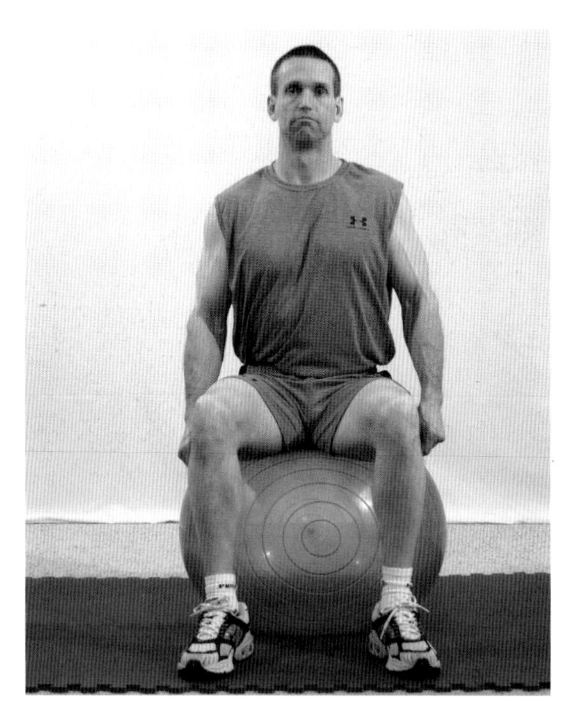

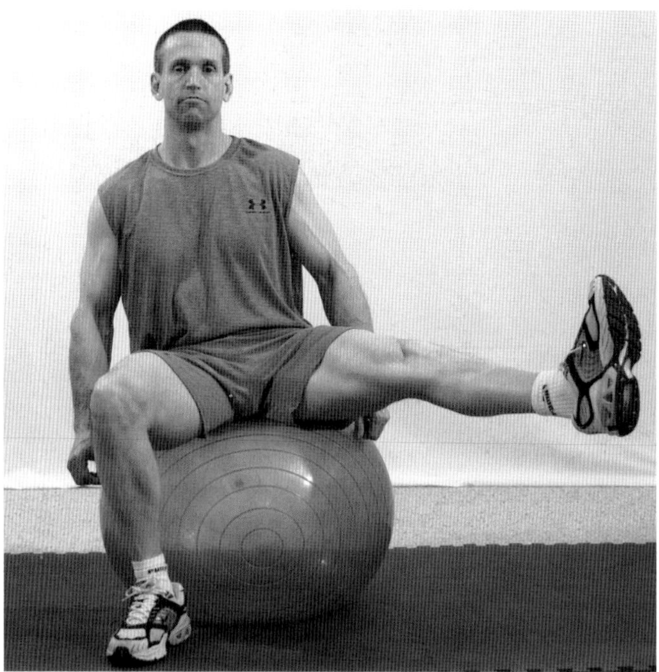

**STARTING POSITION:** Sit on the ball with your upper thighs parallel to the ground, feet flat on the floor, and arms at your sides.

**THE MOVEMENT:** Slowly extend your right leg out to a 45 degree angle, keeping it horizontal with the floor. Return to starting position and repeat.

### TRAINING TIPS

- Extend legs slowly and in a controlled manner.
- Keep inner core activated.
- Breathe naturally; don't hold your breath.

# EXERCISE: ON THE BALL—TORSO CORKSCREW

DIFFICULTY: **3** LOWER BACK: **HIGH RISK**

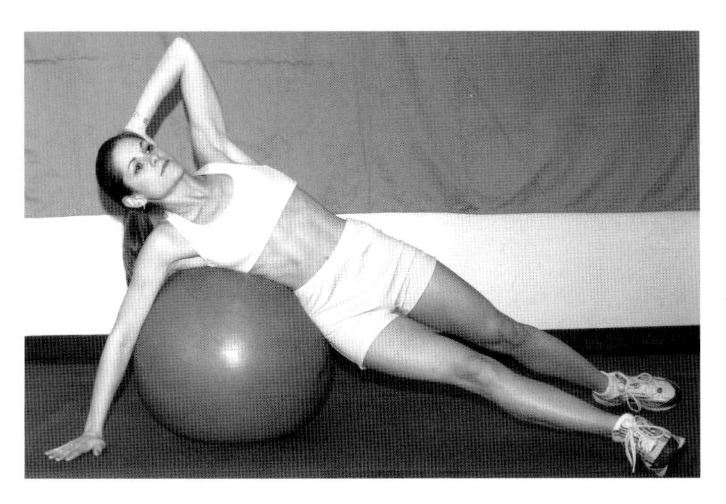

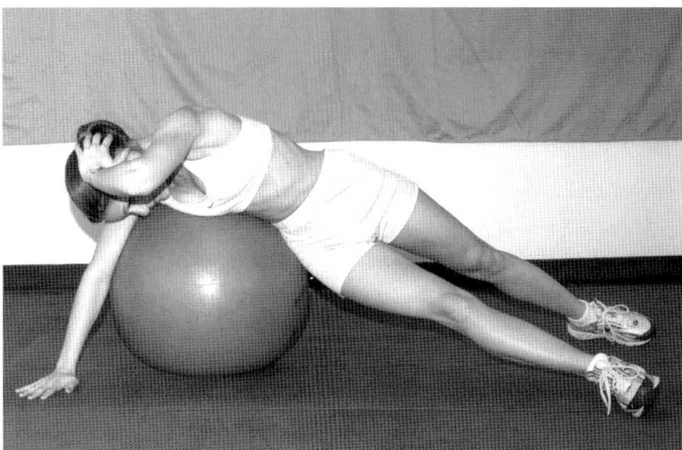

**STARTING POSITION:** Lie sideways on the ball and scissor your legs wide with your feet on the floor for support. Place your left hand behind your ear and your right arm on the floor for support.

**THE MOVE:** Lower and turn your upper body toward the ball. Then raise and rotate your torso back to the starting position.

### TRAINING TIPS

- Don't let the ball move.
- Raise and twist your torso in one motion.
- Keep your inner core activated.
- Keep your neck lengthened and in alignment with your spine.
- Don't look up or tuck in your chin.

# EXERCISE: ON THE BALL—DOUBLE LEG LIFT

DIFFICULTY: **3**  LOWER BACK: **LOW RISK**

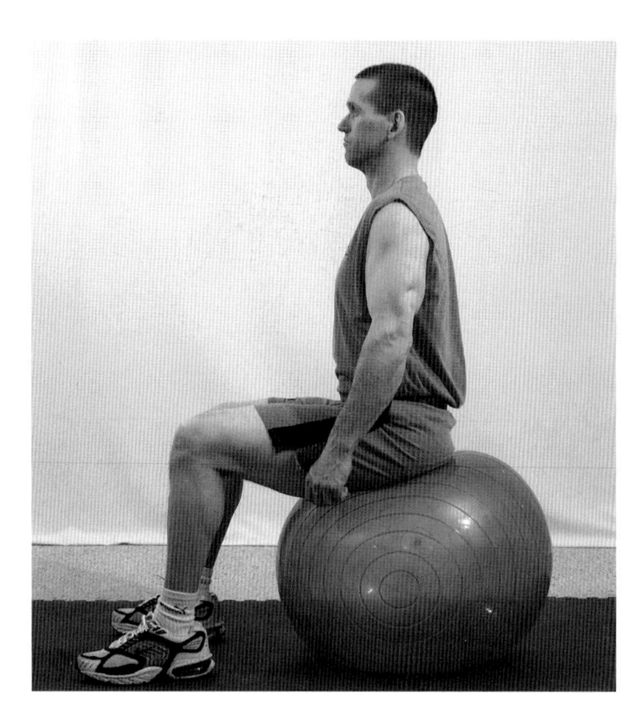

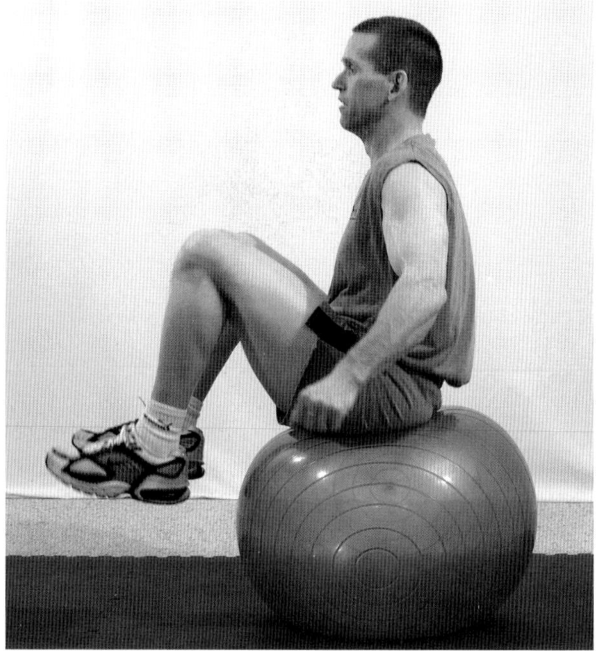

**STARTING POSITION:** Sit on the ball with your spine in the neutral position and feet flat on the floor shoulder-width apart.

**THE MOVEMENT:** Tighten your inner core muscles. Slowly lift your feet from the floor, using your arms to stabilize yourself. Try to hold for a few seconds, then return to the starting position.

### TRAINING TIPS

- Make the exercise harder by crossing your arms over your chest or holding them above your head.
- Keep your inner core activated.
- Keep your eyes focused straight ahead.

# EXERCISE: ON THE BALL—FORWARD AND BACKWARD TILT

DIFFICULTY: **1**  LOWER BACK: **LOW RISK**

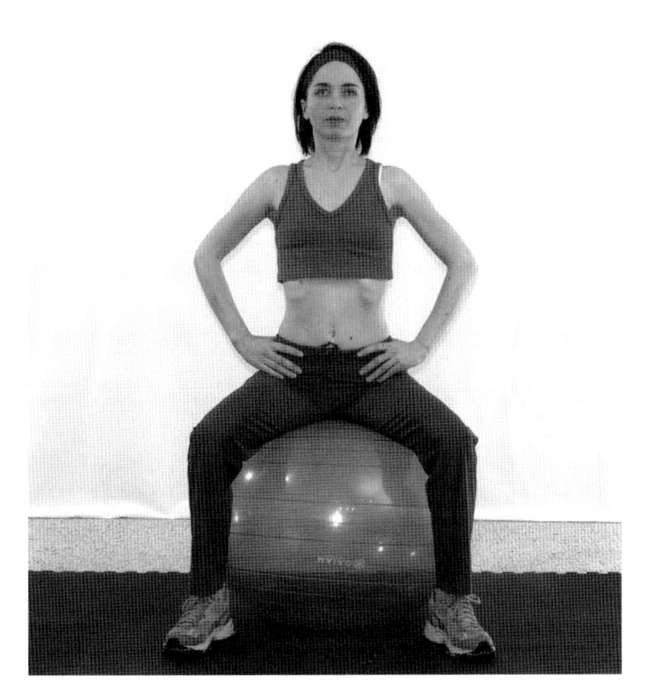

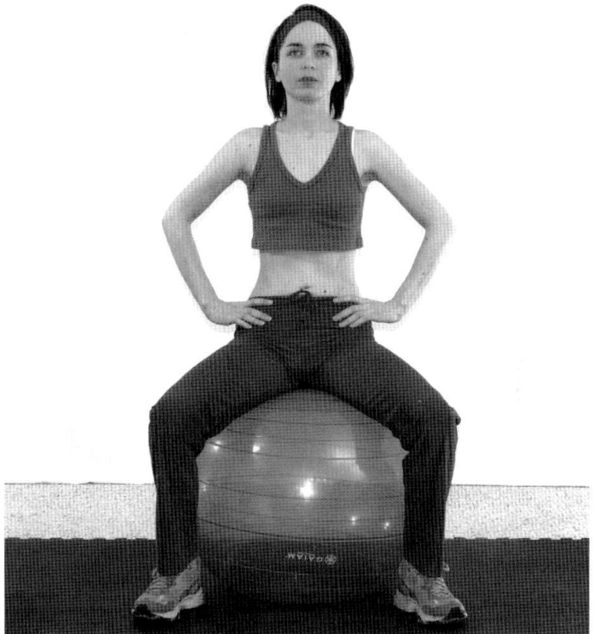

**STARTING POSITION:** Sit on the peak of the ball, feet flat on the floor, hands on your hips. Contract your inner core.

**THE MOVEMENT:** Tilt your pelvis forward, rounding your back. Then tilt your pelvis backward, arching your back. Continue alternating forward and backward moves.

### TRAINING TIPS

- Breathe naturally.
- Keep the motion fluid.
- Initiate the movement from your deep inner muscles.
- Keep your inner core activated.
- This exercise can be made more difficult by raising your hands above your head.

# EXERCISE: ON THE BALL—HIP FLEXION

DIFFICULTY: **2**  LOWER BACK: **LOW RISK**

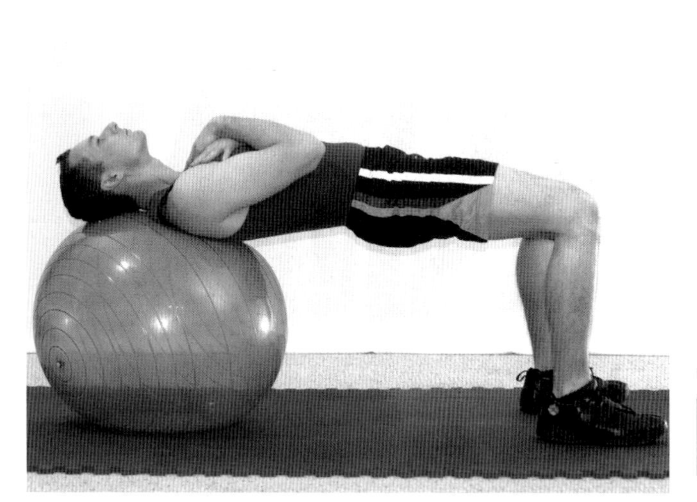

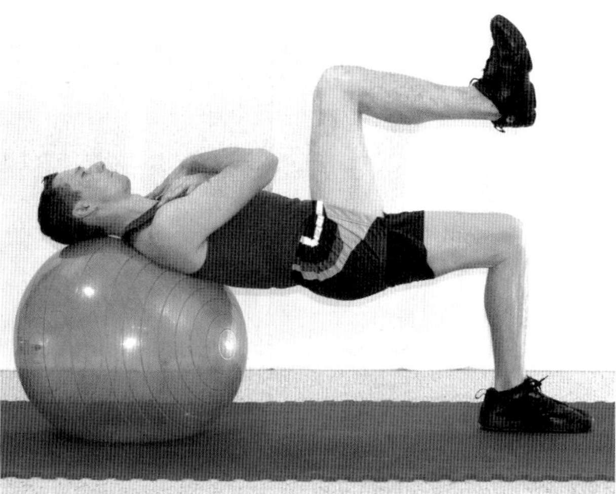

**STARTING POSITION:** Lie with the ball under your shoulders and your feet flat on the floor shoulder-width apart.

**THE MOVEMENT:** Activate your inner core and flex one leg at the hip to 90 degrees (perpendicular with your upper body). Hold, then return your leg to the floor and repeat using the other leg.

### TRAINING TIPS

- Do not allow your back to arch or sag during this exercise.
- Remain stable and still on the ball.
- Breathe naturally; don't hold your breath.

# EXERCISE: ON THE BALL—INNER CORE LEG EXTENSION

DIFFICULTY: **1**   LOWER BACK: **LOW RISK**

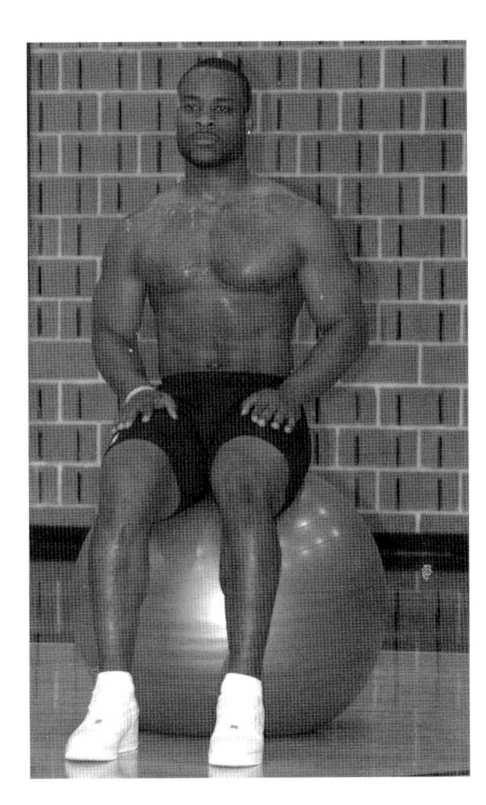

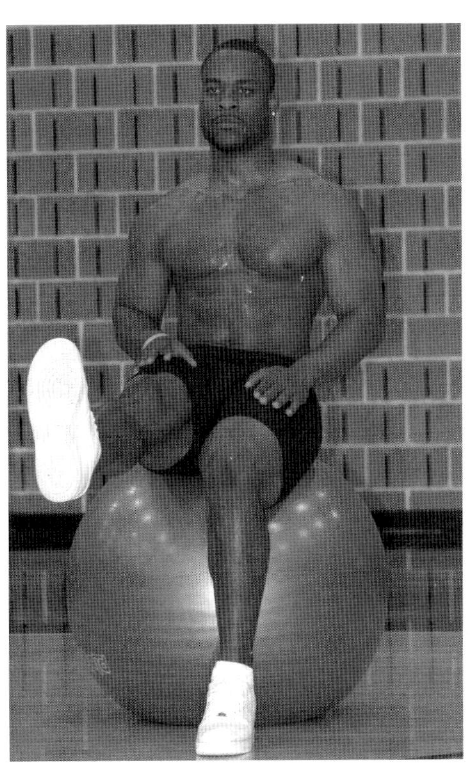

**STARTING POSITION:** Sit on the ball with upper thighs parallel to the ground, feet flat on the floor, hands on your thighs.

**THE MOVEMENT:** Slowly extend right leg straight out to a position horizontal with the floor. Hold, then repeat with other leg.

### TRAINING TIPS

- Extend legs slowly and in a controlled manner.
- Feel the movement initiate from your center.
- Breathe naturally; don't hold your breath.
- Keep your inner core activated.
- The exercise can be made more difficult by raising your hands above your head.

# EXERCISE: PLANK SERIES

DIFFICULTY: **2** LOWER BACK RISK: **LOW RISK**

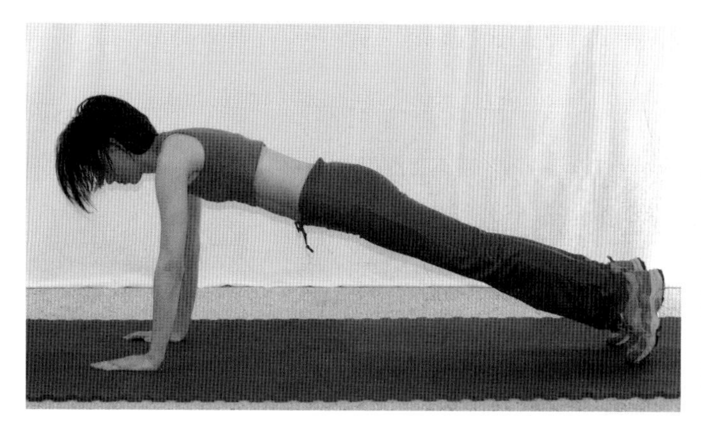

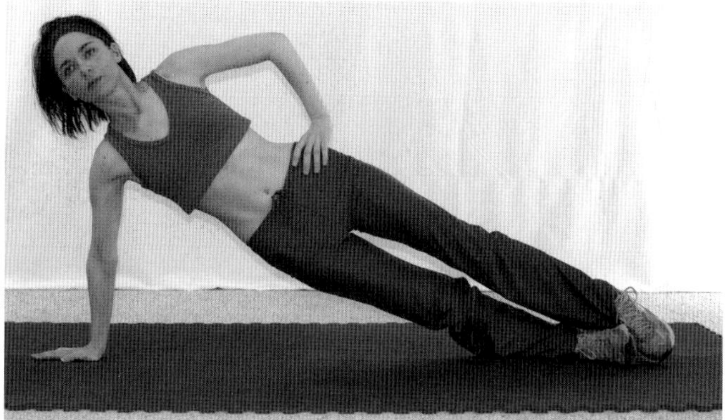

**POSITION ONE:** Down plank. Lie on your stomach, raise your body off the floor, supporting yourself on your forearms (or hands) and your toes. Raise your hips so your body is straight like a board. Hold for prescribed time.

**POSITION TWO:** Side plank. Rest on your right forearm or hand and the outside edge of your right foot. Raise your hips so your body is straight like a board. Hold for prescribed time, then switch sides.

**POSITION FOUR:** Up plank. Lie on your back, resting on your forearms (or hands) and your heels. Raise your hips so your body is straight like a board. Hold for prescribed time.

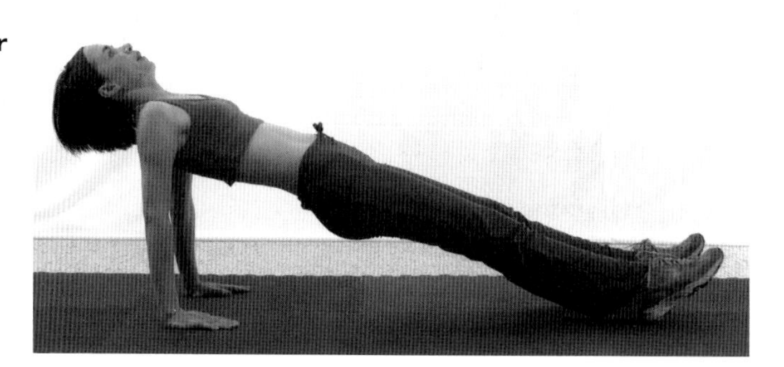

### TRAINING TIPS FOR ALL POSITIONS

- Focus on keeping your body as straight as a board.
- Don't let your hips sag.
- Keep your neck lengthened and in line with your spine.
- Keep your inner core activated.

# EXERCISE: PLANK—SWIMMING

DIFFICULTY: **3** LOWER BACK RISK: **MODERATE RISK**

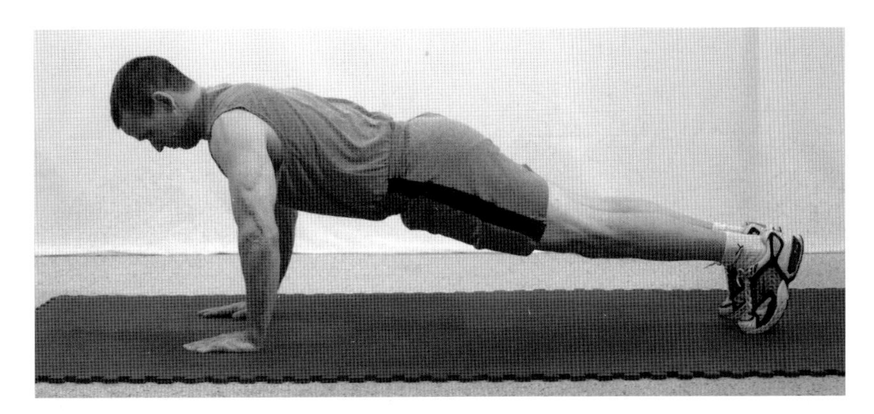

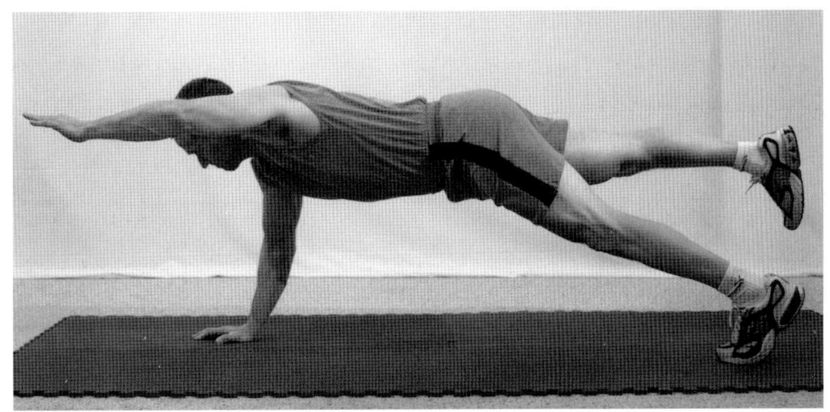

**STARTING POSITION:** Lie on your stomach, then raise your body off the floor, supporting yourself on your hands and your toes in plank position.

**THE MOVE:** Simultaneously raise your left arm and right leg off the floor. Then lower your foot and arm back to the floor. Repeat with right arm and left leg.

### TRAINING TIPS

- Focus on keeping your body as straight as a board.
- Don't let your hips sag.
- Keep your neck lengthened and in line with your spine.
- Maintain a steady balance.
- Keep your inner core activated.

# EXERCISE: PLANK—SWINGING GATE

DIFFICULTY: **3** LOWER BACK RISK: **MODERATE RISK**

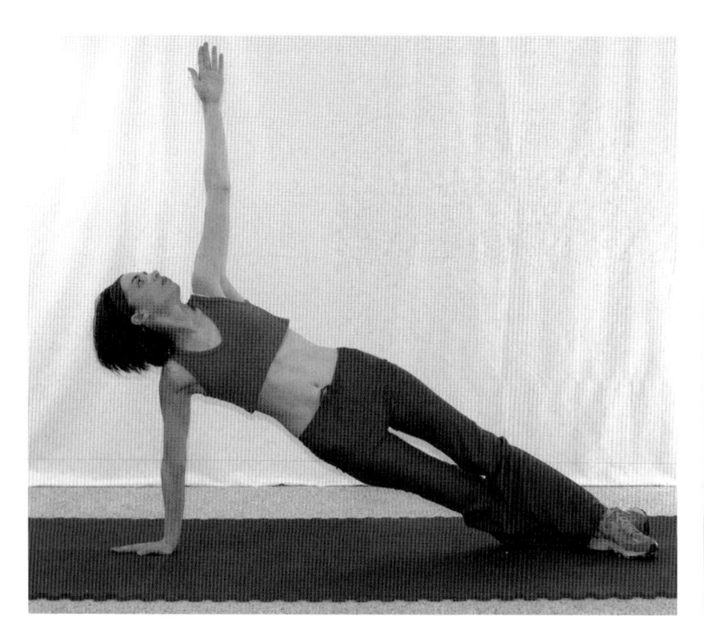

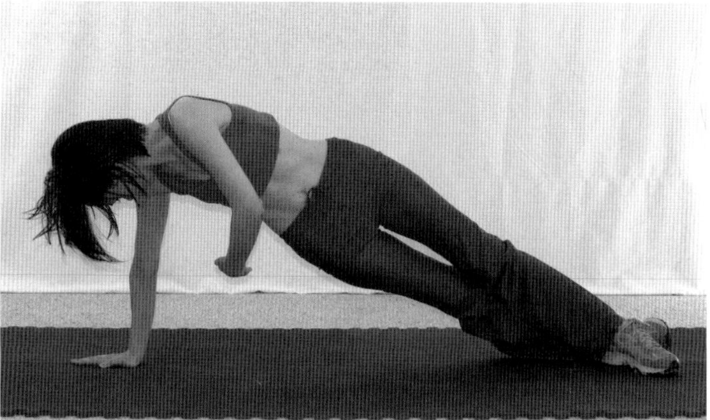

**STARTING POSITION:** Assume a side plank position, supporting your body with your right arm and the outside edges of your feet. Extend your left arm straight up, in line with your supporting arm.

**THE MOVE:** Rotate your entire body toward the floor, bringing your free arm underneath and through. Then rotate back up to the starting position.

### TRAINING TIPS

- Focus on keeping your body as straight as a board.
- Don't let your hips sag.
- Keep your neck lengthened and in line with your spine.
- Maintain a steady balance.
- The finish position is the same as a side plank (with your arm raised).
- Keep your inner core activated.

# EXERCISE: ON THE BALL: PLANK—HANDS ON BALL

DIFFICULTY: **3** LOWER BACK: **MODERATE TO HIGH RISK**

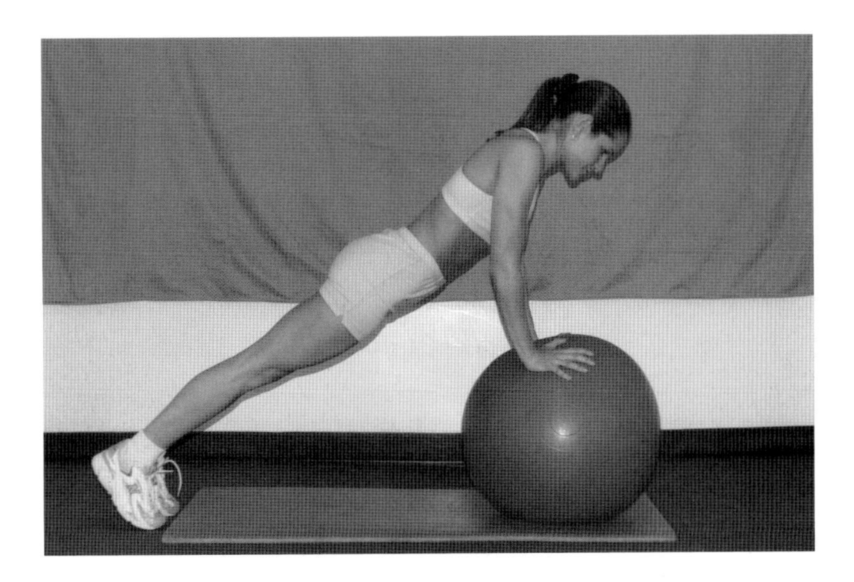

**POSITION:** Balance on the ball in a down plank position.

**VARIATIONS:** Rest your knees on the ground, instead of your feet. Or to make the exercise more difficult, balance on one foot.

**TRAINING TIPS**

- Keep the ball from moving.
- Focus your mind on feeling your core do the work.
- Activate your inner core.
- Keep your neck lengthened and aligned with your spine; don't look up or tuck in your chin.

# EXERCISE: ON THE BALL—DOWN PLANK

DIFFICULTY: **2** LOWER BACK: **MODERATE RISK**

**POSITION:** Start from a push-up position, with your feet on top of the ball and your arms extended directly under your shoulders. Your body should form a straight line.

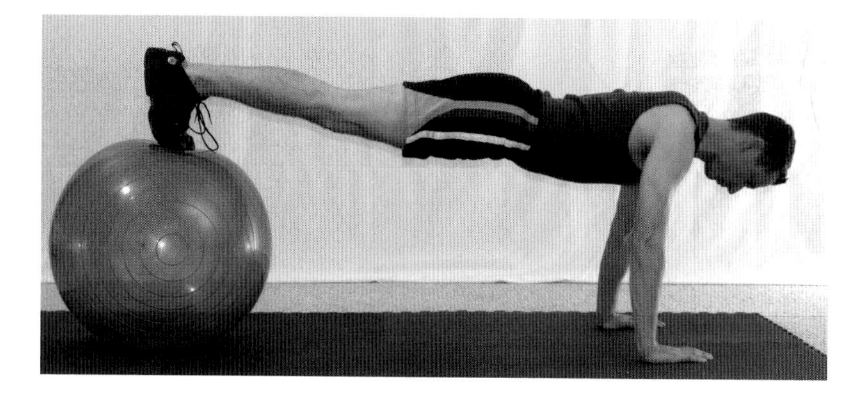

**VARIATIONS:** You can make this exercise easier by moving your legs on top of the ball. Or you can make the move more difficult by placing one foot on top of the other, balancing on one leg.

**TRAINING TIPS**

- Keep the ball from moving.
- Focus your mind on feeling your core do the work.
- Activate your inner core.
- Keep your neck lengthened and aligned with your spine; don't look up or tuck in your chin.
- Keep your hands under your shoulders for the entire movement.

# EXERCISE: ON THE BALL—
# REVERSE BRIDGE WITH LEG EXTENSION

DIFFICULTY: **2** LOWER BACK: **LOW RISK**

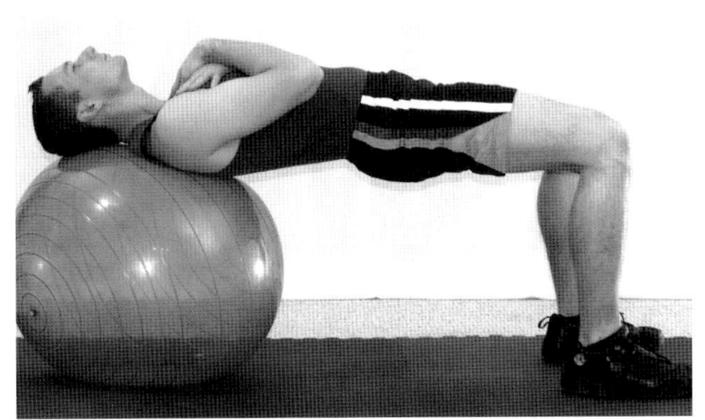

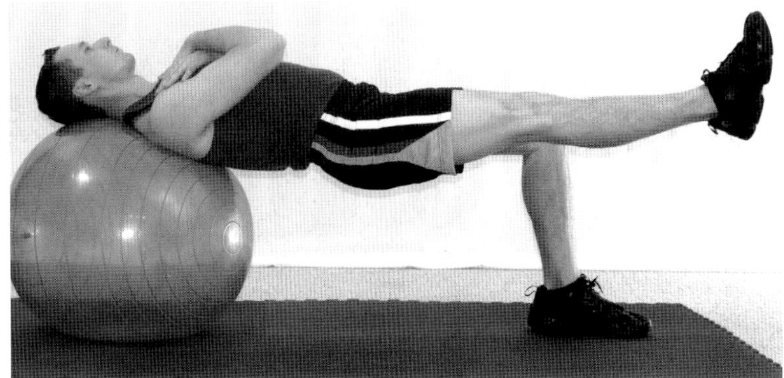

**STARTING POSITION:** Lie with the ball under your shoulders and your feet shoulder-width apart.

**THE MOVEMENT:** Lift one leg off the floor, extending it straight. Repeat using the other leg.

### TRAINING TIPS

- Do not allow your hips to sag.
- Keep the ball from moving.
- Breathe naturally; don't hold your breath.
- Keep your inner core activated.

# EXERCISE: ON THE BALL—ROLL IN WITH A CROSS

DIFFICULTY: **3** LOWER BACK: **HIGH RISK**

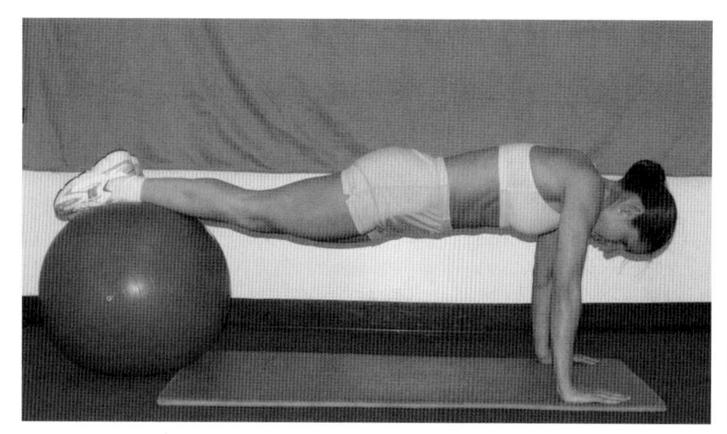 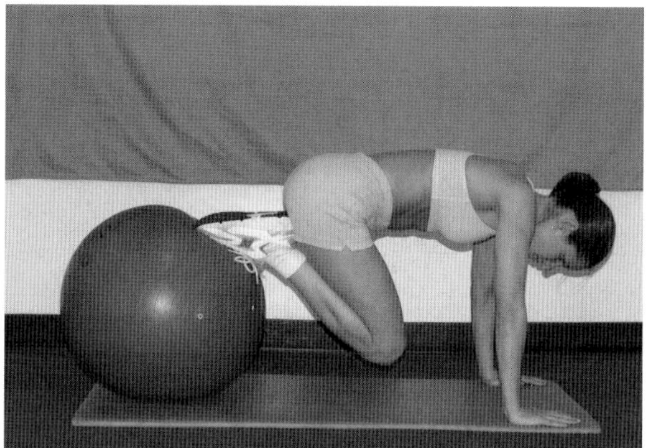

**STARTING POSITION:** From a push-up position, place your lower legs and/or feet on top of the ball. Place your hands directly under your shoulders.

**THE MOVE:** Bring your knees toward your chest as you slowly roll the ball forward. Then extend your legs and the ball back at an angle. Repeat to the other side, rolling the ball out in the opposite direction, drawing a V shape.

### TRAINING TIPS

- Draw a V shape as you roll the ball back and forth.
- Keep the ball's movement under control.
- Focus your mind on feeling your core do the work.
- Look straight down and keep your neck lengthened.
- Keep your hands under your shoulders for the entire movement.

# EXERCISE: ON THE BALL—ROLL OUT WITH A CROSS

DIFFICULTY: **3** LOWER BACK: **HIGH RISK**

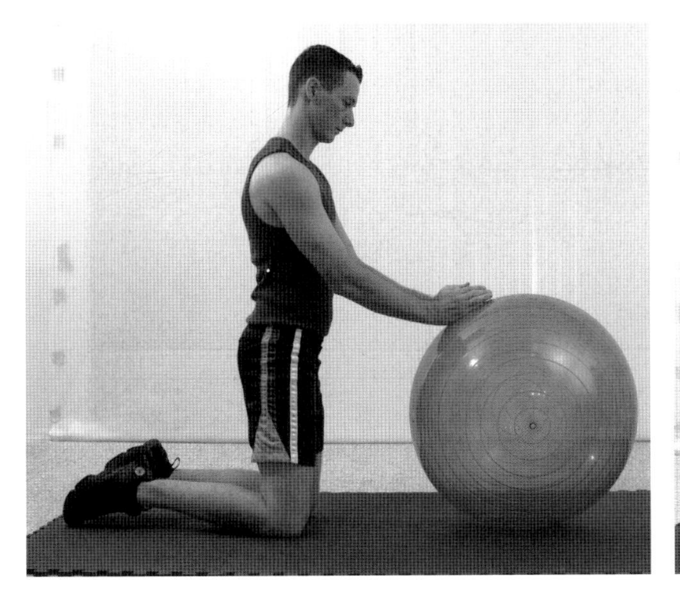

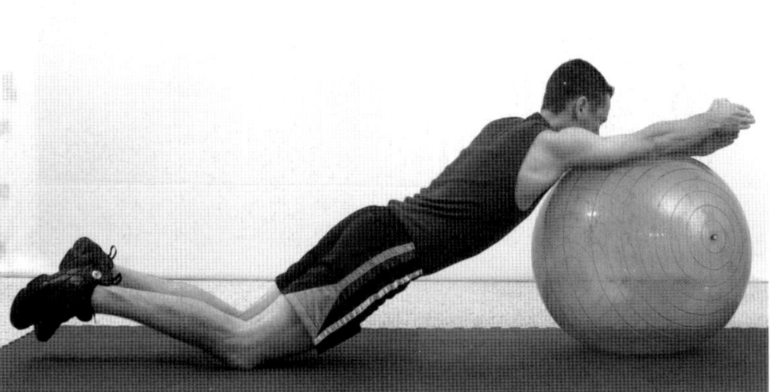

**STARTING POSITION:** Kneel in front of the ball, placing your hands in prayer position on top of the ball.

**THE MOVE:** Roll the ball forward and at an angle to your left until your arms and shoulders are fully extended. Then roll the ball back to the starting position. Then extend the ball out at an angle to your right. Extending your hips forward will make the exercise more difficult.

### TRAINING TIPS

- It's like you're making the letter V.
- Focus your mind on your core.
- Keep your neck lengthened and look straight down.
- Keep your buttocks contracted to protect your lower back.

# EXERCISE: ON THE BALL— SINGLE-LEG CRUNCH WITH A CROSS

DIFFICULTY: **3** LOWER BACK: **MODERATE RISK**

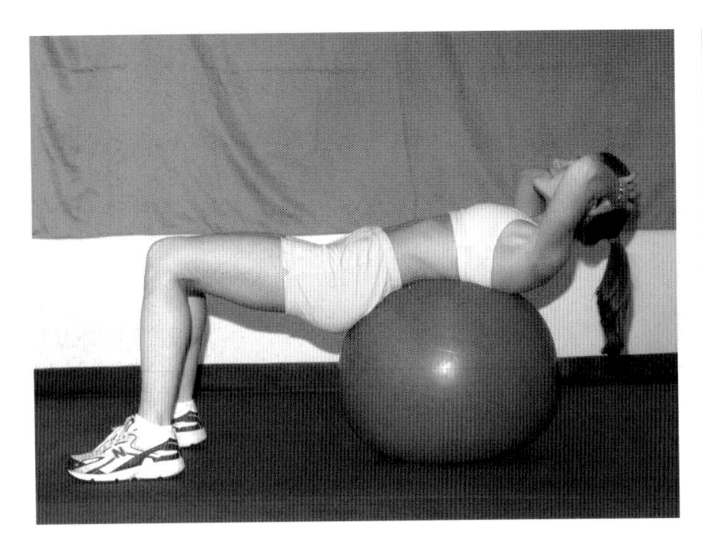

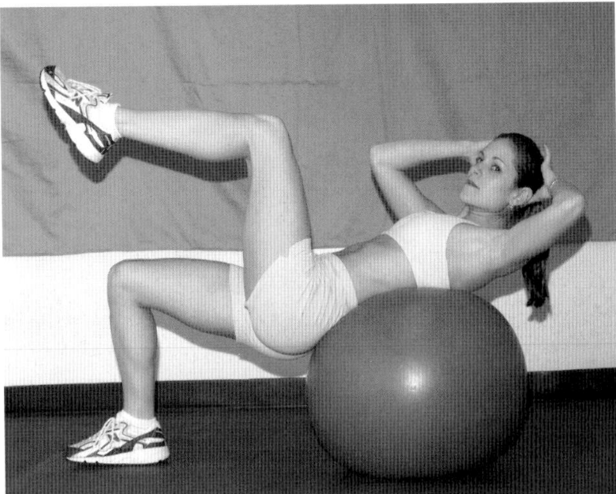

**STARTING POSITION:** Sit on top of the ball, your feet flat on the floor for support.

**THE MOVE:** Curl up and cross your right shoulder over the peak of the ball as you raise your left knee toward your right shoulder. Lower both your torso and leg back to the starting position, then repeat the movement to the opposite side.

### TRAINING TIPS

- Keep the ball stable.
- Move the leg only slightly toward the opposite shoulder.
- Focus your mind on feeling your core do the work.
- Make sure you are far enough back on the ball so your shoulder blades come over the peak of the ball.

# EXERCISE: UP PLANK—FLUTTER

DIFFICULTY: **2** LOWER BACK RISK: **LOW RISK**

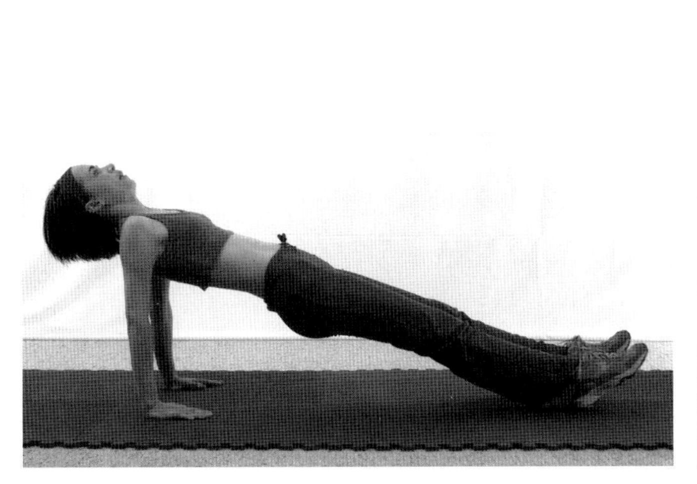

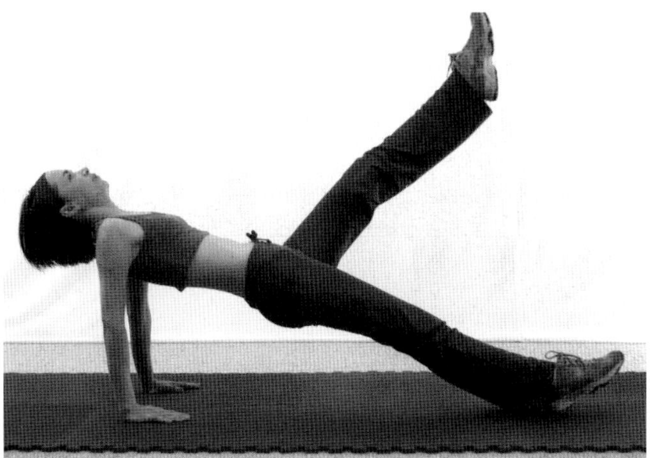

**STARTING POSITION:** Get in an up-plank position, resting on your forearms and elbows (or your hands) and your heels, so your body is straight like a board. Your hands should point toward your feet.

**THE MOVE:** Raise your left foot and hold. Repeat with the right foot.

**TRAINING TIPS**

- Focus on keeping your body as straight as a board.
- Don't let your hips sag.
- Keep your neck lengthened and in line with your spine.
- Maintain a steady balance.

# EXERCISE: DIAGONAL BALL RAISE

DIFFICULTY: **2** LOWER BACK: **MODERATE RISK**

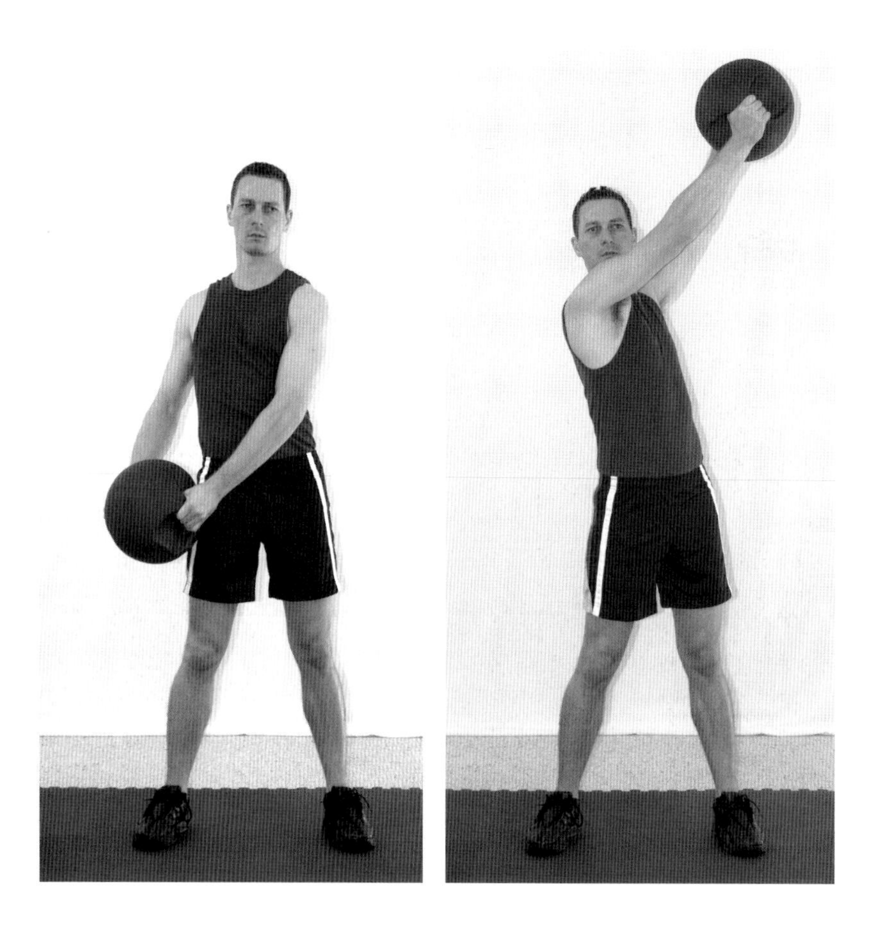

**STARTING POSITION:** Starting from a standing ready position, hold a medicine ball, dumbbell, or weight plate at the outside of your hip, arms fully extended.

**THE MOVEMENT:** Raise your arms across your body over your head. Lower back to the starting position and repeat.

### TRAINING TIPS

- Feel your feet planted firmly on the ground.
- Feel the rotational power initiate from the center of your body.
- Keep your inner core activated.

# EXERCISE: BALL REACH—KNEE AND OVERHEAD

DIFFICULTY: **1** LOWER BACK: **LOW RISK**

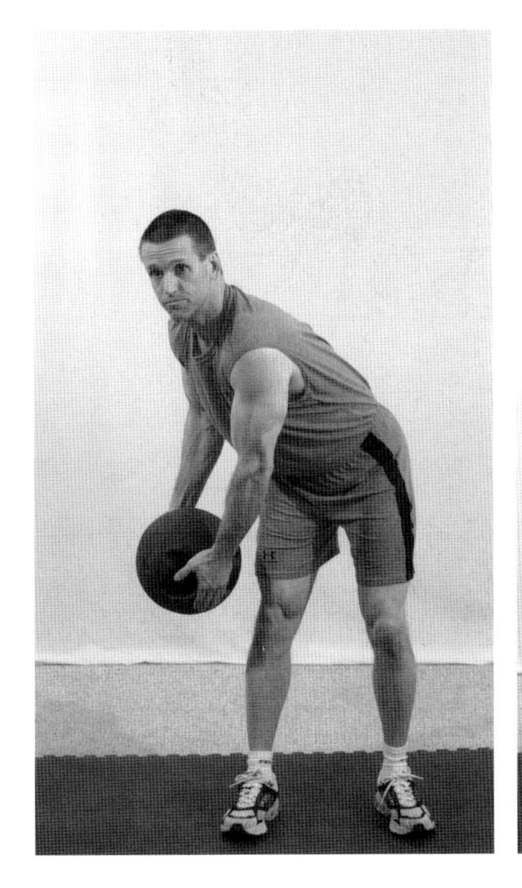

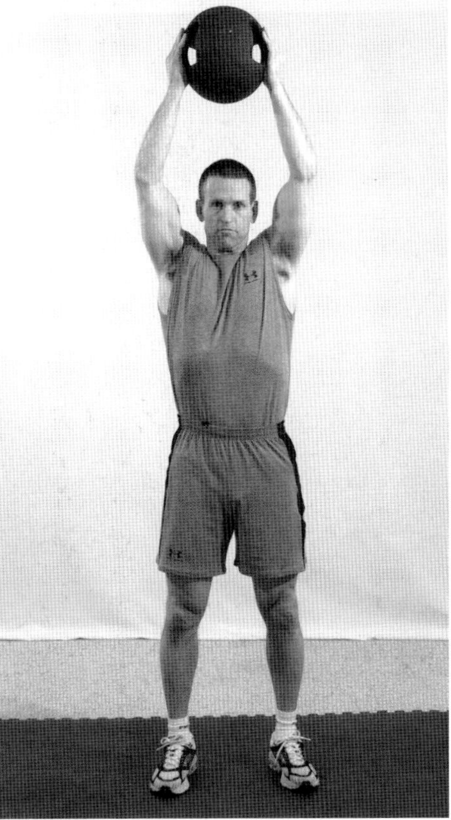

**STARTING POSITION:** Stand in ready position. You can do this movement with a weighted exercise ball, a weight plate, a dumbbell, or with no weight. If you aren't using anything, it is helpful to imagine that you are holding a basketball. Lower your body, bringing your hands to the outside of your right knee.

**THE MOVE:** In a diagonal crossing motion, bring your hands directly above your head. Repeat to other side, alternating.

### TRAINING TIPS

- Keep your inner core activated.
- Initiate the movement from the center of your body, not your arms and legs.
- Maintain spinal alignment.
- Feel the motion transfer from your lower body to your upper body through your core.

# EXERCISE: SUN SALUTE WITH CROSS

DIFFICULTY: **2** LOWER BACK RISK: **MODERATE RISK**

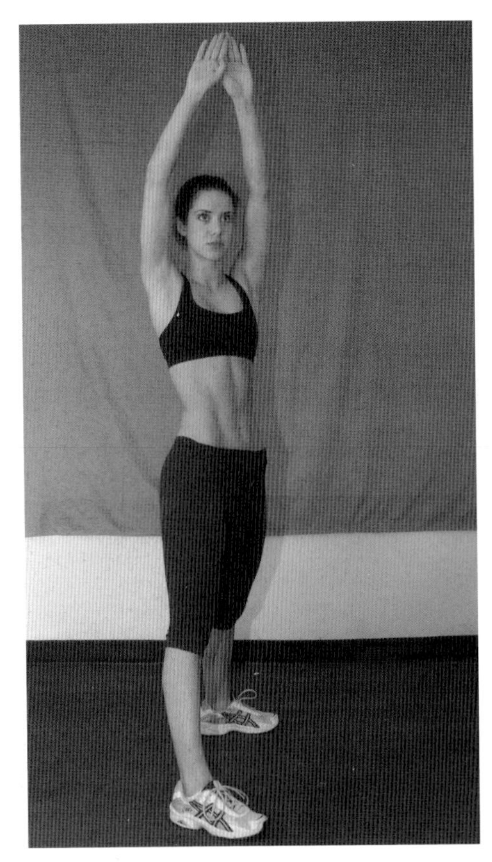

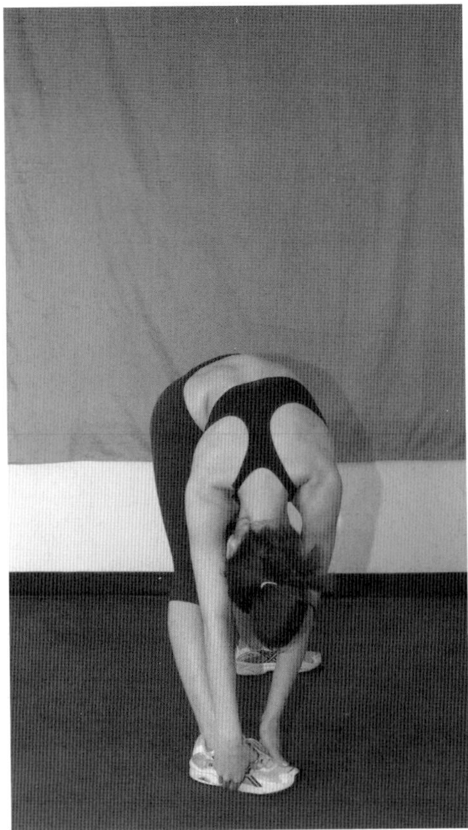

**STARTING POSITION:** Stand with your legs spread wider than shoulder width and your arms extended above your head.

**THE MOVE:** Bend at the waist and reach down and touch your right foot, keeping your torso straight and moving as one unit. Straighten your back to the starting position. Repeat to the other side.

### TRAINING TIPS

- Focus on keeping your body as straight as a board.
- Keep your neck lengthened and in line with your spine.
- Maintain a steady balance.
- Initiate the movement from the center of your body.
- Keep your inner core activated throughout the exercise.

# EXERCISE: BALANCE T-BEND

DIFFICULTY: 3 LOWER BACK: **MODERATE RISK**

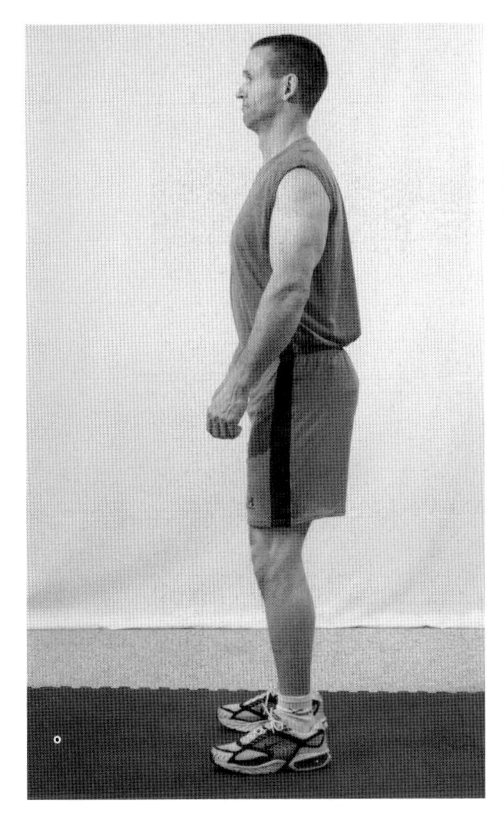

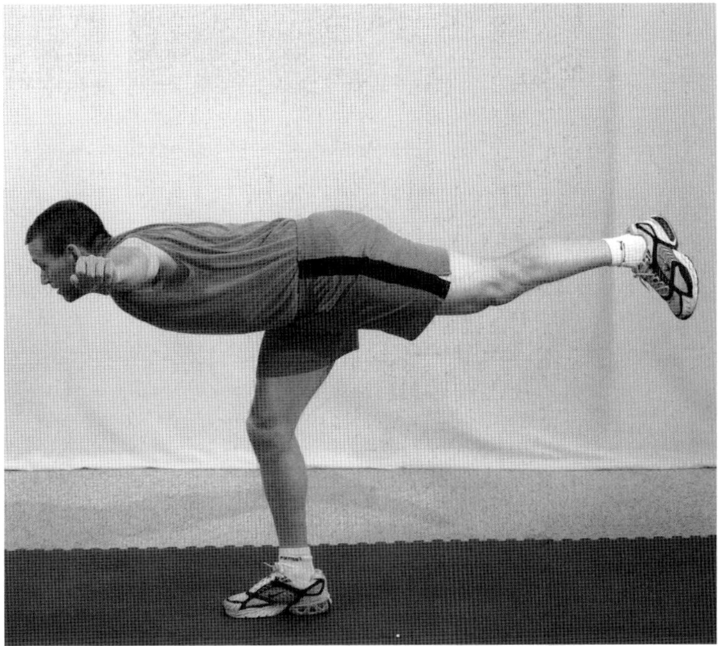

**STARTING POSITION:** Start from the ready position, hands at your sides.

**THE MOVE:** Balance on your right foot, then bend at the waist, making a T shape with your body. You can extend your arms straight overhead or spread them out to your sides like wings.

### TRAINING TIPS

- Keep your inner core activated.
- Keep a neutral spine.
- Initiate the movement from the center of your body, not your arms and legs.
- Strive for the perfect T shape.
- Extending your arms straight above your head makes the move more difficult.

# EXERCISE: BALL REACH TOE AND OVERHEAD

DIFFICULTY: **2** LOWER BACK: **MODERATE RISK**

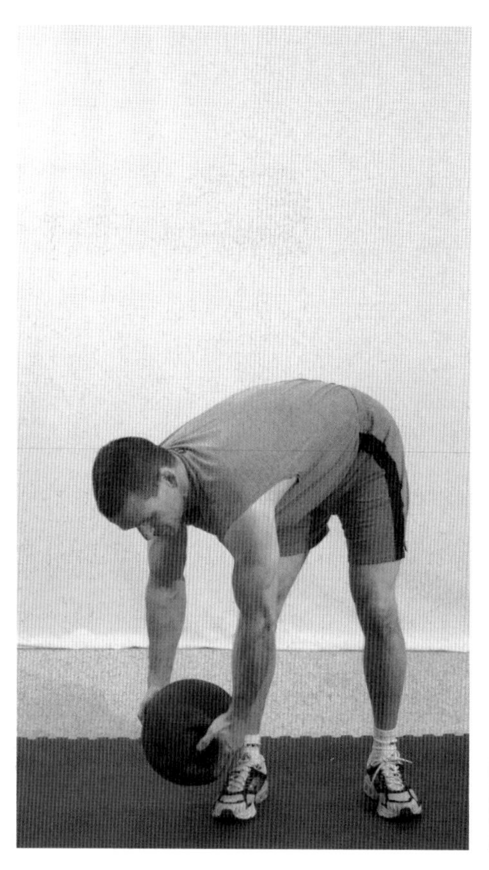

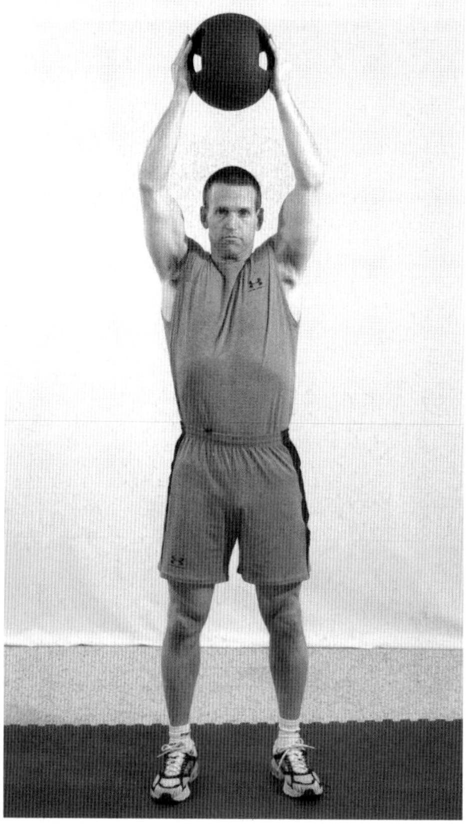

**STARTING POSITION:** Stand in ready position, arms at your sides. You can do this movement with a weighted exercise ball, a weight plate, a dumbbell, or with no weight. If you aren't using anything, it is helpful to imagine that you are holding a basketball. Lower your body, bringing your hands to the outside of your little toe.

**THE MOVE:** In a diagonal crossing motion, bring your hands directly above your head. Repeat to other side, alternating.

### TRAINING TIPS

- Keep your inner core activated.
- Initiate the movement from the center of your body, not your arms and legs.
- Maintain spinal alignment.
- Feel the motion transfer from your lower body to your upper body through your core.

# EXERCISE: STANDING FLEXION WITH ROTATION

DIFFICULTY: **2**  LOWER BACK: **MODERATE RISK**

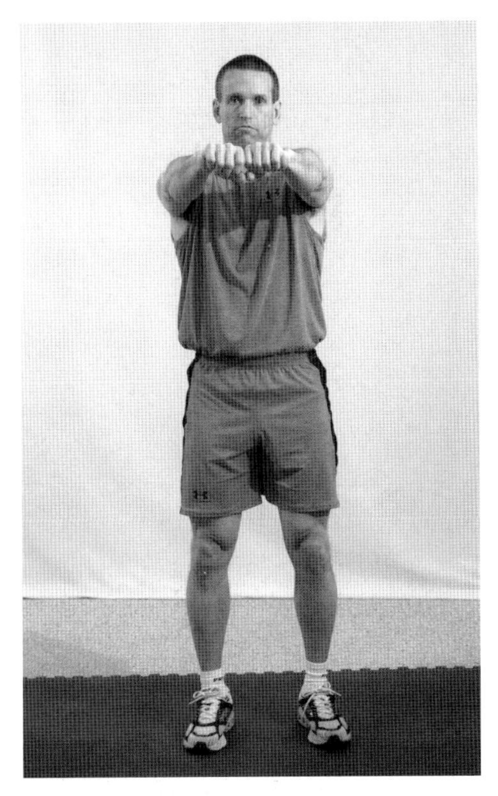

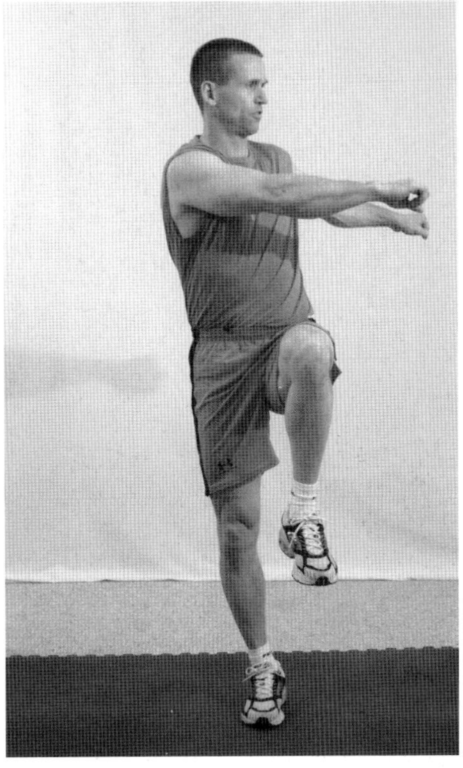

**STARTING POSITION:** Stand in ready position, arms raised to shoulder level.

**THE MOVE:** Bring your left knee up perpendicular to your upper body as you rotate your torso to the left. Repeat the other side, raising your right knee and rotating to your right.

### TRAINING TIPS

- Keep your inner core activated.
- Keep a neutral spine.
- Initiate the movement from the center of your body, not your arms and legs.

# EXERCISE: BALL REACH—HEEL AND OVERHEAD

DIFFICULTY: **3**    LOWER BACK: **MODERATE RISK**

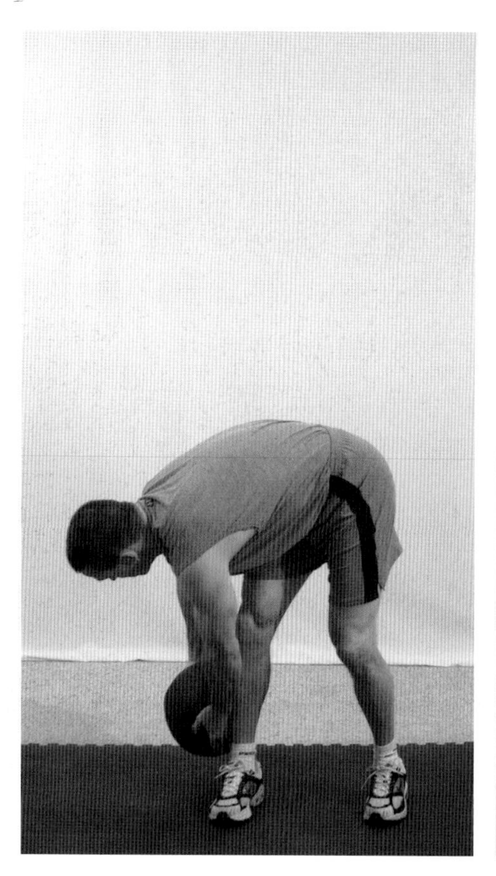

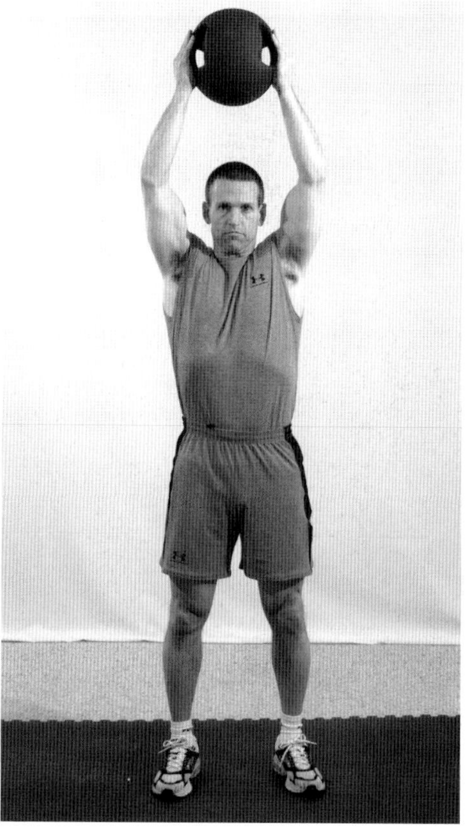

**STARTING POSITION:** Stand in ready position. You can do this movement with a weighted exercise ball, a weight plate, a dumbbell, or with no weight. If you aren't using anything, it is helpful to imagine that you are holding a basketball. Lower and rotate your body backward, bringing your hands to the back and outside of your heel.

**THE MOVE:** In a diagonal crossing motion, bring your hands directly above your head. Repeat to other side, alternating.

### TRAINING TIPS

- Keep your inner core activated.
- Initiate the movement from the center of your body, not your arms and legs.
- Maintain spinal alignment.
- Feel the motion transfer from your lower body to your upper body through your core.

# EXERCISE: DYNAMIC FLEXION AND EXTENSION

DIFFICULTY: **2** LOWER BACK: **MODERATE RISK**

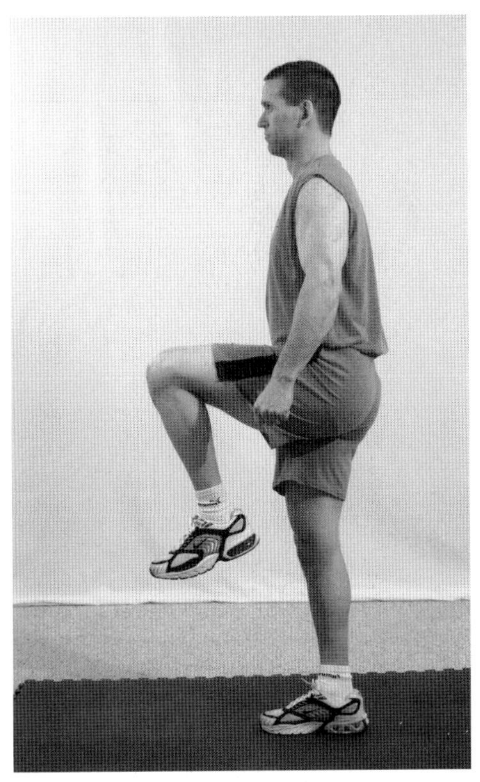

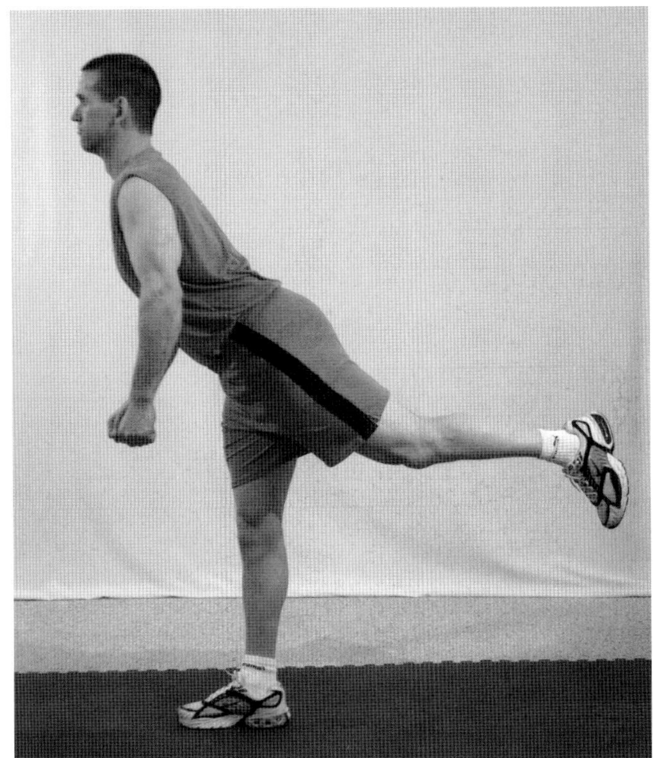

**STARTING POSITION:** Stand in ready position, arms at your sides.

**THE MOVE:** Raise your knee above your waist and then straighten your leg as you extend it behind your body. Finish set and repeat with the other leg.

### TRAINING TIPS

- Keep your inner core activated.
- Initiate the movement from the center of your body, not your arms and legs.
- Maintain spinal alignment.
- Keep your upper body stable.

# EXERCISE: WOODCHOP—LOW CABLE

DIFFICULTY: **2** LOWER BACK: **MODERATE RISK**

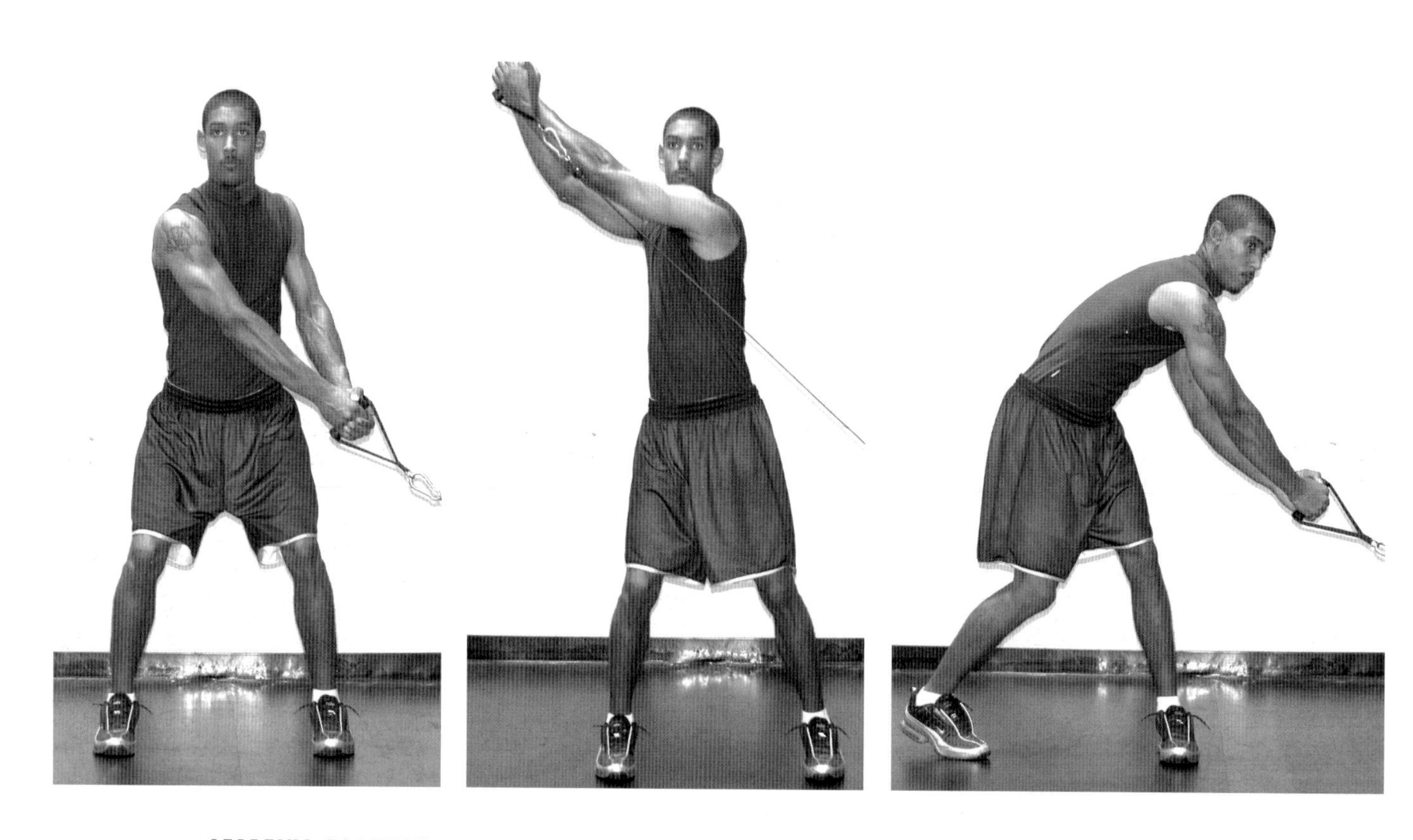

**STARTING POSITION:** Stand with your side facing the weight stack. Grab the handle attachment from the low cable pulley with both hands, arms fully extended.

**THE MOVE:** Rotate your torso as you raise the cable up and diagonally across your body. Complete the set and repeat to the other side.

**VARIATION:** Start with your hips rotated toward the weight stack. (photo right)

**TRAINING TIPS**

- Use a light weight.
- Focus your mind on feeling your core do the work.
- Initiate the movement from the center of your body, not your arms.
- Keep your inner core activated.

# EXERCISE: WOODCHOP—HIGH CABLE

DIFFICULTY: **2** LOWER BACK: **MODERATE RISK**

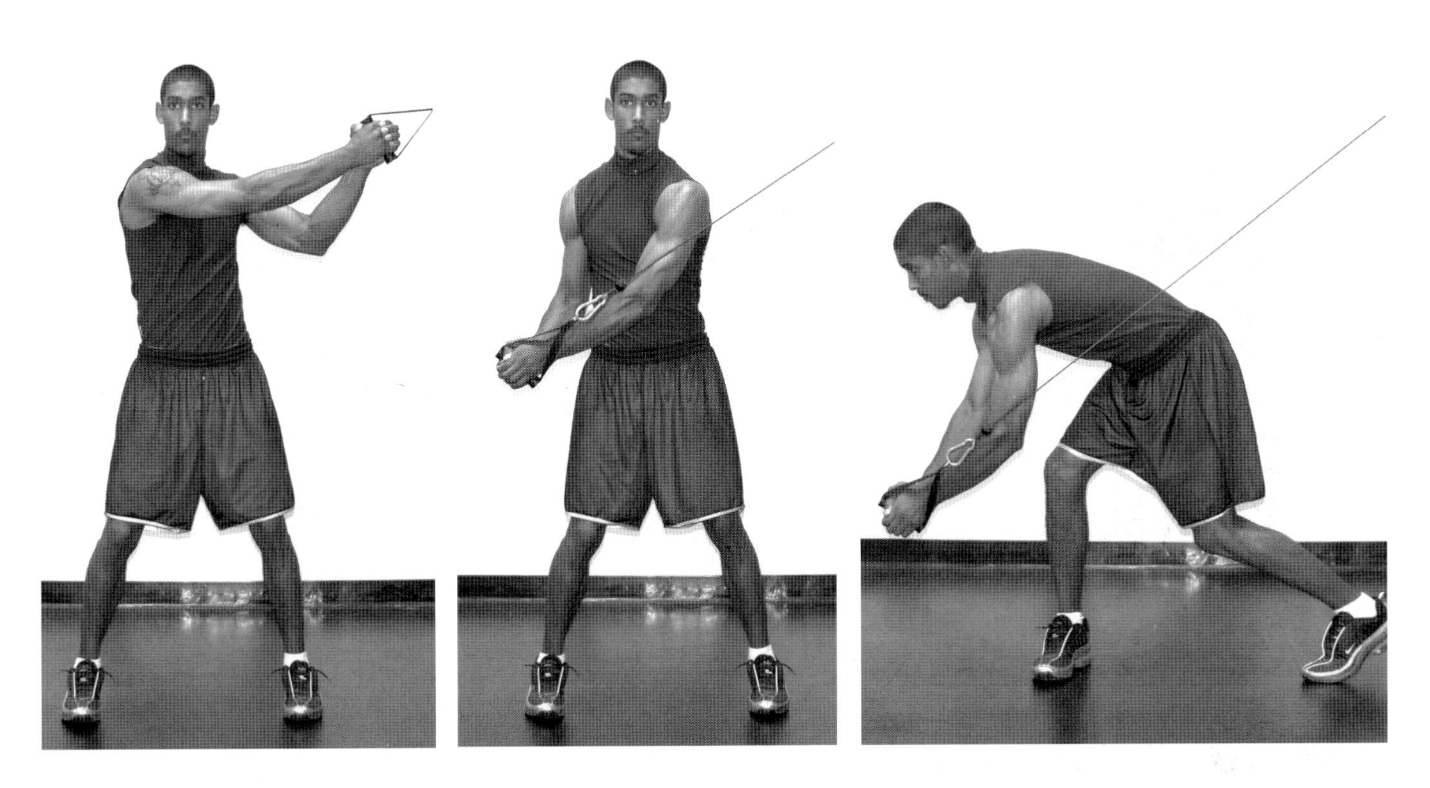

**STARTING POSITION:** Stand with your side facing the weight stack. Grab the handle attachment from the high cable pulley with both hands.

**THE MOVE:** Rotate your torso as you lower the cable down and diagonally across your body. Complete the set and repeat to the other side.

**VARIATION:** You can finish with your hips rotated away from the weight stack. (photo right)

### TRAINING TIPS

- Use a light weight.
- Focus your mind on feeling your core do the work.
- Initiate the movement from the center of your body, not your arms.
- Have the cable adjustment above your head if possible.
- Keep your inner core activated.

# EXERCISE: STANDING BICYCLES

DIFFICULTY: **2** LOWER BACK RISK: **MODERATE RISK**

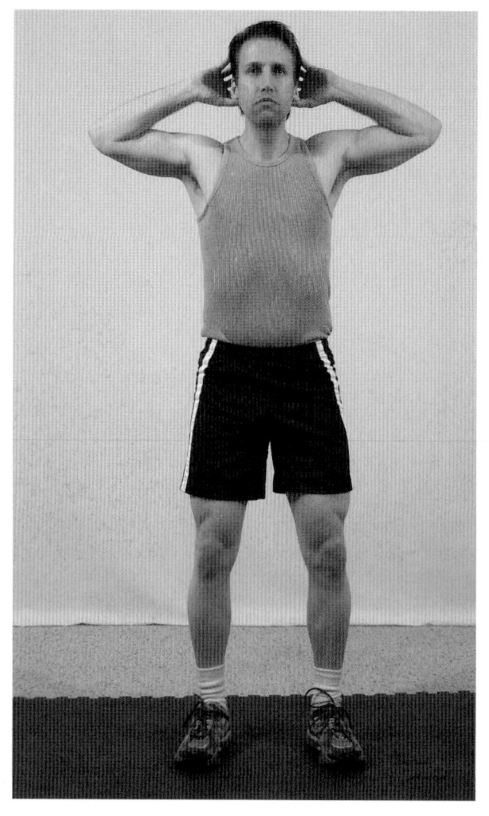

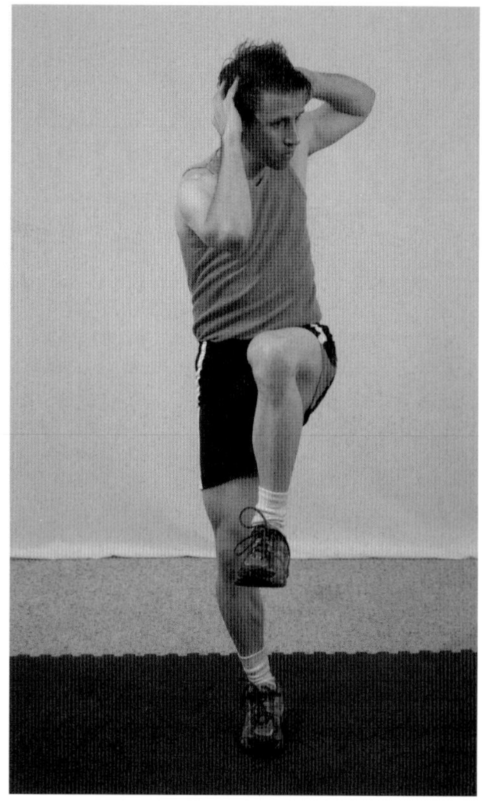

**STARTING POSITION:** Standing in the ready position, place your hands behind your ears.

**THE MOVE:** Simultaneously move your left leg up and across your body, as you bring your right shoulder and elbow down and across your body. Return to the starting position and repeat to the other side.

### TRAINING TIPS

- Feel the movement initiating from the center of your body.
- Keep your inner core activated throughout the movement.
- Imagine your opposite knee and elbow meeting in the center of your body.

# EXERCISE: ON THE BALL—BACK EXTENSION WITH ROTATION

DIFFICULTY: **2** LOWER BACK RISK: **MODERATE RISK**

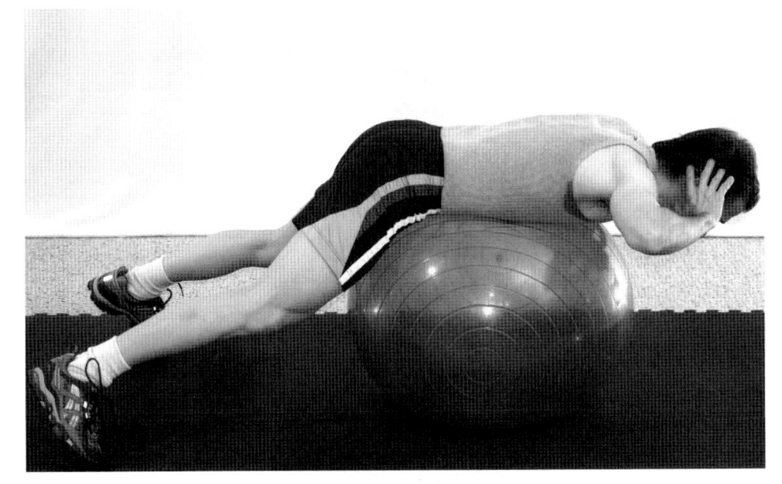

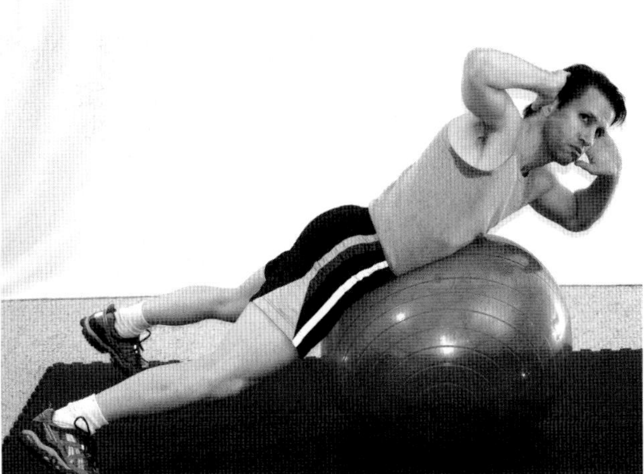

**STARTING POSITION:** Lie on your belly across an exercise ball, drape your torso over the peak of the ball, placing your hands behind your ears.

**THE MOVE:** Lengthening your spine, as you raise your torso off the ball, simultaneously rotate your right shoulder and torso upward. Return to the starting position and repeat to the other side.

**TRAINING TIPS**

- Keep your butt muscles contracted to protect your lower back.
- Keep your inner core activated throughout the movement.
- Throughout the movement, continue to lengthen your spine, making your torso longer.
- You can brace your feet against a wall to increase your range of motion.

# EXERCISE: ON THE BALL: KNEE RAISE

DIFFICULTY: **2** LOWER BACK RISK: **LOW RISK**

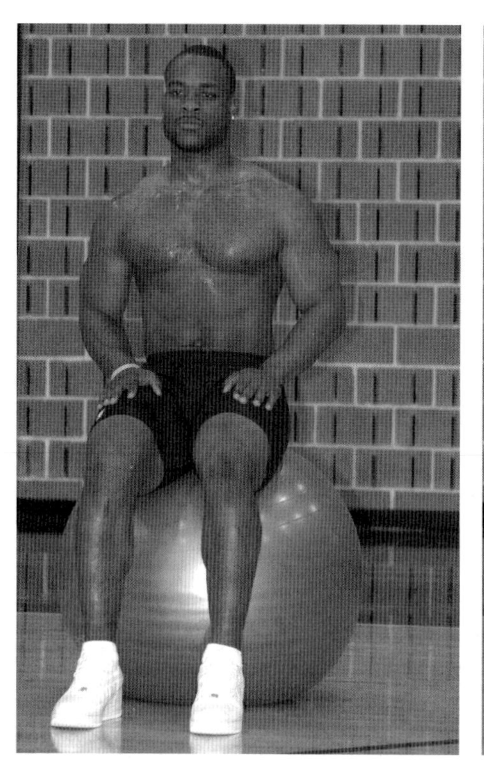

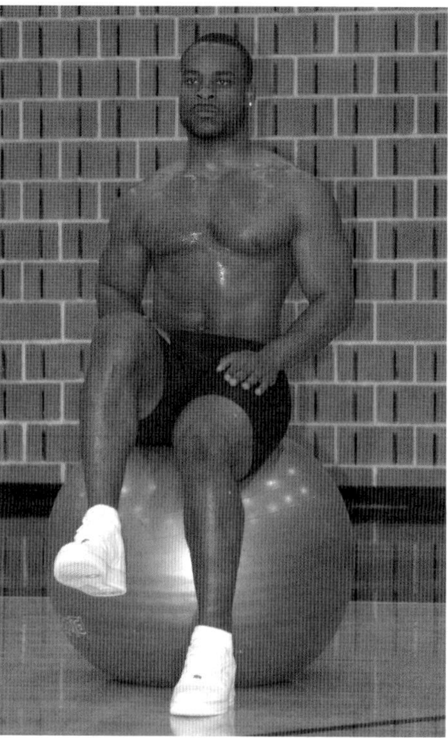

**STARTING POSITION:** Sit on top of an exercise ball, hands lightly resting on top of your thighs.

**THE MOVE:** Raise your right leg about two inches off the floor, then lower it back to the starting position and repeat. Alternate legs with each repetition.

### TRAINING TIPS

- Keep your inner core activated throughout the movement.
- Initiate the movement from the center of your body.
- Use your deep inner core muscles to raise the leg.

# EXERCISE: ON THE BALL: SIDE-TO-SIDE TILT

DIFFICULTY: **1**  LOWER BACK RISK: **LOW RISK**

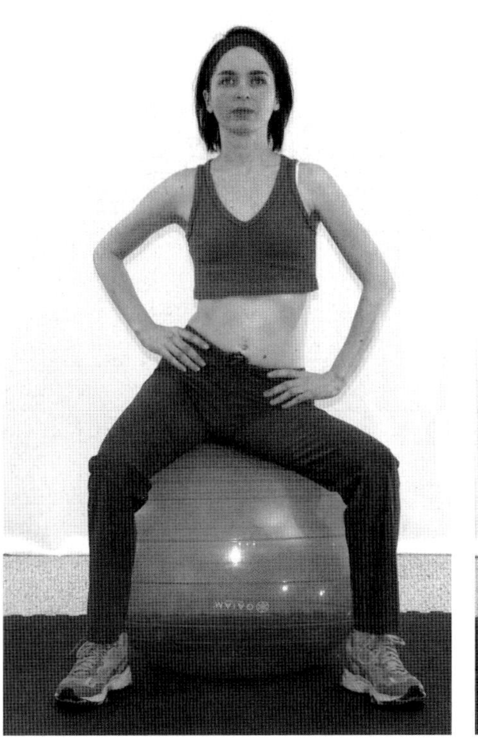

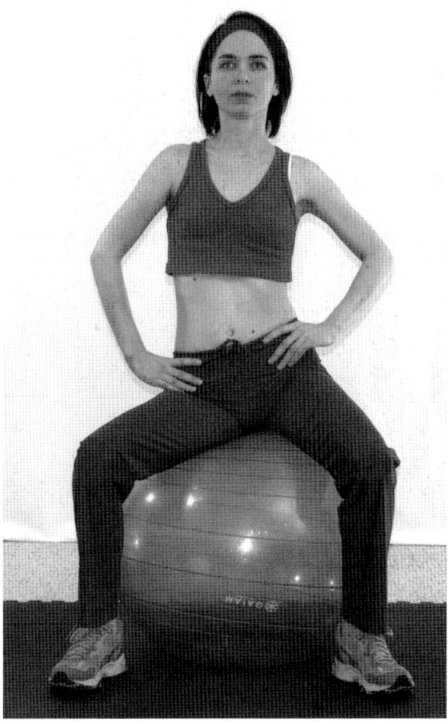

**STARTING POSITION:** Sit on top of an exercise ball, hands on top of your hips.

**THE MOVE:** Use your inner core muscles to tilt your pelvis from side to side.

**TRAINING TIPS**

- Keep your inner core activated throughout the movement.
- Initiate the movement from the center of your body.
- Use your deep inner core muscles.
- Raise your hands above your head to increase difficulty.

# EXERCISE: UP PLANK—FLUTTERS

DIFFICULTY: **3** LOWER BACK RISK: **HIGH RISK**

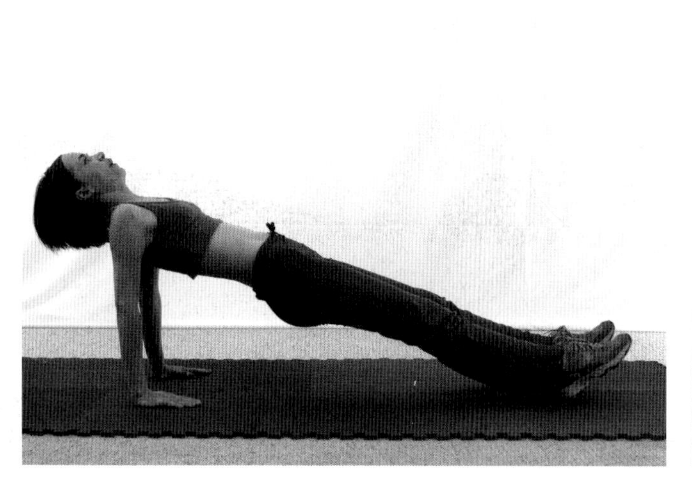

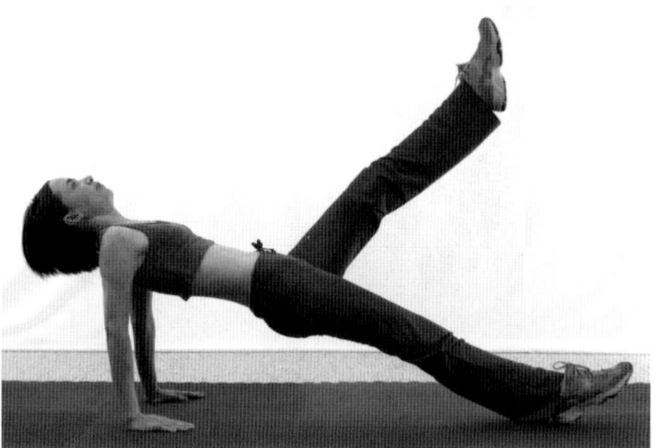

**STARTING POSITION:** Assume an up plank position: rest on your heels and elbows (or hands), making your body as straight as a board.

**THE MOVE:** Raise your left foot as high as you can, then lower it. Raise your right foot. Alternate legs until you complete your set.

**TRAINING TIPS**

- Keep your inner core activated throughout the movement.
- Initiate the movement from the center of your body.
- Keep your body straight and stable.

# EXERCISE: SIDE PLANK—LEG RAISE

DIFFICULTY: **3** LOWER BACK RISK: **HIGH RISK**

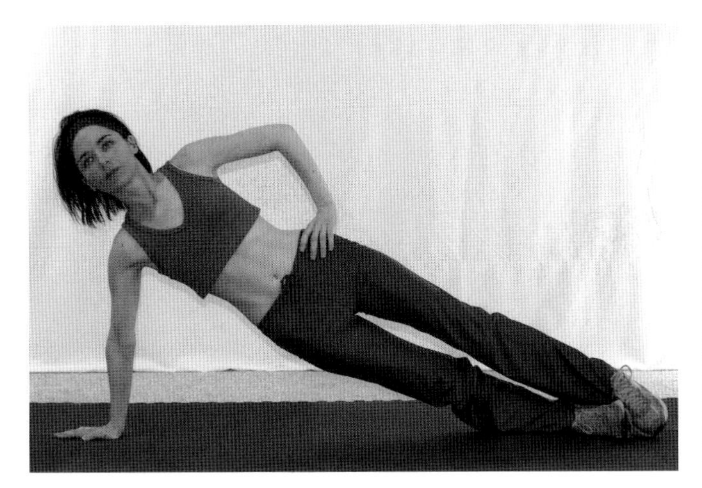

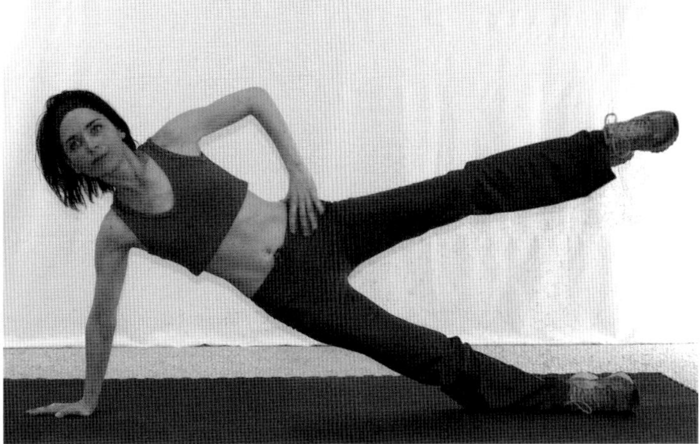

**STARTING POSITION:** Assume a side plank position: rest on the sides of your feet and your elbow or hand.

**THE MOVE:** Raise your top as high as you can, then lower it. Repeat.

### TRAINING TIPS

- Keep your inner core activated throughout the movement.
- Initiate the movement from the center of your body.
- Keep your body straight and stable.

# EXERCISE: MOTTA EXTENSION AND ROTATION

DIFFICULTY: **2** LOWER BACK RISK: **MODERATE RISK**

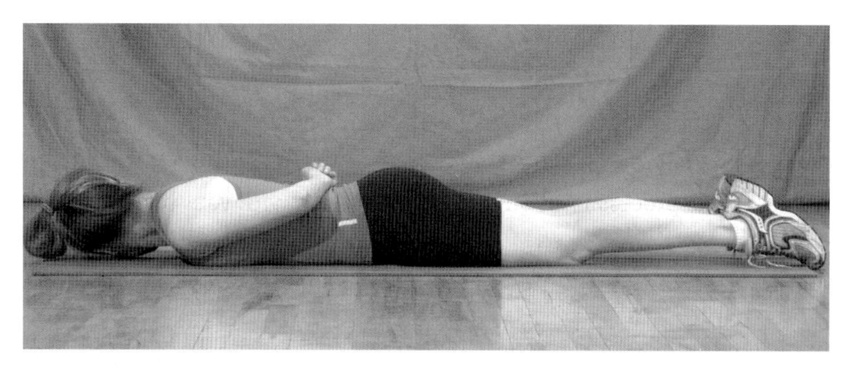

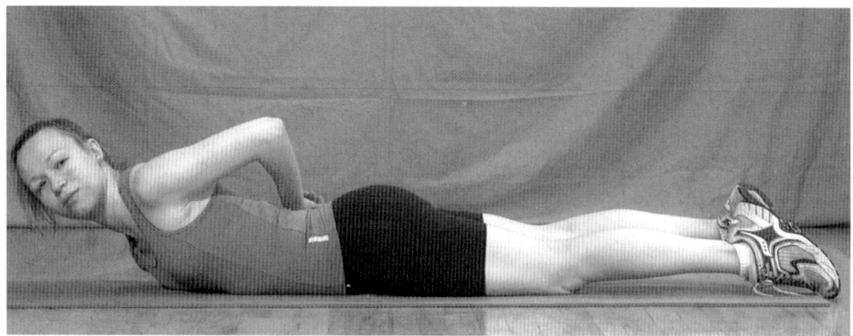

**STARTING POSITION:** Lie on your belly, looking to the right (left cheek on the ground), right arm extended straight and at your side, tight against your body. Then place your left arm, bent at the elbow, behind your back.

**THE MOVE:** Simultaneously lift and turn your head to the left as you raise your torso and rotate it in the direction you are looking. Return to the starting position and repeat.

### TRAINER'S TIPS

- Initiate the movement from your core.
- Don't rest at the bottom of the movement.
- Keep your inner core activated throughout the movement.
- Contract your buttocks to anchor your lower body.

# FINAL WORD: TO THE CORE

Integrating core work into your fitness program is an essential step in a healthy and active lifestyle. Core work strengthens and supports the way the body naturally moves. There is a reason why core work has been a key part of training for sports, martial arts, and dance. A strong core area allows your body to function with greater ease, grace, and power. Then, of course, there's that other benefit, you'll also look better. Core work tones your abs, butt, and thighs.

As you continue your program, remember consistency over time is the key. Be patient and commit to the process. This process is an ongoing conversation with your body. It's the only body you're ever going to have, so you need to develop a strong and healthy relationship with it. This relationship can be one of the most joyful and satisfying parts of your life.

But like any relationship it takes time and work. With your body the commitment truly is for better and for worse, no breakups, no divorce. It is until death do you part. There's no getting out of it. So there is only one rational choice; nurture the relationship. This nurturing will pay health and wellness benefits, both physically and mentally, for the rest of your life. And, as the relationship evolves, the conversation will deepen and become more profound. You will begin to understand your body's strengths and weaknesses. You will be able to respond to your body's needs quickly and intuitively. You will become an artist in the creation of your body. Starting your core workout program will be the beginning of a beautiful and productive friendship.

# CONTRIBUTORS

**STEVE FALK** is an owner of Bikram Yoga San Antonio in San Antonio, Texas. He is also a certified strength and conditioning specialist and the strength and conditioning coach for the Trinity University Men's and Women's basketball teams and the Women's soccer team. For more information, check out *www.bikramyogasa.com* or email Steve at *steve@bikramyogasa.com*.

**GAIL GIOVANNIELLO** is a certified Pilates instructor. She started her own studio, Mind Your Body Fitness, in 1995 on New York's Upper East Side. She also has a BFA in Dance from SUNY Purchase. You can contact her at mindyourbodyfitness.com.

**SCOTT HALL** is a producer and director. He studied theater and film at Arizona State University. He lives in Phoenix, Arizona.

**BRYON HOLMES** is an expert in lower back care: prevention and rehabilitation. He is the cofounder of America's Back, a chain of fitness centers located in Wal-Mart Stores. The centers specialize in lower back care. He is the owner of the MedX of Estes Park (Colorado), which offers a unique circuit program for wellness and performance. He has a Master's Degree in Exercise Physiology from the University of Florida, and he is a member of the American College of Sports Medicine. Bryon has authored and/or co-authored over thirty articles and sixty abstracts on fitness and lower back health.

**DEBBIE HOLMES** is the owner with her husband Bryon of MedX of Estes Park. She specializes in family fitness. She has a Master's Degree in health science and education from the University of Florida. She is a member of the American College of Sports Medicine and I.D.E.A. She writes a weekly column, *High Altitude Health*, and hosts a weekly radio show.

**DAVE JOHNSON** has been a personal trainer in New York City for over ten years. He is a motivational specialist and trains clients from kids to senior citizens.

**MARTIN KAMMLER** is one of New York's top personal trainers. He is a master instructor for Nautilus (Europe). He is the project manager and master instructor for the International Academy of Sports, Culture, and Art. He gives fitness and health seminars throughout the world.

**TRACY MARX** is a nutritional counselor and writer. She is a graduate of the School of Integrative Nutrition. She lives in New York City.

**BAY McCLINTON** is a personal trainer and fitness consultant. He is the owner of All Sports Speed and Fitness, a training facility in San Antonio, Texas. He works with a wide variety of athletes, ranging from aspiring teenagers to all pro running back and NFL rushing champion Priest Holmes.

**WINSLOW SWART** is the first non-Japanese Shihan of Kenseido in the world. He has studied Kenseido for forty years and taught for over twenty. He has trained professional athletes, corporate executives, and kids. Former athletes include such luminaries as NBA All-stars David Robinson and Sean Elliot. He has a B.A. in psychology. He leads corporate seminars in leadership and management. You can reach him at *www.kenseido.com.*

**STEVEN WILDE** has over 18 years of experience as a personal trainer. His clients have included Emmy and Grammy winners, Fortune 500 members, supermodels, professional athletes and both Disney and Warner Bros. executives. As a proponent of functional fitness and overall wellness, Mr. Wilde draws upon his background as an athlete to craft a program of exercise and nutrition that is tailored to meet the individual needs of each client.

# INDEX

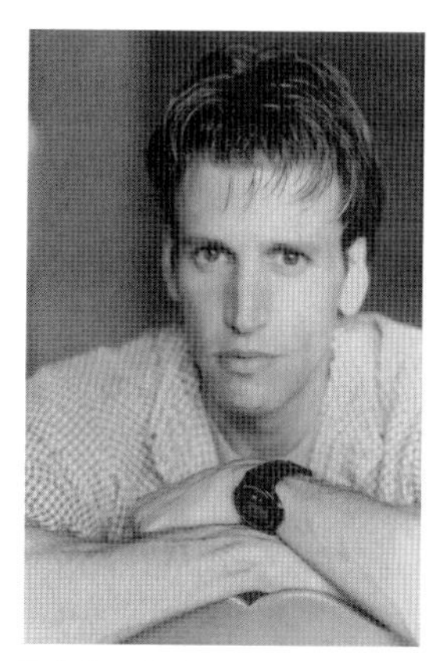

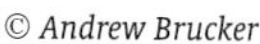

© Andrew Brucker

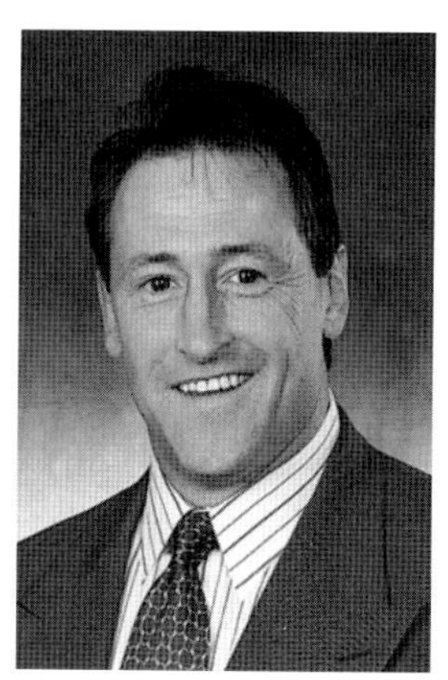

© San Antonio Spurs

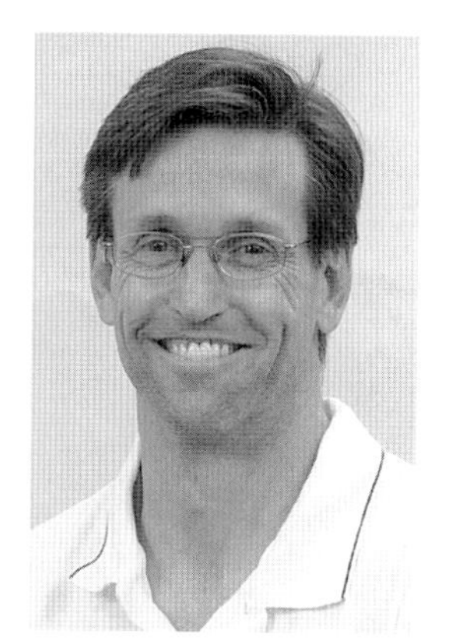

© Bruce Terami

**Kurt Brungardt** (left) is one of America's top personal trainers and fitness writers. The author of eight books, he has appeared on the *Today* show, *Good Morning America*, and more, and has repeatedly been featured in *Men's Health, Vogue, Newsweek, The Wall Street Journal, USA Today*, and *The New York Times*. He is also the host and writer of the bestselling video *Abs of Steel for Men*. **Mike Brungardt** (middle) is the Strength and Conditioning Coach for the San Antonio Spurs. During his tenure, the Spurs have won three NBA championships and have had three league MVPs. He has also served as President of the NBA Strength Coaches Association. He is the co-author of *The Strength Kit, The Complete Book of Butt and Legs, The Complete Book of Shoulders and Arms,* and the kids' workout video *Action Sports Camp,* and has written for *The Austin American Statesman.* **Brett Brungardt** (right) is the Strength and Conditioning Coach for the University of Washington. He is the co-author of *The Strength Kit, The Complete Book of Butt and Legs, The Complete Book of Shoulders and Arms,* and the kids' workout video *Action Sports Camp.* He has also been a strength and conditioning coach with the University of Kentucky and in the NBA with the Dallas Mavericks. He has a Master's Degree in Exercise Science from the University of Houston, and is a Certified Strength and Conditioning Specialist with the National Strength and Conditioning Association.

For more about Core Training, DVDs to supplement the book, camps for athletes and kids, performance supplements, and core training products, go to:

WWW.COMPLETECORE.COM

You will find information on:

One-on-One Core Training

A Full Motion DVD of the Exercises in this Book

The Dynamic Warm-Up DVD

The Complete Core DVD Box Set

- **Beginning, intermediate, and advanced workouts**
- **Sports workouts: golf, tennis, and basketball**
- **Pre- and post-pregnancy routines**
- **Core strength training**
- **Core prime time: routines for seniors**